Skin and Soft Tissue Injuries and Infections: A Practical Evidence Based Guide

Skin and Soft Tissue Injuries and Infections:
A Practical Evidence Based Guide

Adam J. Singer, MD
Professor and Vice Chairman for Research
Department of Emergency Medicine
Stony Brook University and Medical Center
Stony Brook, NY

Judd E. Hollander, MD
Professor and Clinical Research Director
Department of Emergency Medicine
University of Pennsylvania
Philadelphia, PA

Robert M. Blumm, MA, PA-C, DFAAPA
Course Instructor, Surgery and Emergency Medicine
Hofstra University
Hempstead, NY
Chairman, PA Advisory Board, clinician1.com

2010
PEOPLE'S MEDICAL PUBLISHING HOUSE—USA
SHELTON, CONNECTICUT

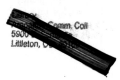

People's Medical Publishing House–USA
2 Enterprise Drive, Suite 509
Shelton, CT 06484
Tel: 203-402-0646
Fax: 203-402-0854
E-mail: info@pmph-usa.com

PMPH-USA

09 10 11 12 13/PMPH/9 8 7 6 5 4 3 2 1

ISBN-13: 978-1-60795-029-5
ISBN-10: 1-60795-029-4
Printed in China by People's Medical Publishing House of China
Copyeditor/Typesetter: Spearhead Global, Inc.
Cover Design: Mary Mckeon

Library of Congress Cataloging-in-Publication Data

Skin and soft tissue injuries, and infections : a practical evidence based guide / [edited by] Adam J. Singer, Judd E. Hollander, Robert M. Blumm.

  p.   ;   cm.

Includes bibliographical references and index.

ISBN-13: 978-1-60795-029-5

ISBN-10: 1-60795-029-4

 1. Skin—Wounds and injuries.   2. Soft tissue injuries.   3. Surgical emergencies.   4. Evidence-based medicine.
I. Singer, Adam J.   II. Hollander, Judd E., 1960- III. Blumm, Robert M.

 [DNLM: 1. Soft Tissue Injuries—therapy.   2. Evidence-Based Medicine.   3. Skin—injuries.

4. Soft Tissue Infections—therapy.   5. Wound Healing. WO

 700 S628 2010]

 RD93.S58 2010

 617.4′77044—dc22

2010025068

Notice: The authors and publisher have made every effort to ensure that the patient care recommended herein, including choice of drugs and drug dosages, is in accord with the accepted standard and practice at the time of publication. However, since research and regulation constantly change clinical standards, the reader is urged to check the product information sheet included in the package of each drug, which includes recommended doses, warnings, and contraindications. This is particularly important with new or infrequently used drugs. Any treatment regimen, particularly one involving medication, involves inherent risk that must be weighed on a case-by-case basis against the benefits anticipated. The reader is cautioned that the purpose of this book is to inform and enlighten; the information contained herein is not intended as, and should not be employed as, a substitute for individual diagnosis and treatment.

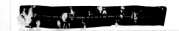

Sales and Distribution

Canada
McGraw-Hill Ryerson Education
Customer Care
300 Water St
Whitby, Ontario L1N 9B6
Canada
Tel: 1-800-565-5758
Fax: 1-800-463-5885
www.mcgrawhill.ca

Foreign Rights
People's Medical Publishing House
Suzanne Robidoux, Copyright Sales Manager
International Trade Department
No. 19, Pan Jia Yuan Nan Li
Chaoyang District
Beijing 100021
P.R. China
Tel: 8610-59787337
Fax: 8610-59787336
www.pmph.com/en/

Japan
United Publishers Services Limited
1-32-5 Higashi-Shinagawa
Shinagawa-ku, Tokyo 140-0002
Japan
Tel: 03-5479-7251
Fax: 03-5479-7307
Email: kakimoto@ups.co.jp

United Kingdom, Europe, Middle East, Africa
McGraw Hill Education
Shoppenhangers Road
Maidenhead
Berkshire, SL6 2QL
England
Tel: 44-0-1628-502500
Fax: 44-0-1628-635895
www.mcgraw-hill.co.uk

Singapore, Thailand, Philippines, Indonesia,
Vietnam, Pacific Rim, Korea
McGraw-Hill Education
60 Tuas Basin Link
Singapore 638775
Tel: 65-6863-1580
Fax: 65-6862-3354
www.mcgraw-hill.com.sg

Australia, New Zealand
Elsevier Australia
Locked Bag 7500
Chatswood DC NSW 2067
Australia
Tel: 161 (2) 9422-8500
Fax: 161 (2) 9422-8562
www.elsevier.com.au

Brazil
SuperPedido Tecmedd
Beatriz Alves, Foreign Trade Department
R. Sansao Alves dos Santos, 102 | 7th floor
Brooklin Novo
Sao Paolo 04571-090
Brazil
Tel: 55-16-3512-5539
www.superpedidotecmedd.com.br

India, Bangladesh, Pakistan, Sri Lanka, Malaysia
CBS Publishers
4819/X1 Prahlad Street 24
Ansari Road, Darya Ganj, New Delhi-110002
India
Tel: 91-11-23266861/67
Fax: 91-11-23266818
Email:cbspubs@vsnl.com

People's Republic of China
People's Medical Publishing House
International Trade Department
No. 19, Pan Jia Yuan Nan Li
Chaoyang District
Beijing 100021
P.R. China
Tel: 8610-67653342
Fax: 8610-67691034
www.pmph.com/en/

Acknowledgments

This book is dedicated to my wife Ayellet, and my three children Daniel, Lee, and Karen, without whose support this book never would have been written.

AJS

This book is dedicated to Jeanne, Greg, and David, who allowed me the time to write this book.

JEH

My gratitude to my wife Celia for editing my contributions to this book as well as to Dr. Singer for impressing upon me that three creative sentences, joined together, is no longer considered evidence based medicine.

RMB

Foreword

Skin and soft tissues injuries and infections are among the most common ailments affecting mankind. While most heal uneventfully, skin and soft tissue injuries and infections may result in significant morbidity and mortality. Early and proper evaluation and management of these injuries and infections will help optimize care and minimize the risk of serious complications.

Skin and soft tissue injuries and infections are managed by a large number of health care practitioners including nurses, nurse practitioners, physician assistants, and physicians. In addition, a wide variety of medical specialties are involved in their care including primary care practitioners, emergency practitioners, and surgeons.

Over the last two decades a large body of evidence has accumulated allowing many of our practices to be based on sound preclinical and clinical studies. Wherever possible, the recommendations of this book are based on such high-quality evidence. In the absence of such evidence, the recommendations are based on expert opinion and consensus. It is our hope that this book will be helpful for both junior practitioners, including students and residents, as well as for more experienced practitioners.

Adam J. Singer
Judd E. Hollander
Robert M. Blumm

Contributors

Joel M. Bartfield, MD, FACEP
Professor, Emergency Medicine
Associate Dean for Graduate Medical Education
Albany Medical College
Albany, NY

Subhasish Bose, MD, MRCP
Resident, Internal Medicine
Pennsylvania Hospital
University of Pennsylvania
Philadelphia, PA

Martin Camacho, MSN, ACNP-BC
Acute Care Nurse Practitioner
Department of Emergency Medicine
Hospital of the University of Pennsylvania
Philadelphia, PA

Guy Cassara, RPA-C
Clinical Instructor, Department of Emergency
   Medicine
School of Medicine
Stony Brook University
Stony Brook, NY

Esther H. Chen, MD
Associate Professor
University of California, San Francisco
San Francisco, CA

Richard A.F. Clark, MD
Professor, Department of Biomedical
   Engineering, Dermatology, and Medicine
Director, Center for Tissue Engineering
Stony Brook University
Stony Brook, NY

**Alexander B. Dagum, MD, FRCS(C),
FACS**
Clinical Professor of Surgery and Orthopaedic
   Surgery
Chief of Plastic Surgery
Stony Brook University Medical Center
Stony Brook, NY

Anthony J. Dean, MD
Associate Professor of Emergency Medicine,
   Assistant Professor of Emergency Medicine -
   Radiology
Director, Division of Emergency
   Ultrasonography
Department of Emergency Medicine
University of Pennsylvania Medical Center
Philadelphia, PA

Mary Farren, RN, MSN, CWOCN
Visiting Nurse Service of New York
New York, NY

David F. Gaieski, MD
Assistant Professor, University of Pennsylvania
   School of Medicine; Department of
   Emergency Medicine
Clinical Director, Center for Resuscitation
   Science
Philadelphia, PA

Mark Gelfand, MD
Assistant Professor, Plastic and Reconstructive
   Surgery
Stony Book University
Stony Brook University Medical Center
Stony Brook, NY

Hans R. House, MD, FACEP
Associate Professor
Department of Emergency Medicine
University of Iowa
Iowa City, Iowa

Patrick Luib, MSN, APRN, BC
Manager, Geriatric Clinical Services
VNS CHOICE
Brooklyn, NY

Mary Jo McBride, PA
Instructor, Stony Brook University
Stony Brook, NY

James R. Miner, MD
Associate Professor of Emergency Medicine
University of Minnesota Medical School
Research Director, Department of Emergency
    Medicine
Hennepin County Medical Center
Minneapolis, MN

Gregory J. Moran, MD
Professor of Medicine
UCLA School of Medicine
Department of Emergency Medicine and
    Division of Infectious Diseases
Olive View-UCLA Medical Center
Sylmar, CA

**Rose M. Moran-Kelly, RN, MSN,
APRN, FNP-BC**
Visiting Nurse Service of New York
New York, NY

Charlene M. Morris, MPAS, PA-C, DFAAPA
Pamlico Medical Medical Center, PA
Bayboro, NC
Carolina East Medical Center
New Bern, NC
Urgent Care Clinic
Marine Air Corps Station Cherry Point
Havelock, NC

Ronald Moscati, MD, FACEP
Research Director, Department of Emergency
    Medicine
Attending Physician, Erie County Medical
    Center
Buffalo, NY

**Charles V. Pollack, Jr, MD, MA, FACEP,
FAAEM, FAHA**
Professor and Chairman, Department of
    Emergency Medicine
Pennsylvania Hospital
University of Pennsylvania
Philadelphia, PA

Lior Rosenberg, MD
Professor and Chair
Department of Plastic and Reconstructive
    Surgery
Soroka University Medical Center
Faculty of Health Sciences
Ben Gurion University
Beer Sheba, Israel

Steven Sandoval, MD
Assistant Professor
Director of the Burn Unit
Department of Surgery
Stony Brook University
Stony Brook, NY

Harry S. Soroff, MD
Professor Emeritus
Former Chairman of Surgery and
    Director of the Burn Unit
Department of Surgery
Stony Brook University
Stony Brook, NY

Breena R. Taira, MD, MPH
Affiliate Faculty, Graduate Program in
    Public Health
Stony Brook University
Stony Brook, NY

Contents

The Epidemiology of Cutaneous Wounds

Patrick Luib, MSN, APRN, BC

There are many types of acute and chronic wounds that are treated in a wide variety of settings from hospitals and nursing homes to home care. Chronic wounds include pressure, venous, arterial, and diabetic neuropathic ulcers. According to a descriptive study of home care patients with wounds, the prevalence of chronic ulcerated skin lesions ranges from 120 per 100,000 persons aged 45 to 64 years to more than 800 per 100,000 persons aged 75 years and older.[1] In contrast, there are a wide variety of acute wounds that include lacerations, animal bites, plantar punctures, cutaneous and subcutaneous abscesses, and burns. The purpose of this chapter is to review the most current epidemiologic data concerning acute cutaneous wounds.

LACERATIONS

A secondary analysis of the National Hospital Ambulatory Medical Care Survey (NHMACS) data set estimated the number of lacerations treated in the United States between 1992 and 2002.[2] Approximately 8% of 300,715 patient encounters had lacerations resulting in an estimated 90 million lacerations. Although the number of emergency department (ED) visits increased by more than 30%, the number of patients being treated for lacerations decreased. As shown in Figure 1-1b, there was a 20% decrease in the total number of lacera-

tions. According to the latest nationally representative data on visits to hospital emergency departments in the United States this trend persists from 2005 to 2006.[3] Singer et al. purported that this decrease cannot be explained by an age shift in the overall population because of an increase in age-adjusted estimates.[2]

There was a relatively constant distribution of characteristics of patients who presented to the ED as well as a constant distribution of lacerations by anatomic sites over time.[2] The estimated frequency of anatomic sites is illustrated in Figure 1-2. About two thirds of patients who came to an ED with a laceration were men, about one third were aged younger than 18 years, and more than three quarters were White. More than 10% of patients reported work-related injuries; less than 5% of all lacerations were caused by assaults; and less than 2% were self-inflicted wounds. Alcohol and drug abuse was cited as a contributing factor in less than 3% of cases. Almost 70% of all lacerations were accidents caused by cutting and piercing instruments, falls, and motor vehicle collisions.

SKIN TEARS

Skin tears are lacerations of the epidermis that occur more than 1.5 million times each year in health care facilities across the United States.[4]

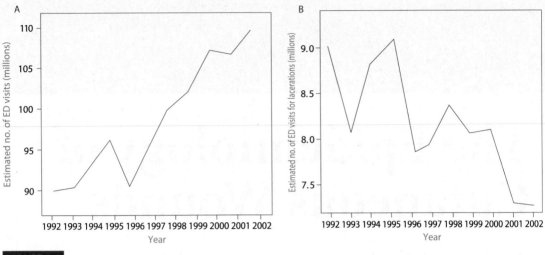

FIGURE 1-1

(A) Trend in emergency department visits (1991–2002). (B) Trend in laceration visits (1991–2002).
Source: Singer et al. (2005).[2]

A retrospective review of incident reports at a large, urban long-term-care facility conducted by Malone et al. revealed an incident rate of less than one skin tear per resident per year.[5] The overall incidence of skin tears significantly increased with the resident's age (P=.043); and although the incidence rate for females increased with age (P=.012), it did not for males (P=.938).[5]

ANIMAL BITES

There was no ongoing national surveillance system for animal bites until the Centers for Disease Control and Prevention conducted an Injury Control and Risk Survey (ICARIS) in 1994. Sacks et al. summarized ICARIS data and concluded that dog bites occurred at an incidence rate of 18 per 1000.[6] According to this

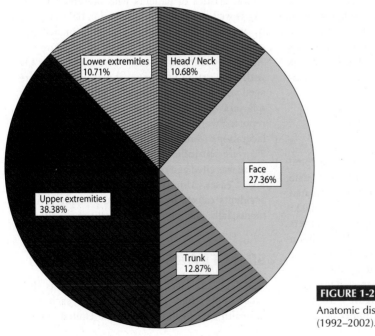

FIGURE 1-2

Anatomic distribution of lacerations (1992–2002). Source: Singer et al. (2005).[2]

TABLE 1–1	Types of Animal Exposure Among Emergency Department Patients by Patient Age		
Animal, *n* (%)	Pediatric Patients (*n* = 687) *n* (%)	Adult Patients (*n* = 1,339) *n* (%)	OR (95% CI)
Dogs, 1,528 (75)	597 (87)	931 (70)	2.9 (2.2, 3.8)
Police dogs, 103 (5.1)	15 (2.2)	88 (6.6)	0.32 (0.17, 0.57)
Cats, 267 (13)	49 (7.1)	218 (16)	0.39 (0.28, 0.55)
Rats/mice, 49 (2.4)	11 (1.6)	38 (2.8)	0.56 (0.27, 1.1)
Squirrels, 20 (1.0)	4 (0.6)	16 (1.2)	N/A
Hamsters/gerbils/ rabbits, 14 (0.7)	8 (1.2)	6 (0.4)	2.6 (0.79, 9.2)
Raccoons, 10 (0.5)	0 (0.0)	10 (0.7)	N/A
Other wild carnivores, 8 (0.4)	0 (0.0)	8 (0.6)	N/A
Gophers, 5 (0.2)	1 (0.1)	4 (0.3)	N/A
Bats, 5 (0.2)	1 (0.1)	4 (0.3)	N/A
Livestock, 8 (0.4)	1 (0.1)	7 (0.5)	N/A
Monkeys, 9 (0.4)	0 (0.0)	9 (0.7)	N/A

Odds ratios and 95% confidence intervals are not reported when at least one of the categories contained fewer than five patients because their validity is questionable or they are undefined when there are no patients in a category.

N/A = not applicable.

Source: Steele et al. (2007).

study almost 2% of the US population has been bitten by a dog and less than half a percent sought care for more than 4 million bites. Patronek and Slavinski analyzed specific aspects of animal bites (dog and cat bites in particular) that were novel or noteworthy with respect to previously unrecognized injuries or cause of death.[7] Dog and cat bites are the most common bite-related injuries associated with vertebrate animals in the United States, Australia, and Italy.[7] Although infrequent in comparison, bites from wildlife, farm animals, rodents, and pets other than dogs and cats make up the remainder of reported bite-related injuries. Table 1-1 shows types of mammalian animal exposures among ED patients by patient age based on an epidemiological study conducted by Steele et al.[8] Pediatric ED patients were more likely to have an exposure because of a dog and less likely to be exposed to a cat than were adults.

Weiss et al. analyzed the NHMACS data set from 1992 to 1994 to determine the frequency of dog bite injuries requiring medical attention at a hospital or hospital admission.[9] New dog bite–related injury visits to US EDs was estimated to occur at a rate of about 13 per 10,000 persons, which comprised less than half a percent of all ED visits.[9] Almost all cases

that were assigned an injury severity score were deemed low severity. Ninety-six percent of patients with dog bite–related injuries were treated and released from the ED and the remainder were admitted to the hospital or transferred to another facility.

PUNCTURE WOUNDS OF THE FOOT

A majority of puncture wounds of the foot are caused by nails and less commonly by glass, wood, or other metal objects besides nails.[10] A survey of 200 ED patients with a history of a plantar puncture wound revealed 44% sustained at least one plantar puncture wound with an infection rate of approximately 11%.[11]

CUTANEOUS AND SUBCUTANEOUS ABSCESSES

A prospective study conducted by Davis et al. indicated skin and soft tissue as the most common site of infection for 80% of patients with community-associated methicillin-resistant *Staphylococcus aureus* (CA-MRSA) and 90% of patients with community-associated methicillin-susceptible *S aureus* (CA-MSSA).[12] In another prospective prevalence study, the only factor that was significantly associated with MSSA was the presence of abscess at enrollment (odds ratio=2.3; 95% confidence interval=1.2 to 4.4).[13]

BURNS

Nearly half a million persons with burns are treated in the ED each year.[14–16] The National Burn Repository[17] is the largest collection of patient care data from 70 burn centers across the United States and Canada. Key findings from its most recent report include but are not limited to the following[17]:

- Nearly 70% of the burn patients were men. Mean age for all cases was 33 years. Infants accounted for 10% of the cases and patients aged 60 years or older represented 14% of the cases.
- Sixty-two percent of the reported total burn sizes were less than 10% TBSA. Sixty-eight percent of the full thickness burns (third degree) were less than 10%. Inhalation injury was present in 7% of the total

reported cases, but played an important role in increasing hospital length of stay and risk of death.
- Forty-three percent of the burn injuries were reported to have occurred in the home.
- Ninety-five percent of patients survived hospitalization. The cause of death for those who died was recorded in 51% of the cases. The leading cause of death was multiple organ failure.
- Hospital length of stay increased significantly with total burn size and presence of inhalation injury.

As illustrated in Figure 1-3, the most commonly reported etiologies were flame burns and scalds. There were 6283 scald injuries in the group aged younger than 2 years, making up 28% of all scald injuries and 70% of all reported injuries to the population aged younger than 2 years.

According to the National Burn Repository, deaths from burn injury increased with advancing age, burn size, and presence of inhalation injury. This finding was consistent with Bessey et al. who purported older adults as being the most vulnerable to the morbidity and mortality of burn injury (see Figure 1-4).[18]

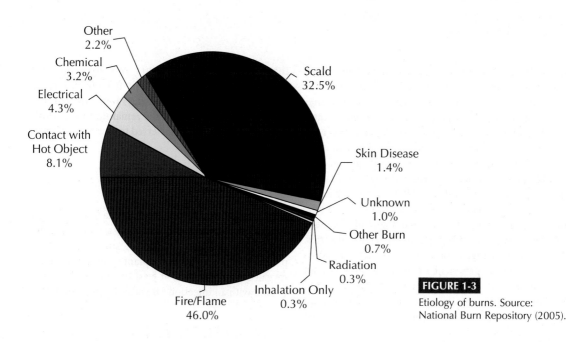

FIGURE 1-3

Etiology of burns. Source: National Burn Repository (2005).

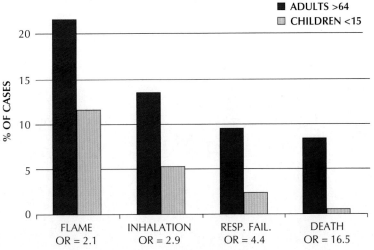

FIGURE 1-4

Burn injuries in children and older adults. Source: Bessey et al. (2006).[18]

REFERENCES

1. Pieper B, Templin TN, Dobal M, Jacox A. Wound prevalence, types and treatments in home care. *Adv Wound Care.* 1999;12(3):117–126.

2. Singer AJ, Thode HC Jr, Hollander JE. National trends in ED lacerations between 1992 and 2002. *Am J Emerg Med.* 2005;24(2):183–188.

3. Nawar EW, Niska RW, Xu J. National hospital ambulatory medical care survey: 2005 emergency department summary. *Advance Data From Vital Health Statistics.* No. 386. Hyattsville, MD: National Center for Health Statistics; 2007. Available at: http://www.cdc.gov/nchs/data/ad/ad386.pdf. Feb 23, 2010.

4. LeBlanc K, Christensen D, Orsted HL, Keast DH. Prevention and treatment of skin tears. *Wound Care Canada.* 2008;6(1):14–30.

5. Malone ML, Rozario N, Gavinski M, Goodwin J. The epidemiology of skin tears in the institutionalized elderly. *J Am Geriatr Soc.* 1991;39(6):591–595.

6. Sacks JJ, Kresnow M, Houston B. Dog bites: how big a problem? *Inj Prev.* 1996;2(1):52–54.

7. Patronek GJ, Slavinski SA. Animal bites. *J Am Vet Med Assoc.* 2009;234(3):336–245.

8. Steele MT, Ma OJ, Nakase J, Moran GJ, et al. Epidemiology of animal exposures presenting to emergency departments. *Acad Emerg Med.* 2007;14(5):398–403.

9. Weiss HB, Friedman DI, Coben JH. Incidence of dog bite injuries treated in emergency departments. *JAMA.* 1998;279(1):51–53.

10. Baddour LM. Puncture wounds to the plantar surface of the foot. In: Baron EL, ed. *UpToDate.* Waltham, MA: UpToDate; 2009.

11. Weber EJ. Plantar puncture wounds: a survey to determine the incidence of infections. *J Accid Emerg Med.* 1996;13(4):274–277.

12. Davis SL, Perri MB, Donabedian SM, et al. Epidemiology and outcomes of community-associated methicillin-resistant Staphylococcus aureus infection. *J Clin Microbiol.* 2007;45(6):1705–1711.

13. Moran GJ, Krishnadasan A, Gorwitz RJ, et al. Methicillin-resistant S. aureus infections among patients in the emergency department. *N Engl J Med.* 2006;355 (7):667–674.

14. Pitts SR, Niska RW, Xu J, Burt CW. National hospital ambulatory medical care survey: 2006 emergency department summary. *National Health Statistics Reports.* No. 7. Hyattsville, MD: National Center for Health Statistics; 2008. Available at: http://www.cdc.gov/nchs/data/nhsr/nhsr007.pdf. Feb 23, 2010.

15. McCaig LF, Burt CW. National hospital ambulatory medical care survey: 2003 emergency department summary. *Advance Data From Vital and Health Statistics.* No. 358. Hyattsville, MD: National Center for Health Statistics; 2005. Available at: http://www.cdc.gov/nchs/data/ad/ad358.pdf. (Accessed July 13, 2009)

16. McCaig LF, Nawar EW. National hospital ambulatory medical care survey: 2004 emergency department summary. *Advance Data From Vital and Health Statistics.* No. 372. Hyattsville, MD: National Center for Health Statistics; 2006. Available from: http://www.cdc.gov/nchs/data/ad/ad372.pdf. (Accessed July 13, 2009)

17. National Burn Repository: 2005 Report (version 2.0). Chicago, IL: American Burn Association. Available at: http://www.ameriburn.org/NBR2005.pdf. Accessed July 10, 2009.

18. Bessey PQ, Arons RR, DiMaggio CJ, Yurt RW. The vulnerabilities of age: burns in children and older adults. *Surgery.* 2006;140(4):705–717.

The Biology of Wound Healing

Adam J. Singer, MD, and Richard A.F. Clark, MD

THE FUNCTION AND STRUCTURE OF THE SKIN

The skin is the largest organ in the body and is composed of three layers: the epidermis, dermis, and hypodermis (Figure 2-1). The thickness of the skin varies based on location and age. Although the skin has many functions (Table 2-1), its primary function is to serve as a barrier between the organism and the external environment. This function reduces the risk of infection and evaporative fluid losses. The barrier function is mainly attributed to the outermost epidermal layer, and in particular to the stratum corneum. The importance of the skin is demonstrated by the fact that loss of large areas of the skin caused by disease or injury (as in extensive burns) results in significant morbidity and mortality. The main function of the dermis is to support the structural integrity of the skin giving it both its durability and its elasticity. The hypodermis or subcutaneous layer contains mostly adipose tissue, which functions as a thermal insulator and also helps to cushion or protect the underlying structures. Recent evidence suggests that the adipose layer may also be a source of multipotent stem cells that help regenerate the skin after disease or injury.[1]

The epidermis is the most superficial layer of the skin and provides the first barrier of protection from the invasion of foreign substances into the body. The epidermis is subdivided into four layers or strata, the stratum germinatum (basal layer), the stratum spinosum, the stratum granulosum (granular cell layer), and the stratum corneum in which keratinocytes terminally differentiate and are pushed upward to the surface and slough off the skin. The basal layer provides the precursor rapidly proliferating cells necessary for the regeneration of the layers of the epidermis. These basal cells are separated from the dermis by a thin basement membrane. After mitotic division, newly formed epidermal cells undergo progressive differentiation or keratinization as they are pushed toward the surface. The dermis is divided into two zones, the papillary dermis and the reticular dermis. The dermis contains mostly fibroblasts, which are responsible for secreting collagen, elastin, and ground substance that give support and elasticity to the skin. The dermis also contains blood vessels that supply the epidermis and help regulate body temperature, as well as epithelial appendages including hair follicles, sebaceous glands, and apocrine glands. Immune cells are also present, which defend against foreign invaders passing through the epidermis. The lower reticular layer of the dermis consists of dense irregular connective tissue that is important in giving the skin it overall strength and elasticity.

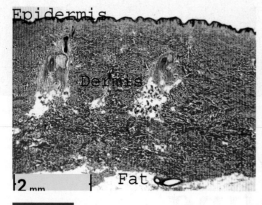 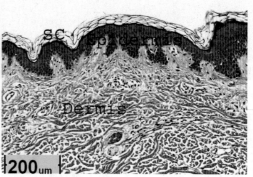

FIGURE 2-1

Structure of the skin. SC = Stratum corneum.

THE PATHOPHYSIOLOGY OF WOUND HEALING

A wound is defined as a defect in the structural or functional integrity of the skin. Wounds to the skin may be caused by a wide range of insults including mechanical (e.g., abrasions and lacerations), thermal, chemical, electrical, ischemic, and irradiation-induced. With all types of wounds, the original insult results in the activation of multiple cellular and molecular processes intended to restore the integrity of the skin.[2,3] Except for with very superficial wounds and in early fetal life,[4] the regenerative capacity of the skin is limited and most wounds are replaced with various amounts of scar tissue. Both underhealing (as with chronic diabetic ulcers) and overhealing (as with hypertrophic scars and keloids) are fairly common.

The well orchestrated process of wound healing is complex and dynamic and involves many different types of cells, soluble mediators, and extracellular matrix (Figure 2-2).[2,3] For example, the protein fragments in the provisional blood clot serve as chemoattractants for monocytes, stimulate phagocytosis, and direct the expression of multiple growth factors.[5] Wound healing generally requires the migration, pro-liferation, and differentiation of the skin cells. These processes are regulated by multiple cell signaling pathways that control the expression of many genes with vital functions. For purposes of simplicity, wound healing is divided into four overlapping temporal stages: hemostasis, inflammation, tissue formation, and re-modeling. A deep mechanical abrasion is a classical example in which all four stages play a significant role.

Hemostasis

Mechanical injuries (such as lacerations, abrasions, and surgical incisions and excisions) result in the disruption of blood vessels and bleeding. Immediate vasoconstriction helps to slow blood loss. Hemostasis is initially achieved by the formation of a platelet plug quickly followed by a fibrin clot. The fibrin clot not only serves to prevent further blood loss, but also functions as a scaffold or provisional matrix for the influx of inflammatory and tissue cells. The platelets themselves are also a source of multiple soluble mediators (such as platelet-derived growth factor) that play a vital role in wound healing.

Inflammation

The main purpose of the inflammatory stage is to clean the wound by removing dead or dying tissues and to prevent infection.[6] Wound infection has many deleterious effects including delayed healing, excessive scarring, and systemic dissemination of microorganisms. The inflammatory cells are also a source of mediators that promote the later stages of wound healing (Table 2-2). The earliest inflammatory cells are the neutrophils, which are recruited to the wound within minutes to hours in response to substances released by

TABLE 2–1	Functions of the Skin

Protective barrier against the external environment
Fluid homeostasis
Thermoregulation
Immune surveillance
Sensory detection
Self healing

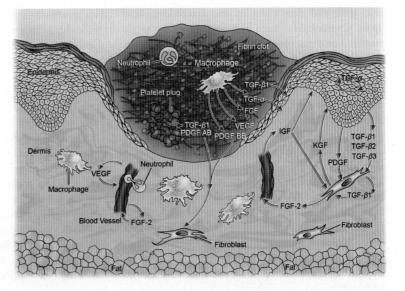

FIGURE 2-2

Schematic Illustration of Wound Healing Process Approximately 3 Days after Injury.

the activated coagulation and complement systems. Within 2 or 3 days, blood-derived monocytes enter the wound and differentiate into tissue macrophages, which serve as major producers of a large number of mediators that coordinate later stages of healing such as granulation tissue formation.

The earliest signals for recruitment of inflammatory cells are small molecules including ATP, adenosine,

TABLE 2–2	Selected Wound Mediators	
Mediator	**Source**	**Main Function(s)**
PDGF	Platelets, macrophages, keratinocytes, endothelial cells, fibroblasts	Stimulates inflammation, granulation tissue formation, reepithelialization, matrix formation, and remodeling
VEGFA	Keratinocytes, endothelial cells, fibroblasts, smooth muscle cells	Stimulates angiogenesis
EGF	Kidneys, salivary glands	Stimulates reepithelialization
HB-EGF	Keratinocytes	Stimulates reepithelialization
TGF-α	Platelets, keratinocytes, macrophages, fibroblasts, lymphocytes	Stimulates reepithelialization
FGF2	Keratinocytes, fibroblasts, endothelial cells, smooth muscles, mast cells	Stimulates angiogenesis, fibroblast proliferation
FGF7	Keratinocytes, fibroblasts, endothelial cells, smooth muscles, mast cells	Stimulates reepithelialization
TGF-β	Platelets, keratinocytes, macrophages, fibroblasts, lymphocytes	Stimulates fibrogenesis, inhibits reepithelialization
TNF-α	Neutrophils, macrophages	Stimulates inflammation, reepithelialization
IL-1	Neutrophils, macrophages, keratinocytes	Stimulates inflammation, reepithelialization
IL-6	Neutrophils, macrophages	Stimulates inflammation, reepithelialization

Note: PDGF=platelet-derived growth factor; VEGFA=vascular endothelial growth factor A; EGF=epithelial growth factor; HB-EGF=heparin binding epidermal growth factor; TGF-α=transforming growth factor alpha; FGF=fibroblast growth factor; TGF-β=transforming growth factor beta; TNF-α=tumor necrosis factor alpha; IL=interleukin.

uric acid, and derivatives of the arachidonic-acid lipids. Chemokines,[7] such as monocyte chemotactic protein-1 and macrophage-inflammatory protein-1α, are also very potent chemoattractants for inflammatory cells. The ability of the leukocytes to exit the systemic bloodstream and enter the wound is dependent on their ability to adhere to and cross the blood vessel wall. The leukocytes stick to the endothelial cell surface by attaching to adhesion molecules called selectins that are expressed on endothelial cells after injury.[8] These adhesion molecules are upregulated by inflammatory cytokines such as tumor necrosis factor alpha (TNF-α) that are released in response to injury. The release of inflammatory mediators is dependent on upregulation of several signal transduction pathways.[9] The resolution of the inflammatory phase is dependent on self-destruction of the neutrophils in a process termed apoptosis.[10] Although neutrophils and macrophages play a major role in wound healing, their individual absence is not crucial to wound healing, possibly because of considerable redundancy. When both cells types are absent, only small wounds can heal.

New Tissue Formation

For the wound to heal, the gap remaining after injury that is initially occupied by the blood clot needs to be replaced with scar tissue and resurfaced with a new epidermal surface layer. One of the earliest stages of new tissue formation is reepithelialization that results from the proliferation and migration of keratinocytes. With small and superficial wounds, the main source of these keratinocytes is the surrounding basal layer of uninjured epidermis. With deep wounds a major source of keratinocytes is the bulge area located in the infundibulum, or upper portion of the hair follicle located between the epidermis and the sebaceous gland.[11-13]

The proliferation and migration of the keratinocytes is stimulated in part by a number of mediators, the most important of which include the hepatocyte growth factor and members of the epidermal growth factor and fibroblast growth factor (FGF) families (especially FGF7 and FGF10).[14,15] In contrast, transforming growth factor beta (TGF-β) inhibits reepithelialization. Other regulators of reepithelialization include acetylcholine,[16] catecholamines,[17] and a variety of fatty acid derivatives.[18] Electrical signals generated by the injury may also help direct the migration of keratinocytes.[19] The ability of keratinocytes to migrate along the wound edge and through the provisional extracellular matrix is also dependent on the expression of proteolytic enzymes (e.g., metalloproteinases) that help pave a pathway.[20] The ability of keratinocytes to migrate also requires a change in their phenotype to allow detachment from the underlying structures. In addition, the migrating keratinocytes express cell surface molecules (termed integrins) that interact with substances in the provisional matrix (such as fibronectin) that serve as navigation beacons directing the advancing epithelial cells.[3]

For the wound to heal new blood vessels are formed in a process called angiogenesis that helps deliver vital oxygen and nutrients to the healing wound.[21] The sprouting of new blood vessels from existing blood vessels is stimulated mostly by vascular endothelial growth factor A and basic FGF, also known as FGF2. Platelet-derived growth factors also work synergistically with the other mediators in stimulating angiogenesis. These mediators are released from surrounding cells (such as the platelets, macrophages, keratinocytes, and endothelial cells) in response to various stimuli, including hypoxia,[22] which induces the formation of a transcriptional complex termed hypoxia-inducible factor-1.[23] New blood vessels may also arise from endothelial progenitor or stem cells derived from the bone marrow. The ingrowth of blood vessels into the wound is accompanied by fibroblasts and macrophages that together are referred to as granulation tissue. The migration of endothelial cells into the wound is guided by a series of receptors expressed on the cell surface (integrins) that interact with the components of the extracellular matrix, including fibrin, fibronectin, and vitronectin. For example, the integrin alpha V beta 3 is only expressed on endothelial cells during wound healing and after interacting with the extracellular matrix initiates endothelial cell migration.[24]

Most acute wounds are hypoxic and hypoxia is a major stimulus for wound healing.[22] Hypoxia is secondary to reduced wound perfusion that results from the initial injury as well as from an increase in cell metabolism and oxygen consumption. Hypoxia probably stimulates repair by creating an oxygen gradient between the injured tissue and the surrounding normal tissues. However, oxygen is essential for wound healing. For example, oxygen is necessary for fibroblast proliferation and collagen synthesis. A certain amount of oxygen is also necessary for phagocytes to produce reactive oxygen species during the respiratory burst that is crucial for oxidative killing of bacteria.

The majority of the wound is filled in by scar tissue or collagen that is formed by the entering fibroblasts. A major stimulator of collagen formation (fibrogenesis) is TGF-β.[25] Some of the fibroblasts undergo functional and structural transformation to myofibroblasts that supply the contractile force that helps shrink the size of the wound and bring the wound edges together. The transition from fibroblasts to myofibroblasts is under the influence of TGF-β, mechanical stress, and cellular fibronectin.[26] The entry of endothelial cells and fibroblasts into the wound is aided by the elaboration of metalloproteinases that help digest the extracellular matrix and the interaction of cell surface molecules (integrins) between the entering cells and the extracellular matrix proteins.

Wound Remodeling

The final and longest phase of wound healing is the remodeling phase, which lasts months to years. During this phase very little if any collagen is added to the wound with the formation of new collagen being balanced by its degradation by various matrix metalloproteinases.[27] Increased formation of cross links between the various collagen fibrils results in a steady increase in the wound's tensile strength that is most rapid between the second to sixth week after injury. Even after complete healing, the resulting scar is only about 80% as strong as the original skin (Figure 2-3).[28] During this process the majority of the collagen is transformed from type I to type III and the majority of the cells (including blood vessels, fibroblasts, and macrophages) exit the wound or undergo a process of apoptosis or programmed cell death. Thus, the original wound is replaced by a mostly acellular collagenous scar. Continuous regulation of the skin's integrity also requires complex interactions between the epithelial and mesenchymal elements of the skin.[29]

HEALING OF RAT SKIN WOUNDS

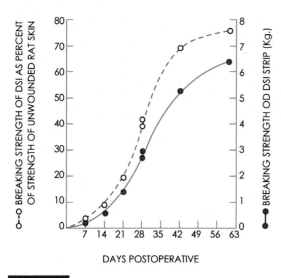

DAYS POSTOPERATIVE

FIGURE 2-3

Change in bursting strength over time.

REFERENCES

1. Ebrahimian TG, Pouzoulet F, Squiban C, et al. Cell therapy based on adipose tissue-derived stromal cells promote physiological and pathological wound healing. *Arterioscler Thromb Vasc Biol.* 2009;29(4):503–510.
2. Gurtner GC, Werner S, Barrandon Y, Longaker MT. Wound repair and regeneration. *Nature.* 2008;453(7193):314–321.
3. Singer AJ, Clark RA. Cutaneous wound healing. *N Engl J Med.* 1999;341(10);738–746.
4. Ferguson MW, O'Kane S. Scar-free healing: from embryonic mechanisms to adult therapeutic intervention. *Philos Trans R Soc Lond B Biol Sci.* 2004;359(1445):839–850.
5. Schultz GS, Wysocki A. Interactions between extracellular matrix and growth factors in wound healing. *Wound Repair Regen.* 2009;17(2):153–162.
6. Martin P, Leibovich SJ. Inflammatory cells during wound repair: the good, the bad and the ugly. *Trends Cell Biol.* 2005;15(11):599–607.
7. Thelen M. Dancing to the tune of chemokines. *Nat Immunol.* 2001;2(2):129–134.
8. Muller WA. Leukocyte-endothelial-cell interactions in leukocyte transmigration and the inflammatory response. *Trends Immunol.* 2003;24(6):327–334.
9. Thuraisingam T, Xu YZ, Eadie K, et al. MAPKAPK-2 signaling is critical for cutaneous wound healing. *J Invest Dermatol.* 2010;130(1):278–286.
10. Savill J. Phagocyte recognition of apoptotic cells. *Biochem Soc Trans.* 1996;24(4):1065–1069.
11. Stappenbeck TS, Miyoshi H. The role of stromal stem cells in tissue regeneration and wound repair. *Science.* 2009;324(5935):1666–1669.
12. Taylor G, Lehrer MS, Jensen PJ, Sun TT, Lavker RM. Involvement of follicular stem cells in forming not only the hair follicle but also the epidermis. *Cell.* 2000;102(4):451–461.
13. Cotsarelis G. Epithelial stem cells: a folliculocentric view. *J Invest Dermatol.* 2006;126(7):1459–1468.
14. Werner S, Grose R. Regulation of wound healing by growth factors and cytokines. *Physiol Rev.* 2003;83(3):835–870.
15. Chmielowiec J, Borowiak M, Morkel M, et al. c-Met is essential for wound healing in the skin. *J Cell Biol.* 2007;177(1):151–162.
16. Chernyavsky AI, Arredondo J, Wess JR, Karlsson E, Grando SA. Novel signaling pathways mediating reciprocal control of keratinocyte migration and wound epithelialization through M3 and M4 muscarinic receptors. *J Cell Biol.* 2004;166(2):261–272.
17. Pullar CE, Rizzo A, Isseroff RR. beta-Adrenergic receptor antagonists accelerate skin wound healing: evidence for a catecholamine synthesis network in the epidermis. *J Biol Chem.* 2006;281(30):21225–21235.

18. Icre G, Wahli W, Michalik L. Functions of the peroxisome proliferator-activated receptor (PPAR)α and β in skin homeostasis, epithelial repair, and morphogenesis. *J Investig Dermatol Symp Proc.* 2006;11 (1):30–35.

19. Zhao M, Song B, Pu J, et al. Electrical signals control wound healing through phosphatidylinositol-3-OH kinase-gamma and PTNE. *Nature.* 2006;442(7101): 457–460.

20. Sternlicht MD, Werb Z. How metalloproteinases regulate cell behavior. *Annu Rev Cell Dev Biol.* 2001;17: 463–516.

21. Chan LK. Current thoughts on angiogenesis. *J Wound Care.* 2009;18(1):12–14, 16.

22. Bishop A. Role of oxygen in wound healing. *J Wound Care.* 2008;17(9):399–402.

23. Pugh CW, Ratcliffe PJ. Regulation of angiogenesis by hypoxia: role of the HIF system. *Nat Med.* 2003;9(6): 677–684.

24. Serini G, Valdembri D, Bussolino F. Integrins and angiogenesis: a sticky business. *Exp Cell Res.* 2006; 312(5):651–658.

25. Barrientos S, Stojadinovic O, Golinko MS, Brem H, Tomic-Canic M. Growth factors and cytokines in wound healing. *Wound Repair Regen.* 2008;16(5): 585–601.

26. Gabbiani G. The myofibroblast in wound healing and fibrocontractive diseases. *J Pathol.* 2003;200 (4);500–503.

27. Stamenkovic I. Extracellular matrix remodeling: the role of matrix metalloproteinases. *J Pathol.* 2003;200 (4):448–464.

28. Levenson SM, Geever EF, Crowley LV, Oates JF III, Berard CW, Rosen H. The healing of rat skin wounds. *Ann Surg.* 1965;161:293–308.

29. Werner S, Krieg T, Smola H. Keratinocyte-fibroblast interactions in wound healing. *J Invest Dermatol.* 2007;127(5):998–1008.

Patient and Wound Assessment

Judd E. Hollander, MD

Evaluation of the patient with a traumatic wound begins with an expeditious, comprehensive assessment of the patient. This initial assessment can be divided into primary and secondary surveys, following Advanced Trauma Life Support Algorithms. Before focusing attention on the laceration, the clinician must exclude less obvious but more serious life-threatening injuries.

External bleeding can usually be controlled by direct pressure over the site of bleeding. Application of a tourniquet is seldom necessary and is not recommended for routine wound care. When possible, skin flaps should be returned to their original position prior to application of pressure. This will prevent further vascular compromise of the injured area. Amputated extremities should be covered with a moist, sterile, protective dressing, placed in a waterproof bag, and then placed in a container of ice water for preservation and consideration of future reattachment.

Remove any constricting rings or other jewelry from the injured body part as soon as possible to prevent circumferential objects from acting as constricting bands and causing distal ischemia.

Patient comfort should be a priority. In most cases, pain can be reduced by compassionate and professional evaluation of the patient. Before wound preparation, many patients will need some form of anesthesia (see Chapter 5). Preparing the local anesthetic out of the patient's sight may reduce anxiety caused by seeing a needle.

MEDICAL HISTORY

Many patients may have already attempted to cleanse or care for their wound. The clinician should inquire about any treatments or home remedies that the patient has used to self-manage the laceration, including solutions or cleansing agents that may have been applied.

A history of any allergies to anesthetic agents or antibiotics should be obtained. With the increased incidence of severe reactions to latex products, one should also review any prior allergies to latex. The need for further tetanus vaccination should be determined, following the recommendations of the Centers for Disease Control and Prevention.[1] (See Chapter 23.)

Proper wound management begins with a thorough patient history, especially emphasizing the various factors that can have adverse effects on wound healing. Host factors such as the extremes of age, diabetes mellitus, chronic renal failure, obesity, malnutrition, and the use of immunosuppressive medications such as steroids and chemotherapeutic agents all increase the risk of wound infection and can impair wound healing.[2] Wound healing may also be impaired by inherited or acquired connective tissue disorders such as Ehlers–Danlos syndrome, Marfan's syndrome, osteogenesis imperfecta, and protein and vitamin C deficiencies.[1] The tendency of patients to form keloids should be ascertained, as this may result in a poor scar. Black and Asian populations are more prone to keloid formation.[1]

The anatomic location of the injury helps predict the likelihood of infection as well as the long-term cosmetic result. In general, the body can be divided into separate anatomic areas according to the composition of the skin microflora:

- On the body surface of the upper arms, and legs, the density of the bacterial population is low.
- Moist areas of the body, such as the axilla, perineum, toe webs, and intertriginous areas, contain millions of bacteria per square centimeter.
- The exposed areas of the body may also have a bacterial density in the millions per square centimeter but the flora will be more homogeneous.
- Organisms are normally sparse on the palms and dorsa of the hands, in the hundreds per square centimeter.
- Most organisms on the hands (10,000 to 100,000 per square centimeter) reside beneath the distal end of the fingernail plate or adjacent to the fingernail folds.
- The oral cavity is usually heavily contaminated with facultative species and obligate anaerobes.

Obviously, any wounds with human or animal fecal contaminants run a high risk of infection, even with therapeutic intervention.

In addition to bacterial flora, anatomical variation in regional blood flow also plays a role in determining the likelihood of infection (Table 3-1). Wounds located on highly vascular areas, such as the face or scalp, are less likely to be infected than wounds located in less vascular areas.[3] The increased vascularity of the area more than offsets the high bacterial inoculum found in the scalp. Lacerations of the scalp and face have a very low infection rate regardless of the intensity of cleansing (Table 3-1).[4]

Identification of the mechanism of injury helps identify the presence of any potential wound contaminants and foreign bodies that can result in chronic infection and delayed healing. Visible contamination of the wound doubles the risk of infection.[5] Organic and inorganic components of soil are infection-potentiating: wounds contaminated by these fractions will become infected with lower doses of bacterial inoculum. The major inorganic infection-potentiating particles are the clay fractions, which are most concentrated in the subsoil rather than the topsoil. Injuries that occur in swamps or excavations are at high risk of being contaminated by these fractions. Some soil contaminants, such as sand grains, are relatively innocuous. The black dirt on the surface of highways appears to have minimal chemical reactivity.

The type of forces applied at the time of injury also helps predict the likelihood of infection.[6] The most common mechanism of injury is application of a blunt force such as bumping the head against a coffee table. Such contact crushes the skin against an underlying bone, causing the skin to split. Crush injuries, which tend to cause greater devitalization of tissue, are more susceptible to infection than wounds resulting from shearing forces. Mammalian bites are a relatively infrequent cause of lacerations, but the management of bite wounds differs from that of other lacerations (see Chapter 15).

Impact injuries with low energy levels may not result in division of the skin but they can disrupt vessels, leading to an ecchymosis. Disruption of vessels in the underlying tissue results in hematoma formation. Some hematomas spontaneously resorb. Those that become encapsulated usually require treatment to prevent permanent subcutaneous deformity. While still gelatinous, a hematoma may be treated by incision and drainage. As further liquefaction occurs, aspiration with a large-bore needle (18-gauge or larger) with sterile technique may be possible.

WOUND EXAMINATION AND EXPLORATION

Adequate wound examination should optimally be conducted under good lighting conditions with minimal bleeding. Cursory examination under poor lighting or when the depths of the wound are obscured by blood will ultimately result in underdetection of

TABLE 3–1	Risk of Wound Infection as a Function of Anatomic Location
Location	**Risk of Infection**
Head and neck	1%–2%
Upper extremity	4%
Lower extremity	7%

embedded foreign bodies and damage to important structures such as tendons, nerves, or arteries. One way to minimize the possibility of missing an injury to a vital structure is to start the wound examination with a careful neurovascular assessment of pulses, motor function, and sensation distal to the laceration. Finger tourniquets may be used to obtain a bloodless field, but they should not be used for more than 30 to 60 minutes. The use of sterile technique is addressed in Chapter 4, on wound preparation.

The presence of a foreign body is associated with a threefold increase in risk of infection.[5] In fact, failure to diagnose foreign bodies is the fifth leading cause of litigation against emergency physicians. Missed tendon and nerve injuries and failure to prevent infection are other common wound-related causes of litigation.

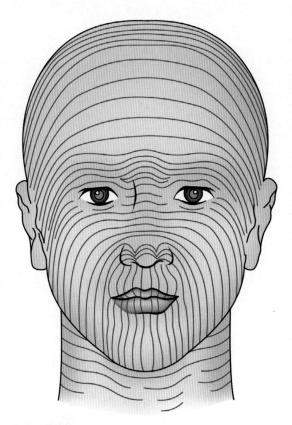

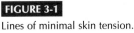

FIGURE 3-1
Lines of minimal skin tension.

PREDICTING COSMETIC OUTCOME

Patients should be educated regarding the expected cosmetic outcome. They should be explicitly told that they will have some scarring. The maximal width of the scar can often be predicted based upon wound location and alignment with lines of minimal tension. Wound location contributes to the cosmetic appearance of the scar by affecting static and dynamic skin tensions. Lacerations over joints are subject to large dynamic skin tensions and will have a wider scar than similar lacerations that are subject to less tension. Wounds that run perpendicular to the lines of minimal skin tension will also be prone to the development of wider scars (see Figure 3-1). Minimally modifiable to nonmodifiable factors associated with a suboptimal cosmetic outcome include the location of the laceration (larger scars on extremities), presence of tissue trauma, patient age, and wound width.[7] Patients should be educated about the expected outcome before wound closure to reduce the likelihood that the result will not meet their expectations. They should clearly understand that all traumatic lacerations result in some scarring.

REFERENCES

1. Singer AJ, Hollander JE, Quinn JV. Evaluation and management of traumatic lacerations. *N Engl J Med.* 1997;337(16):1142–1148.
2. Cruse PJ, Foord R. A five-year prospective study of 23,649 surgical wounds. *Arch Surg.* 1973;107(2):206–209.
3. Hollander JE, Singer AJ, Valentine S, Henry MC. Wound registry: development and validation. *Ann Emerg Med.* 1995;25(5):675–685.
4. Hollander JE, Richman PB, Werblud M, Miller T, Huggler J, Singer AJ. Irrigation in facial and scalp lacerations: does it alter outcome? *Ann Emerg Med.* 1998;31(1):73–77.
5. Hollander JE, Singer AJ, Valentine SM, Shofer FS. Risk factors for infection in patients with traumatic lacerations. *Acad Emerg Med.* 2001;8(7):716–720.
6. Cardany CR, Rodeheaver G, Thacker J, Edgerton MT, Edlich RF. The crush injury: a high risk wound. *JACEP.* 1976;5(12):965–970.
7. Singer AJ, Quinn JV, Thode HC Jr, Hollander JE; TraumaSeal Study Group. Determinants of poor outcome after laceration and surgical incision repair. *Plast Reconstr Surg.* 2002;110(2):429–435.

CHAPTER 4

Wound Preparation

Ronald Moscati, MD, FACEP

Open wounds continue to be a common presenting complaint to the emergency department (ED), with Centers for Disease Control and Prevention statistics for 2004 reporting 11.7 million visits for wound care and 6.4 million visits for open wounds.[1] For many wounds that do not involve damage to underlying structures, the most important complication to avoid is the development of a wound infection. Studies of wounds undergoing primary closure in the ED give overall infection rates of less than 5% in the United States.[2–4] Many factors influence the likelihood of infection. These include wound characteristics such as contamination, presence of foreign material, devitalized tissue, anatomic location, and timing of closure. Host factors such as immune competence, perfusion of the affected area, age, and other medical comorbidities also influence the rate of infection. In general, wounds in highly vascular areas such as the face and scalp have a low likelihood of infection whereas those in the distal extremities are at higher risk. The practitioner can reduce the likelihood of infection by good wound preparation prior to closure as well as by choosing the best closure technique for the given wound.

Preparing the wound for closure often begins during the initial assessment of the wound. This requires a controlled environment with good lighting. For optimal wound care, the patient needs to be calm and cooperative as well. The provider should explain the process and provide appropriate analgesia. If circumstances preclude patient cooperation, such as with small children or individuals with cognitive impairment, sedation should be considered. Wound preparation for closure is best performed with the wound anesthetized. This allows the wound to be thoroughly examined without the examination causing patient discomfort.

Bleeding control and removal of clotted blood, foreign material, and devitalized tissue is necessary for evaluation of the extent of the wound and involvement of deeper structures. Wounds need to be explored in their entirety. Deeper wounds, especially in the presence of significant subcutaneous adipose, can make the identification of deep structure injury or contamination difficult. These wounds may require extension to achieve adequate visualization. Gross contamination, foreign bodies, damage to structures beneath the cutaneous injury, devitalized tissue, and large areas of missing tissue should be identified. For extremity lacerations, the practitioner should also assess distal motor and sensory function and distal perfusion. Significant deep structure damage, missing tissue, or loss of distal function may necessitate consultation with other surgical services.

USE OF STERILE TECHNIQUE

Traditionally lacerations have been closed with sterile technique. This necessitates the use of sterile gloves, sterile saline for irrigation, and sterile supplies. A study comparing the use of sterile technique versus clean technique showed no benefit with the former.[5] Several studies have been

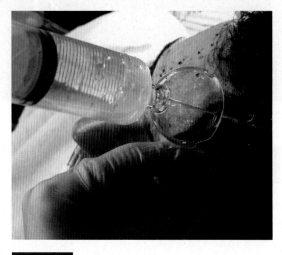

FIGURE 4-1

Wound irrigation with a syringe and splash shield.

published regarding the use of tap water rather than sterile saline.[3,4,6–10] The use of sterile gloves has also been challenged recently.[11] These studies support the idea that clean technique is likely reasonable for most simple laceration closures.

Wounds require an inoculum of more than 10^5 bacteria per gram of tissue to initiate infection.[12–14] The number of bacteria required to cause infection is lower if foreign materials are present. Such debris may serve as a nidus for bacteria. Many if not most wounds do not contain this level of bacterial contamination. Clean technique does not introduce sufficient bacteria into the wound to result in infection. Cost savings in supplies and health provider time are another argument in favor of clean technique.

Providers preparing to clean and close wounds must protect themselves from blood and body fluid exposure. Gloves and face shields are necessities. Gloves that are powder- and latex-free reduce the risk of contamination or allergic reactions. Hair covers and protective gowns should be used when appropriate. When one is using syringes for irrigating, splash guards help to contain contaminated irrigating fluids (Figure 4-1).[15]

FOREIGN BODIES

Foreign material should be removed from wounds if possible prior to closure. Such materials may carry bacteria into the wound or serve as a nidus for other bacterial contamination. Retained foreign bodies may also cause additional injury and inflammation in the future. In instances where the removal of inert foreign

material may cause more damage, patients should be informed of the decision to forgo removal.[16]

For wounds with suspected large foreign bodies, an attempt to explore and remove these should precede any imaging. Imaging after removal of obvious foreign bodies will confirm that additional material is not present. In cases where multiple smaller foreign bodies are present, removal before imaging may eliminate the need for multiple attempts at imaging to confirm removal.

Plain radiography will identify radiopaque materials such as metallic objects, stone or gravel, bone, teeth, and glass.[17] The ability to identify objects also depends upon the size, shape, and location of the foreign body. Overlying bone may obscure less radiodense objects. Placement of surface markers can facilitate pinpointing the location of foreign bodies. Wood and other vegetable matter are typically not well visualized on plain radiographs.

Ultrasound has been studied to identify radiolucent objects such as plastics, wood, and other organic materials.[18–20] It is also capable of detecting metals and other radiopaque objects. Because most foreign bodies being sought in the ED are fairly superficial, a high-frequency probe is most useful. Ultrasound has advantages in cost and time in EDs with bedside ultrasound capability.

HAIR REMOVAL

Removal of hair around a wound is not absolutely necessary for wound closure. In fact, it has been suggested that scalp wounds can be reapproximated by using long straight hair adjacent to the wound to tie across the wound as a suture would be.[21,22] Hair is also useful as a landmark when reapproximating wound edges. This is particularly true in areas where hair density changes abruptly such as scalp margins, eyebrows, and some areas of truncal hair. Hair removal of the eyebrows in particular should not be done because it may not regrow and can leave an obvious cosmetic defect.

Hair can get into wounds or obscure good visualization of the wound, however. When this is the case, hair should be clipped or alternatively can be wetted to slick it away from the laceration. Clipping hair is preferred over shaving because the latter causes small abrasions to skin around the wound that may allow bacterial contamination during the healing process and increase the likelihood of infection.[23]

HEMOSTASIS

In wounds with arterial bleeding or significant persistent venous bleeding, hemostasis is a priority for patient stabilization. On the extremities, tourniquets can be applied proximal to the wound to control bleeding and identify the source of bleeding. In other areas, clamps or clips may be used to initially control and identify bleeding sources. Bleeding from large arteries or extensive deep structure damage warrants consultation with other surgical services. Further ED patient care should be directed at fluid resuscitation and possibly transfusion with correction of clotting deficiencies if indicated.

For most wounds in the ED, hemostasis is necessary during the initial wound assessment to adequately visualize the wound. Bleeding can also occur as a result of debridement, scrubbing, or irrigation. Applying pressure may be adequate to control minor bleeding. The use of epinephrine in local anesthetics can also help control bleeding because of its vasoconstrictive effects. As is mentioned previously, tourniquets on the extremities and clamps or clips in other anatomical areas can facilitate initial control and identification of more significant bleeding sources. Small vessels can be ligated with absorbable suture or cauterized with electrocautery devices. If tourniquets are used on proximal extremities, the time should be kept to less than 30 minutes and should be properly documented.[16] Small rubber bands or a sterile glove rolled back on the affected digit can be used to tourniquet individual fingers.

SCRUBBING

The intact skin in the field surrounding the wound should be cleaned with antiseptic solution to remove bacteria and other contaminants prior to cleaning within the wound. A recent multicenter randomized trial found that preoperative application of chlorhexidine–alcohol was more effective as a skin preparation than povidine–iodine for preventing surgical incisional infections in the operating room setting.[24] If there is dried blood or other embedded debris, the area may need to be scrubbed. Abrading the area, as with shaving, should be avoided because it can allow bacterial contamination of surrounding skin and increase development of wound infections.

Likewise if the wound itself has significant dried debris, scrubbing may be useful to remove it. Vigorous scrubbing causes tissue damage that may delay healing. Therefore scrubbing a wound should be reserved for wounds with visible, adherent debris. High porosity sponges with surfactant are recommended as most efficient for wound scrubbing.[25]

Dried blood can be loosened with water or a mixture of water and hydrogen peroxide. After wetting and loosening adherent debris, removal requires less vigorous scrubbing.

Extensive use of hydrogen peroxide in wound fields is not routinely encouraged because of tissue toxicity. But in wounds that contain large amounts of adherent material, the trade off with less vigorous scrubbing may warrant its limited use.

SURGICAL DEBRIDEMENT

Devitalized tissue needs to be removed from wounds prior to closure. This includes crushed and devascularized or grossly contaminated tissue. This is particularly true at the wound margins where healing will be impaired by the presence of nonviable tissue.[26] Small islands or pedicles of tissue are frequently devascularized and should be removed. Inorganic material left in the dermis or superficial subcutaneous tissue can result in tattooing and should be removed whenever possible.[27] Delayed healing and/or the presence of contaminated tissue increases the risk of developing wound infections.

Sharp excision with a scalpel resulting in clean edges of healthy tissue results in better healing and cosmesis. Irregular wound margins with devitalized tissue can be debrided in an elliptical shape to provide better wound closure. Care should be taken not to remove so much tissue that closure results in excessive skin tension. Subcutaneous tissue may also need to be excised to reduce skin tension. Wounds that require more extensive debridement should be referred to surgical services for debridement in the operating room.

WOUND IRRIGATION

Lacerations in the ED are irrigated to reduce the likelihood of infection. Irrigation techniques have been extensively studied. Many lacerations do not initially contain sufficient bacteria to cause infection. However, this is not always able to be determined by gross inspection. The objective of irrigation is to physically remove bacteria and foreign material present in the wound that can serve as a nidus for bacterial contamination.

The irrigant fluid need not be antiseptic nor even necessarily sterile. Older studies demonstrated that irrigants such as povidine-iodine did not reduce infection rates over sterile saline.[28] This was explained as being because of the tissue toxicity of antiseptics, which delayed healing. The net effect was no decrease in infections. More recent studies comparing sterile saline with tap water also showed no difference in infection rates and some studies even showed improvement in infection rates with tap water.[3,4,6-10]

The important issue in wound irrigation is adequate pressure of the irrigating fluid. The irrigant must be applied throughout the wound with greater than 8 psi.[29] The upper end of irrigant pressure is likely around 70 psi before the pressure itself causes further tissue damage.[30]

The volume of irrigant is likely a secondary factor in good irrigation technique. In general, the greater volume of irrigant applied, the better removal of foreign material, although this has not been well studied.

Adequate irrigating pressure can be achieved with tap water in most municipalities in the United States. Typical irrigant pressures are in the 40 to 50 psi range.[31] Irrigation of wounds in a sink in the ED works well for hands and forearms but can be more impractical for other areas of the body. This also has the added benefit of reducing splash exposure for the ED provider. Connecting tubing to a tap can allow other anatomical areas to be irrigated in this manner. The use of 35 cc syringes with plastic catheters or splash shields also achieves pressures greater than 8 psi (Figure 4-1).[32] These devices can be used with tap water from a basin.

Inadequate pressure is generated by bags of IV saline with IV tubing running by gravity or even when used with pressure on the IV bag. Likewise, squeezing saline from plastic bottles with holes punched in the cap will also not reach 8 psi. Bulb syringes do not generate adequate pressure either.[33] Soaking wounds does little to remove bacteria or foreign material and may allow further bacterial proliferation.[33]

DELAYED PRIMARY CLOSURE

Delayed primary closure should be considered for wounds with gross contamination, preexisting infection, or bite wounds that require closure for functional or aesthetic reasons.[34] These wounds need to be prepared for closure as has been described for wounds being closed immediately. The wound is then packed with saline-soaked gauze and a dressing is applied. The packing and dressing can be changed daily or left intact for several days. Topical antibiotics are not necessary. Systemic antibiotics may be used. The patient then returns in 2 to 5 days to have the wound reassessed. If it is without evidence of infection, it can then be closed in the standard fashion. These wounds have much less risk of infection than they would have had they been closed initially.

SUMMARY

Good wound preparation facilitates wound healing that results in lower risk of wound infection and better cosmetic outcome. Patient cooperation, proper lighting, and appropriate equipment are necessary to prepare wounds for closure. Assessment of the wound requires complete exploration to identify the full extent of injury and exclude involvement of deeper structures.

Wound preparation for closure involves prepping surrounding intact skin and removal of foreign bodies, dried blood, contaminants, and any devitalized tissue. Wound irrigation removes smaller particulate matter and bacteria to reduce the inoculum below levels that lead to infection. Tap water irrigation provides sufficient pressure to clean wounds and has advantages in volume, cost, and potential health provider exposure to body fluid. Clean technique, as opposed to sterile technique, is sufficient for most wounds and has additional advantages in cost and time. Delayed primary closure should be considered for wounds with gross contamination.

REFERENCES

1. McCaig L. National Hospital Ambulatory Medical Care Survey: 2004 emergency department summary. *Advance Data From Vital and Health Statistics.* Hyattsville, MD: National Center for Health Statistics; 2006. DHHS publication no. (PHS) 2006–1250.
2. Rutherford WH, Spence RA. Infection in wounds sutured in the accident and emergency department. *Ann Emerg Med.* 1980;9(7):350–352.
3. Valente JH, Forti RJ, Freundlich LF, Zandieh SO, Crain EF. Wound irrigation in children: saline solution or tap water? *Ann Emerg Med.* 2003;41(5): 609–616.
4. Moscati RM, Mayrose J, Reardon RF, Janicke DM, Jehle DV. A multicenter comparison of tap water versus sterile saline for wound irrigation. *Acad Emerg Med.* 2007;14(5):404–409.
5. Worrall J. Repairing skin lacerations: does sterile technique matter? *Can Fam Physician.* 1987;33: 1185–1187.
6. Bansal BC, Wiebe RA, Perkins SD, Abramo TJ. Tap water for irrigation of lacerations. *Am J Emerg Med.* 2002;20(5):469–472.
7. Godinez FS, Grant-Levy TR, McGuirk TD, Letterle S, Eich M, O'Malley GF. Comparison of normal saline vs tap water for irrigation of minor lacerations in the emergency department. *Acad Emerg Med.* 2002;9:396–397.
8. Griffiths RD, Fernandez RS, Ussia CA. Is tap water a safe alternative to normal saline for wound irrigation in the community setting? *J Wound Care.* 2001;10 (10):407–411.

9. Fernandez R, Griffiths R. Water for wound cleansing [see comment] [update of *Cochrane Database Syst Rev.* 2002;(4):CD003861; PMID: 12519612]. *Cochrane Database of Syst Rev.* 2008;(1):CD003861.

10. Weiss E, Lin M, Oldham G. Tap water is equally safe and effective as sterile normal saline for wound irrigation: a double blind, randomized, controlled, prospective clinical trial. *Acad Emerg Med.* 2007;14: S146–S147.

11. Perelman VS, Francis GJ, Rutledge T, Foote J, Martino F, Dranitsaris G. Sterile versus nonsterile gloves for repair of uncomplicated lacerations in the emergency department: a randomized controlled trial. *Ann Emerg Med.* 2004;43(3):362–370.

12. Edlich RF, Rodeheaver GT, Morgan RF, Berman DE, Thacker JG. Principles of emergency wound management. *Ann Emerg Med.* 1988;17(12):1284–1302.

13. Marshall KA, Edgerton MT, Rodeheaver GT, Magee CM, Edlich RF. Quantitative microbiology: its application to hand injuries. *Am J Surg.* 1976;131(6): 730–733.

14. McManus AT, Kim SH, McManus WF, Mason AD Jr, Pruitt BA Jr. Comparison of quantitative microbiology and histopathology in divided burn-wound biopsy specimens. *Arch Surg.* 1987;122(1):74–76.

15. Pigman EC, Karch DB, Scott JL. Splatter during jet irrigation cleansing of a wound model: a comparison of three inexpensive devices. *Ann Emerg Med.* 1993;22(10):1563–1567.

16. DeBoard RH, Rondeau DF, Kang CS, Sabbaj A, McManus JG. Principles of basic wound evaluation and management in the emergency department. *Emerg Med Clin North Am.* 2007;25(1):23–39.

17. Manthey DE, Storrow AB, Milbourn JM, Wagner BJ. Ultrasound versus radiography in the detection of soft-tissue foreign bodies. *Ann Emerg Med.* 1996; 28(1):7–9.

18. Schlager D. Ultrasound detection of foreign bodies and procedure guidance. *Emerg Med Clin North Am.* 1997;15(4):895–912.

19. Orlinsky M, Knittel P, Feit T, Chan L, Mandavia D. The comparative accuracy of radiolucent foreign body detection using ultrasonography. *Am J Emerg Med.* 2000;18(4):401–403.

20. Hill R, Conron R, Greissinger P, Heller M. Ultrasound for the detection of foreign bodies in human tissue. *Ann Emerg Med.* 1997;29(3):353–356.

21. Karaduman S, Yürüktümen A, Güryay SM, Bengi F, Fowler JR Jr. Modified hair apposition technique as the primary closure method for scalp lacerations. *Am J Emerg Med.* 2009;27(9):1050–1055.

22. Ong MEH, Chan YH, Teo J, et al. Hair apposition technique for scalp laceration repair: a randomized controlled trial comparing physicians and nurses (HAT 2 study). *Am J Emerg Med.* 2008;26(4):433–438.

23. Seropian R, Reynolds BM. Wound infections after preoperative depilatory versus razor preparation. *Am J Surg.* 1971;121(3):251–254.

24. Darouiche RO, Wall MJ Jr, Itani KM, et al. Chlorhexidine-alcohol versus povidine-iodine for surgical-site antisepsis. *N Engl J Med.* 2010;362(1): 18–26.

25. Rodeheaver GT, Smith SL, Thacker JG, Edgerton MT, Edlich RF. Mechanical cleansing of contaminated wounds with a surfactant. *Am J Surg.* 1975;129(3):241–245.

26. Haury B, Rodeheaver G, Vensko J, Edgerton MT, Edlich RF. Debridement: an essential component of traumatic wound care. *Am J Surg.* 1978;135(2):238–242.

27. Singer AJ, Dagum AB. Current management of acute cutaneous wounds. *N Engl J Med.* 2008;359(10): 1037–1046.

28. Dire DJ, Welsh AP. A comparison of wound irrigation solutions used in the emergency department. *Ann Emerg Med.* 1990;19(6):704–708.

29. Rodeheaver GT, Pettry D, Thacker JG, Edgerton MT, Edlich RF. Wound cleansing by high pressure irrigation. *Surg Gynecol Obstet.* 1975;141(3):357–362.

30. Wheeler CB, Rodeheaver GT, Thacker JG, Edgerton MT, Edilich RF. Side-effects of high pressure irrigation. *Surg Gynecol Obstet.* 1976;143(5):775–778.

31. Moscati R, Mayrose J, Fincher L, Jehle D. Comparison of normal saline with tap water for wound irrigation. *Am J Emerg Med.* 1998;16(4):379–381.

32. Singer AJ, Hollander JE, Subramanian S, Malhotra AK, Villez PA. Pressure dynamics of various irrigation techniques commonly used in the emergency department. *Ann Emerg Med.* 1994;24(1):36–40.

33. Lammers RL, Fourré M, Callaham ML, Boone T. Effect of povidone-iodine and saline soaking on bacterial counts in acute, traumatic, contaminated wounds. *Ann Emerg Med.* 1990;19(6):709–714.

34. Edlich RF, Rogers W, Kasper G, Kaufman D, Tsung MS, Wangensteen OH. Studies in the management of the contaminated wound. I. Optimal time for closure of contaminated open wounds. II. Comparison of resistance to infection of open and closed wounds during healing. *Am J Surg.* 1969;117(3):323–329.

CHAPTER 5

Wound Anesthesia

Joel M. Bartfield, MD, FACEP

Patients with lacerations commonly present to the emergency department. Wound repair can be an emotional and traumatic experience even for the most stoic of patients. It is therefore important to maintain a calm, supportive environment during wound treatment. One study reported beneficial effects of allowing patients to listen to music during laceration repair.[1] In this study, patients who listened to music during laceration repair reported less pain and anxiety (though only the former reached statistical significance) than those who did not. Although it may not be possible to provide music for patients in many emergency settings, physicians should make every effort to minimize patient anxiety during wound care. For example, anesthesia preparation including withdrawing anesthetics and needle and syringe preparation should be done out of the eyesight of patients. Minimizing the pain of infiltration of local anesthetics has obvious merit.

MINIMIZING PAIN OF INJECTION

Several factors have been demonstrated to influence the pain of local anesthetic infiltration. These include the type of anesthetic,[2,3] needle size,[4,5] pH[3,6-7] and temperature of the solution,[8-10] and speed and depth of injection.[4,5,11,12] The best studied technique for minimizing pain is buffering. Local anesthetics are weak bases. They are marketed in solutions that are slightly acidic to increase their shelf-life. Several studies have shown that buffering solutions to approximately physiologic pH decreases the pain of infiltration.[3,4,6-10] Appropriate buffering is done by adding sodium bicarbonate (1 mEq/mL) to anesthetic in approximately a 10:1 dilution (10 mL of anesthetic to 1 mL of sodium bicarbonate). This can be accomplished by adding 2 mL of sodium bicarbonate to a 20 mL vial of anesthetic. Buffered lidocaine can be used for up to one week after preparation with no clinical change in efficacy.[13]

Warming local anesthetics has not always been shown to decrease pain of infiltration.[9-14] In contrast, pain has been consistently shown to decrease by slow infiltration and subcutaneous injection as opposed to intradermal injection.[4,5,11,12] Pain of infiltration has also been shown to decrease by infiltration of local anesthetics from within the wound rather through intact skin.[15,16] Pretreatment of wounds with topical tetracaine has been shown to reduce pain of infiltration.[17] Pretreatment with other combination topical anesthetics has also been shown to minimize the pain associated with anesthetic infiltration.[18-20]

LOCAL ANESTHESIA WITHOUT INJECTION

A number of different combinations of agents have been studied as topical anesthetics that completely obviate the need for needle infiltration. The combination that was first studied is TAC, a combination of tetracaine (0.5%), adrenaline (1:2000), and cocaine (11.8%). However, TAC has a number of limitations. It has been found to be inferior to lidocaine infiltration on wounds other than those involving the face and scalp in one study,[21] and inferior to lidocaine in another.[22] It has also been found to be less effective for large lacerations, and in adults compared with children.[21] Like other topical anesthetics, TAC needs to be left in place for at least 10 to 15 minutes to achieve anesthesia. The agent has traditionally been contraindicated on areas supplied by end arterioles because of its vasoconstrictive properties.[21–22] Finally, TAC cannot be used on mucous membrane abrasions and burns because of enhanced cocaine absorption[21] and inappropriate use of TAC on mucous membranes has been associated with seizures and death.[23–27]

Other topical anesthetic combinations have been shown to be effective as local anesthetics. Topical 5% lidocaine with epinephrine[28] and lidocaine, adrenaline, and tetracaine (LET)[29] have both compared favorably to TAC. EMLA™ cream is a eutectic mixture of lidocaine and prilocaine and has been used successfully as an anesthetic on intact skin prior to invasive procedures such as phlebotomy, intravenous insertion, and lumbar puncture.[30–36] Both EMLA™ and LET have been shown to reduce the pain of infiltration of local anesthetics.[18–20]

Traditional local anesthetics can be "infiltrated" into the skin without the use of a needle. This can be accomplished through either jet injection or iontophoresis. Jet injection involves the use of a device that essentially sprays material at high pressure (200 psi) into skin. Small amounts (0.1 mL) of anesthetic can be infiltrated in this way to depths of 1.5 cm. The technique is limited by the fact that only small amounts of anesthetic can be delivered at a time.[37–39]

Iontophoresis takes advantage of the fact that anesthetics exist in solution as salts of weak bases and therefore are positively charged. Anesthetics can therefore be forced into the skin by being exposed to an electric field in which the positively charged anesthetic is repelled by the positive pole. This technique has been shown to be effective in delivering anesthetics in volunteer subjects[40,41] and prior to intravenous catheter placement in pediatric patients.[42] The technique has not been studied as a means of providing anesthesia for lacerations. Widespread use of iontophoresis is limited by the fact that it requires special equipment and several minutes to deliver anesthetic.

DOSAGE CONSIDERATIONS

Local anesthetics have dosage-related toxicities. A weight-based (mg/kg) dosing is useful in pediatric patients. In adult patients the maximum safe dosages are generally expressed in absolute terms, because weight does not correlate well with peak anesthetic drug levels.[43] The maximum safe amount of plain lidocaine in an adult patient is 300 mg. This amount corresponds to 30 cc of a 1% solution because a 1% solution contains 1000 mg per 100 mL or 10 mg/mL. It is important to note that the maximum doses refer to subcutaneous or intradermal injections. Toxicity may occur at a much lower dosage if anesthetics are inadvertently injected intravascularly. Table 5-1 provides generally accepted maximum dosages for commonly used local anesthetics.

Several options are available if volumes that approach toxicity are required. These include selection of a less toxic agent; dilution of the agent; providing anesthesia as a nerve or field block, which often requires less volume than simple local anesthesia; and the addition of epinephrine. Epinephrine at a concentration of approximately 1:100,000 can be added to anesthetics or is commercially available for some anesthetics. The vasoconstrictive properties of epinephrine increase the amount of anesthetic that can be safely injected by decreasing systemic absorption.

TABLE 5–1	**Maximum Safe Dosages for Selected Anesthetics**			
Generic Name	**Trade Name**	**Classification**	**Adult Dosage**	**Pediatric Dosage**
Lidocaine	Xylocaine	Amide	300 mg	4 mg/kg
Lidocaine with epinephrine	Xylocaine with epinephrine	Amide	500 mg	7 mg/kg
Bupivacaine	Marcaine	Amide	175 mg	1.5 mg/kg
Bupivacaine with epinephrine	Marcaine with epinephrine	Amide	225 mg	3 mg/kg
Procaine	Novocain	Ester	500 mg	7 mg/kg
Procaine with epinephrine	Novocain with epinephrine	Ester	600 mg	9 mg/kg

A more bloodless field is also provided by the use of epinephrine. The use of anesthetics with epinephrine has several disadvantages. Though difficult to reference, the vasoconstrictive properties of epinephrine may theoretically increase the risk of wound infections. Anesthetics containing epinephrine or any other vasoconstrictor have traditionally been avoided in regions of the body with end-arteriolar supply such as digits, penis, ear lobes, and nose. However there is a growing body of evidence suggesting that the use of commercially available anesthetic combinations containing epinephrine is safe in most of these areas.[44] Finally, anesthetics containing epinephrine have been shown to be more painful to inject.[2,3]

ALTERNATIVES TO COMMONLY USED LOCAL ANESTHETICS

Local and regional anesthetics are generally either amides or esters of the "caine" family. Esters were the first to be developed, of which procaine is the prototype. Esters are metabolized in plasma by pseudocholinesterases compared with amides, which are metabolized by the liver. Amides such as lidocaine are most often utilized because esters have a relatively high incidence of allergic reactions.

True anaphylaxis to local anesthetics, particularly amides, is extremely rare.[45–47] Skin testing among patients with a reported lidocaine allergy have shown that very few reactions represent true allergies.[46,47] However, it is not uncommon for patients to report an allergy to local anesthetics and, even if it is only a remote possibility, anaphylaxis is a potentially lethal complication, which is obviously best avoided.

The first step in evaluating a patient who states that he or she is "allergic" to local anesthetics is to define the true nature of the previous reaction. This can sometimes be challenging because patients are often unable to distinguish a true allergic reaction from a vasovagal reaction. If a patient is felt to have a true history of an allergic reaction, choosing an alternate class of anesthetics would be a viable option. For instance, if a patient was know to be allergic to lidocaine, an amide anesthetic, an ester anesthetic such as tetracaine could be used safely. However, patients may not be able to identify which anesthetic caused the previous reaction. The situation is further complicated by the fact that patients who report a true allergy to "lidocaine" are most often allergic to methylparaben, the preservative used in multidose vials, rather than allergic to lidocaine itself. Ester anesthetics would not be a good choice in such a scenario because they are degraded to para-aminobenzoic acid, a chemical that is closely related to methylparaben and could possibly induce the same allergic reaction. Single-dose lidocaine (lidocaine for IV use) would be a reasonable alternative to multidose lidocaine if it were possible to determine that an individual patient was allergic to methylparaben rather than lidocaine itself. However, it is often impossible to make this distinction. Therefore, alternatives to traditional anesthetics have been sought.

Diphenhydramine is an antihistamine that has been studied as an alternate anesthetic to lidocaine.[48–51] Though the chemical structure of antihistamines is closely related to that of local anesthetics, it is dissimilar enough that the antigenicity is not the same.[47] A 1% solution of diphenhydramine provides anesthesia comparable to 1% lidocaine, but the solution is considerably more painful to administer than lidocaine.[48–50] In an effort to reduce pain of infiltration, Ernst et al.[49] compared 0.5% diphenhydramine to 1% lidocaine, but found the lower concentration of diphenhydramine was less effective than 1% lidocaine. The clinical utility of diphenhydramine is further limited by side effects including sedation, local irritation, erythema, vesicle formation, tissue necrosis, and prolonged anesthesia.[48,49,51,52] Singer and Hollander[52] attempted to attenuate the pain of injection as well as the local irritant effects of diphenhydramine by buffering the solution. However, they found no significant differences between the pain of infiltration of plain and buffered diphenhydramine solutions. Because of the relative discomfort of diphenhydramine infiltration and potential side effects, other non-"caine" anesthetics have been sought for patients who are allergic to lidocaine.

Benzyl alcohol (as found as a preservative in multidose normal saline) has been studied as a possible alternative local anesthetic.[2,53–55] Wightman and Vaughan[2] compared benzyl alcohol and five other anesthetics and found that benzyl alcohol was the least painful. Novak et al.[56] and Kimura et al.[57] found very low toxicity of benzyl alcohol in parenteral administration. Thomas[54] and Nuttall et al.[55] have reported that benzyl alcohol facilitates intravenous line placement via its anesthetic effect. The utility of benzyl alcohol is limited by its short duration of action, which has been found to be only a few minutes.[2] By adding epinephrine to the solution, Martin and Wilson[53] showed that benzyl alcohol can provide long-term anesthesia, though less adequately than lidocaine with epinephrine.

Bartfield et al.[58] compared benzyl alcohol with epinephrine 1:100,000, 1% diphenhydramine, and 0.9% buffered lidocaine and reported that benzyl alcohol with epinephrine was the least painful of the three anesthetics. Although benzyl alcohol with epinephrine was found to be somewhat less effective than buffered lidocaine, it was generally felt to provide adequate anesthesia for the majority of subjects tested in this volunteer-based study. Bartfield et al. also compared benzyl alcohol with epinephrine to lidocaine with epinephrine in patients with simple lacerations.[59] The benzyl alcohol with epinephrine was found to be less painful. Although not statistically significant, eight of the 26 patients in the benzyl alcohol group with epinephrine needed additional anesthesia compared to two of 26 in the lidocaine group. Two of the 26 patients in the benzyl alcohol group required supplemental anesthesia within 15 minutes.[59] A solution containing benzyl alcohol with epinephrine 1:100,000 can be made by adding 0.2 mL of epinephrine 1:1000 to a 20 mL vial of multidose normal saline containing 0.9% benzyl alcohol.

CLINICAL PRACTICE

Local Versus Regional Anesthesia

For many wounds, anesthesia is accomplished by local infiltration of anesthetics directly into the wound. This technique has the advantage of being easy to perform, reliable, and safe providing proper technique is utilized and toxicity is not exceeded. Local hemostasis is also achieved by direct infiltration of local anesthetics, particularly those containing epinephrine.

Local anesthesia has several noteworthy disadvantages. Infiltration of anesthetics in and around wounds distorts anatomy and can make subsequent repair of lacerations more difficult. Compared with nerve blocks, local anesthesia often requires larger volumes of anesthetic. Additionally, local infiltration requires multiple injections. Table 5-2 summarizes advantages and disadvantages of nerve blocks, topical anesthesia, and local anesthesia.

Field blocks involve infiltration of anesthetic either surrounding an area or interrupting the nerve supply to that area. This technique has the advantage of providing reliable anesthesia without disrupting anatomy. However, field blocks can only be used in certain areas of the body with appropriate sensory innervation. Common areas that can be anesthetized by field blocks include the forehead, ear, and nose. Compared with nerve blocks, or sometimes even local anesthesia, a relatively large volume of anesthetic is required.

Lacerations to several areas of the body can be anesthetized through the use of nerve blocks. For certain clinical situations nerve blocks offer several advantages over local infiltration of anesthetics. Nerve blocks generally require less volume of anesthetic, do not distort anatomy, and can often be accomplished with a single injection. The practitioner must have a good working knowledge of anatomy to successfully perform nerve blocks. Care should be taken to identify landmarks and it is essential to utilize proper sterile technique when performing nerve blocks. Patients should be warned that they might feel paresthesias during the technique. If paresthesias are elicited (indicating that the needle is very close to the target nerve) the needle should be withdrawn slightly and then the anesthetic should be injected. It is important to always aspirate prior to injecting because vascular structures

TABLE 5–2	**Comparison of Types of Anesthesia**	
	Advantages	**Disadvantages**
Topical	■ Painless ■ Does not distort the anatomy	■ Not always reliable (works best on face) ■ Danger of absorption if used on mucous membranes ■ Cannot be used on areas with end-arteriolar circulation ■ Delayed onset
Local	■ Ease of technique ■ Reliability	■ May require high volumes of anesthetic ■ May be excessively painful in certain locations (tips of extremities, palms, soles) ■ May distort anatomy
Nerve/field blocks	■ Does not distort anatomy ■ Requires lower volume of anesthetic	■ Only useful for certain locations ■ Not as reliable as local ■ Somewhat delayed onset

tend to be close to nerves. An adequate amount of anesthetic should be injected in the area of the nerve, and after infiltration, the practitioner should gently massage the area (if possible) to help diffuse the anesthetic into the nerve being blocked. It may take several minutes for nerve blocks to take effect. If a block has been unsuccessful, the practitioner has the option of attempting the block again or resorting to local anesthesia, remembering not to exceed the maximum allowable amount of local anesthetic.

An exhaustive review of all nerve blocks is beyond the context of this text. Several of the most commonly used blocks that are particularly useful will be reviewed. These include digital nerve blocks and blocks involving nerves supplying sensation to the hand, foot, and face.

Digital Nerve Block

Injuries to digits are commonly encountered and performing digital nerve blocks is easily learned. There are two sets (palmar and dorsal) of digital nerves that each run along the lateral aspect of the digit. The palmar nerves supply most of the sensation to the fingertips of the middle three fingers; therefore, a block at this location is generally all that is required. The dorsal nerves must also be blocked to provide good anesthesia for the thumb and fifth finger. Care must be taken to avoid injury to vascular structures when one is performing these blocks.

Buffered lidocaine has been shown to be less painful to administer for digital nerve blocks than plain lidocaine.[7] Several acceptable techniques for performing digital nerve blocks are available. Conventional digital blocks can be performed by introducing the needle through the dorsal or ventral surface of the digit near its base (Figure 5-1). The nerve can be blocked either at the metacarpophalangeal joint or anywhere along its course. Metacarpophalangeal blocks are performed by inserting a needle into the web space between the digits on either side of the digit being blocked and depositing the anesthetic opposite the joint (Figure 5-2). Although the technique is relatively easy to learn, in one study involving 30 volunteers, it was found to be less reliable (23% failure rate vs 3% failure rate) and to have a slower onset (6.35 minutes vs 2.82 minutes) compared with block performed along the digit.[60]

Nerve Blocks of the Hand

A knowledge of the sensory innervation of the hand is essential when one is choosing appropriate nerve blocks for hand injuries. Local infiltration into the

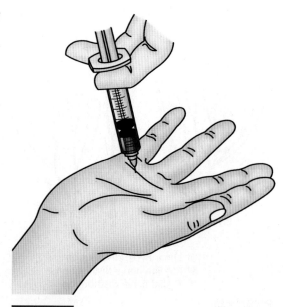

FIGURE 5-1

Metacarpal digital nerve block. The needle is introduced through the palmar aspect of the hand at the level of the distal palmar crease , or in the webspace between the fingers.

hand, particularly into the thick palmar skin, can be particularly painful; therefore, the practitioner is well advised to learn and utilize these blocks when clinically indicated. Figure 5-3 demonstrates the typical sensory innervation of the hand. The practitioner should remember that innervation is variable and, therefore, more than one block may be required for wounds in certain locations.

Ulnar nerve block

The ulnar nerve can be blocked at the wrist or the elbow. The wrist is preferable because the nerve can be easily damaged at the elbow because of its superficial

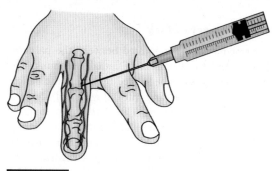

FIGURE 5-2

Conventional digital nerve block. The needle is introduced through the dorsal aspect of the finger at its base.

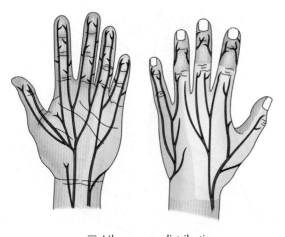

Ulnar nerve distribution
Median nerve distribution
Radial nerve distribution

FIGURE 5-3

The sensory innervation of the hand.

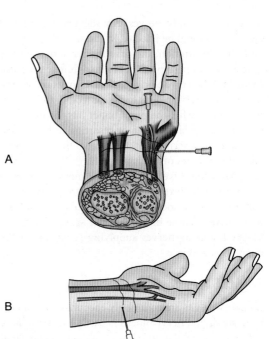

A

B

FIGURE 5-4

Ulnar nerve block. The nerve can be blocked by inserting the needle through the volar (A) or ulnar (B) aspect of the wrist.

location and close proximity to bony structures. At the wrist, the nerve lies between the flexor carpi ulnaris tendon and the ulnar artery. It can be blocked either by introducing the needle between these two structures (Figure 5-4A) or by introducing the needle underneath the flexor carpi ulnaris tendon at the ulnar aspect of the wrist (Figure 5-4B, author's preferred method). With either technique, care should be taken to avoid injection into the ulnar artery by aspirating prior to injection. A total of 5 cc to 7 cc of agent is injected to achieve anesthesia.[61] The ulnar nerve can also be blocked at the elbow by infiltrating small amounts of anesthesia in proximity to the nerve that runs in the groove between the medial epicondyle of the humerus and the olecranon of the ulna.

Median nerve block

The median nerve is located between the palmaris longus and the flexor carpi radialis tendons. The palmaris longus can be located by having the patient oppose the thumb and fifth finger and flex the wrist against resistance. This tendon is congenitally absent approximately 20% of the time. In these instances, the nerve can be found approximately 1 cm ulnar to the flexor carpi radialis. The median nerve is blocked by puncturing the flexor retinaculum between the two wrist creases at the location of the nerve and injecting 5 cc to 8 cc of agent at this site (Figure 5-5).[61]

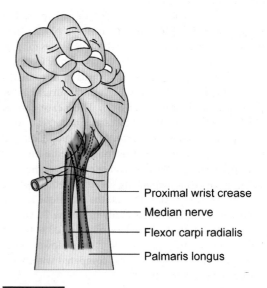

—— Proximal wrist crease
—— Median nerve
—— Flexor carpi radialis
—— Palmaris longus

FIGURE 5-5

Median nerve block. The needle is inserted between the palmaris longus and flexor carpi radialis tendons between the proximal and distal wrist crease. The Palmaris longus can be easily visualized when the patient makes a fist and flexes the wrist.

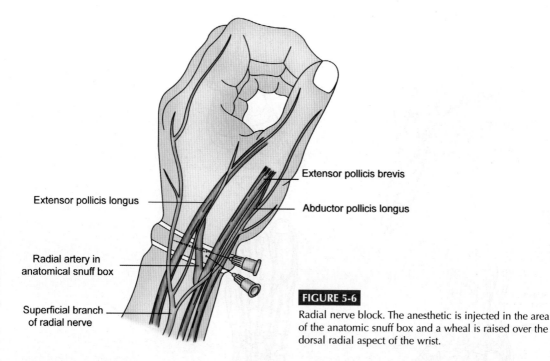

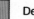

Extensor pollicis brevis

Extensor pollicis longus

Abductor pollicis longus

Radial artery in anatomical snuff box

Superficial branch of radial nerve

FIGURE 5-6

Radial nerve block. The anesthetic is injected in the area of the anatomic snuff box and a wheal is raised over the dorsal radial aspect of the wrist.

Radial nerve block

The radial nerve follows the radial artery and then fans out dorsally distal to the wrist. The nerve is blocked by injecting into the anatomic snuff box and laying a 6 cm to 8 cm wheal of anesthetic as a field block across the dorsal portion of the radial aspect of the wrist (Figure 5-6).

Nerve Blocks of the Ankle

Ankle blocks are somewhat more difficult to accomplish than the other blocks discussed in this chapter. However, because local anesthesia to the sole of the foot is particularly difficult to accomplish and painful to administer because of skin thickness, familiarity with these blocks can be very useful. Anesthesia to the foot can be provided by five different nerve blocks at the ankle. Sensory innervation is somewhat variable; therefore, multiple blocks are often employed. The sole of the foot is supplied by the tibial nerve (which branches into the medial and lateral plantar nerve) and the sural nerve (Figure 5-7). The most lateral aspect of the dorsum of the foot is supplied by the sural nerve with the remainder supplied by the superficial and deep peroneal nerves and the saphenous nerve (Figure 5-7).

Tibial nerve (medial and lateral plantar nerves) block

The tibial nerve is located in close proximity to the tibia between the medial malleolus and the Achilles

Superficial peroneal distribution

Sural nerve distribution

Deep personal distribution

Posterior tribial nerve distribution

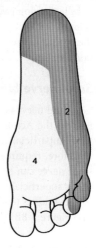
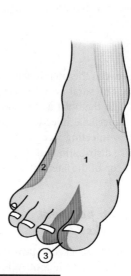

FIGURE 5-7

Sensory innervation of the foot.

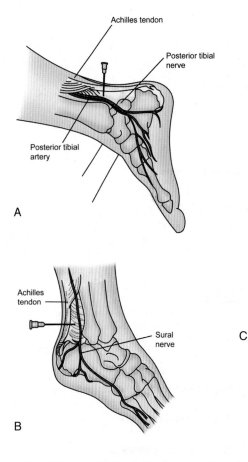

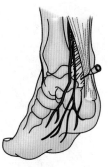

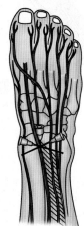

FIGURE 5-8

Nerve blocks of the ankle. Posterior tibial (A), sural (B) and deep perineal (C) blocks. See text for details.

tendon. This nerve is blocked by injecting 5 cc of anesthetic agent between the posterior tibial artery and the Achilles tendon just posterior to the medial malleolus (Figure 5-8A).[61] The block is best accomplished with the patient in the prone position with the foot in slight dorsiflexion.

Sural nerve block

The sural nerve is located between the lateral malleolus and the Achilles tendon. The sural nerve is relatively superficial compared with the tibial nerve, and, therefore, requires a more superficial injection. The sural nerve can be blocked by injecting 5 cc of anesthetic superficially in a fanlike distribution just lateral to the Achilles tendon at the top of the lateral malleolus (Figure 5-8B).[62]

Superficial peroneal, deep peroneal, and saphenous nerve blocks

All three of these nerves should be blocked to provide adequate anesthesia to the dorsum of the foot. With the patient in a supine position, the skin is entered between the extensor hallucis longus and anterior tib-

ial tendons at a point parallel to the superior aspect of the medial malleolus. The deep peroneal nerve is blocked by a deep injection between the two tendons, while the other two nerves are blocked by superficial injections (Figure 5-8C). The needle is then withdrawn and redirected subcutaneously toward the lateral malleolus to block the superficial peroneal nerve and then medially to block the saphenous nerve.[61] A total of 15 cc of agent will usually be required to block all three nerves.

Facial Nerve Blocks

The advantages of nerve blocks are well demonstrated regarding the management of facial lacerations. Meticulous attention to wound repair can often be facilitated by the proper placement of a nerve block, which provides complete anesthesia without distorting the edges of the laceration. The trigeminal nerve supplies sensation to the face. The three branches of this nerve commonly blocked are the supraorbital, infraorbital, and mental nerves. The three nerves exit from foramina that fall along a line that connects the medial aspect of the pupil with the corner of the mouth (Figure 5-9.)

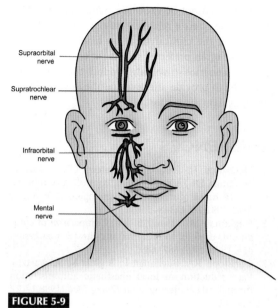

FIGURE 5-9

Sensory innervation of the face.

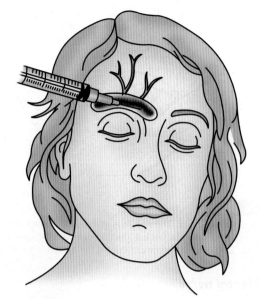

FIGURE 5-10

Supraorbital nerve block. The needle is inserted at the site of the supraorbital notch to block the supraorbital nerve and a wheal is raised medially over the eyebrow to block the supratrochlear nerve as well.

Supraorbital and supratrochlear nerves

The supraorbital nerve supplies sensation to most of the forehead. The area near the bridge of the nose is supplied by the supratrochlear nerve. The supraorbital nerve exits at the supraorbital foramen and the supratrochlear nerve exits 5 mm to 10 mm medial to it. Both nerves can therefore be blocked at this easily identifiable location (Figure 5-10).[62]

Infraorbital nerve

The infraorbital nerve supplies sensation to the medial aspect of the mid-face including the upper lip. The nerve exits through the infraorbital foramen. The foramen is easily palpated just below the inferior border of the orbit along the line previously described. The infraorbital nerve can be blocked either by injection through intact skin or through buccal mucosa (Figure 5-11). This latter technique was shown to be more reliable and less painful in a study involving 12 volunteers.[63] Injection through the buccal mucosa is accomplished by inserting a ³/₄-inch needle to the hub into the buccal–mucosal sulcus opposite the upper canine and palpating the foramen as the anesthetic is introduced. Care must be taken to introduce the needle along the surface of the maxilla to avoid the globe and to not penetrate the skin of the face. Because of the risk of an inadvertent needle stick to the practitioner with the intraoral approach, some prefer the percutaneous approach.

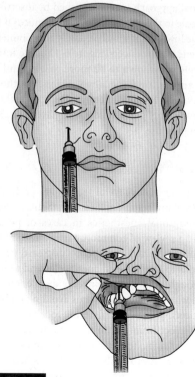

FIGURE 5-11

Infraorbital nerve block. The nerve can be blocked by introducing the needle through the skin at the level of the infraorbital foramen (top) or through the oral mucosa (bottom).

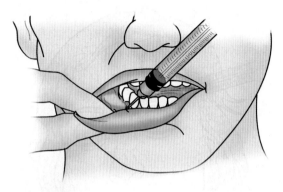

FIGURE 5-12

Mental nerve block. The needle is introduced through the mouth at the alveolar-buccal junction opposite the canine tooth and directed downward toward the mental foramin.

Mental nerve

The mental nerve supplies sensation to the superior chin and lower lip. This nerve exits through the mental foramen, which can be palpated along the previously described line in the lateral chin. Similar to with the infraorbital nerve, there are two approaches to blocking the mental nerve, transcutaneous or intraoral injection. The intraoral approach is accomplished by inserting a $\frac{3}{4}$-inch needle to the hub into the buccal–mucosal fold opposite the lower canine and palpating the foramen as the anesthetic is introduced (Figure 5-12). The intraoral technique was shown to be more reliable and less painful in a study involving 10 volunteers.[64] Although facial blocks can be very effective, their reliability is lower in emergency practitioners who have little experience with their use.[65]

SUMMARY

This chapter describes several techniques of decreasing the pain of infiltration of local anesthetics, alternatives to traditional anesthetics in cases of possible allergy, and a review of commonly used nerve blocks. The author's preferred method to decrease pain of infiltration is to use buffered anesthetics and to inject slowly through a small-gauge needle deep enough so that a skin wheal is not raised (thus avoiding intradermal injection). When administering local anesthesia, I prefer to inject from within the wound rather than through intact skin. Topical anesthetics such as LET provide alternatives to infiltration of anesthetics and are useful either alone or prior to local infiltration. Even if complete anesthesia is not provided with these agents, subsequent pain of infiltration should be lessened. When allergy to amide and/or ester "caine"

anesthetics cannot be excluded, benzyl alcohol with epinephrine offers a relatively painless viable alternative. When the clinical situation lends itself, nerve blocks are often preferred to local anesthesia. For all clinical scenarios involving wound care, the goal should be to provide affective anesthesia while minimizing patient discomfort.

REFERENCES

1. Menegazzi JJ, Paris PM, Kersteen CH, Flynn B, Trautman DE. A randomized, controlled trial of the use of music during laceration repair. *Ann Emerg Med.* 1991;20(4):348–350.
2. Wightman MA, Vaughan RW. Comparison of compounds used for intradermal anesthesia. *Anesthesiology.* 1976;45(6):687–689.
3. Christoph RA, Buchanan L, Begalia K, Schwartz S. Pain reduction in local anesthetic administration through pH buffering. *Ann Emerg Med.* 1988;17(2):117–120.
4. Arndt KA, Burton C, Noe JM. Minimizing the pain of local anesthesia. *Plast Reconstr Surg.* 1983;72(5):676–679.
5. Berk WA, Welch RD, Bock BF. Controversial issues in clinical management of the simple wound. *Ann Emerg Med.* 1992;21(1):72–80.
6. Bartfield JM, Gennis P, Barbera J, Breuer B, Gallagher EJ. Buffered versus plain lidocaine as a local anesthetic for simple laceration repair. *Ann Emerg Med.* 1990;19(12):1387–1389.
7. Bartfield JM, Ford DT, Homer PJ. Buffered versus plain lidocaine for digital nerve blocks. *Ann Emerg Med.* 1993;22(2):216–219.
8. Orlinsky M, Hudson C, Chan L, Deslauriers R. Pain comparison of unbuffered versus buffered lidocaine in local wound infiltration. *J Emerg Med.* 1992;10(4):411–415.
9. Brogan GX Jr, Giarrusso E, Hollander JE, Cassara G, Maranga MC, Thode HC. Comparison of plain, warmed, and buffered lidocaine for anesthesia of traumatic wounds. *Ann Emerg Med.* 1995;26(2):121–125.
10. Mader TJ, Playe SJ, Garb JL. Reducing the pain of local anesthetic infiltration: warming and buffering have a synergistic effect. *Ann Emerg Med.* 1994;23(3):550–554.
11. Krause RS, Moscati R, Filice M, Lerner EB, Hughes D. The effect of injection speed on the pain of lidocaine infiltration. *Acad Emerg Med.* 1997;4(11):1032–1035.
12. Scarfone RJ, Jasani M, Gracely EJ. Pain of local anesthetics: rate of administration and buffering. *Ann Emerg Med.* 1998;31(1):36–40.
13. Bartfield JM, Homer PJ, Fort DT, Sternklar P. Buffered lidocaine as a local anesthetic: an investigation of shelf life. *Ann Emerg Med.* 1992;21(1):16–19.
14. Bartfield JM, Crisafulli KM, Raccio-Robak N, Salluzzo RF. The effects of warming and buffering on pain of infiltration of lidocaine. *Acad Emerg Med.* 1995;2(4):254–258.

15. Kelly AM, Cohen M, Richards D. Minimizing the pain of local infiltration anesthesia for wounds by injection into the wound edges. *J Emerg Med.* 1994;12(5):593–595.

16. Bartfield JM, Sokaris SJ, Raccio-Robak N. Local anesthesia for lacerations: pain of infiltration inside versus outside the wound. *Acad Emerg Med.* 1998; 5(2):100–104.

17. Bartfield JM, Lee FS, Raccio-Robak N, Salluzzo RF, Asher SL. Topical tetracaine attenuates the pain of infiltration of buffered lidocaine. *Acad Emerg Med.* 1996;3(11):1001–1005.

18. Adler AJ, Dubinsky I, Eisen J. Does the use of topical lidocaine, epinephrine, and tetracaine solution provide sufficient anesthesia for laceration repair? *Acad Emerg Med.* 1998;5(2):108–112.

19. Singer AJ, Stark MJ. Pretreatment of lacerations with lidocaine, epinephrine, and tetracaine at triage: a randomized double-blind trial. *Acad Emerg Med.* 2000;7(7):751–756.

20. Singer AJ, Stark MJ. LET versus EMLA for pretreating lacerations: a randomized trial. *Acad Emerg Med.* 2001;8(3):223–230.

21. Grant SA, Hoffman RS. Use of tetracaine, epinephrine, and cocaine as a topical anesthetic in the emergency department. *Ann Emerg Med.* 1992;21(8): 987–997.

22. Hegenbarth MA, Altieri MF, Hawk WH, Greene A, Ochsenschlager DW, O'Donnell R. Comparison of topical tetracaine, adrenaline, and cocaine anesthesia with lidocaine infiltration for repair of lacerations in children. *Ann Emerg Med.* 1990;19(1):63–67.

23. Dailey RH. Fatality secondary to misuse of TAC solution. *Ann Emerg Med.* 1988;17(2):159–160.

24. Jacobson S. Errors in emergency practice. *Emerg Med.* 1987;19(20):106–109.

25. Daya MR, Burton BT, Schleiss MR, DiLiberti JH. Recurrent seizures following mucosal application of TAC. *Ann Emerg Med.* 1988;17(6):646–648.

26. Wehner D, Hamilton GC. Seizures following topical application of local anesthetics to burn patients. *Ann Emerg Med.* 1984;13(6):456–458.

27. Dronen SC. Complications of TAC [letter]. *Ann Emerg Med.* 1983;12(5):333.

28. Blackburn PA, Butler KH, Hughes MJ, Clark MR, Riker RL. Comparison of tetracaine-adrenaline-cocaine (TAC) with topical lidocaine-epinephrine (TLE): efficacy and cost. *Am J Emerg Med.* 1995; 13(3):315–317.

29. Ernst AA, Marvez-Valls E, Nick TG, Weiss SJ. LAT (lidocaine-adrenaline-tetracaine) versus TAC (tetracaine-adrenaline-cocaine) for topical anesthesia in face and scalp lacerations. *Am J Emerg Med.* 1995; 13(2):151–154.

30. Buckley MM, Benfield P. Eutectic lidocaine/prilocaine cream. A review of the topical anaesthetic/analgesic efficacy of a eutectic mixture of local anaesthetics (EMLA). *Drugs.* 1993;46(1):126–151.

31. Michael A, Andrew M. The application of EMLA and glyceryl trinitrate ointment prior to venepuncture. *Anaesth Intensive Care.* 1996;24(3):360–364.

32. Young SS, Schwartz R, Sheridan MJ. EMLA cream as a topical anesthetic before office phlebotomy in children. *South Med J.* 1996;89(12):1184–1187.

33. Vaghadia H, al-Ahdal OA, Nevin K. EMLA patch for intravenous cannulation in adult surgical outpatients. *Can J Anaesth.* 1997;44(8):798–802.

34. Sharma SK, Gajraj NM, Sidawi, Lose K. EMLA cream effectively reduces the pain of spinal needle insertion. *Reg Anesth.* 1996;21(6):561–564.

35. Juárez Gimenez JC, Oliveras M, Hidalgo E, et al. Anesthetic efficacy of eutectic prilocaine-lidocaine cream in pediatric oncology patients undergoing lumbar puncture. *Ann Pharmacother.* 1996;30(11):1235–1237.

36. Lee JJ, Rubin AP. EMLA cream and its current uses. *Br J Hosp Med.* 1993;50(8):463–466.

37. Hingston RA, Hughes JG. Clinical studies with jet injection: a new method for drug administration. *Curr Res Anesth Analg.* 1947;26:221–230.

38. Bennett CR, Mundell RD, Monheim LM. Studies on tissue penetration characteristics produced by jet injection. *J Am Dent Assoc.* 1971;83(3):625–629.

39. Hardison CD. Application of a versatile instrument for the production of cutaneous anesthesia without needle penetration of the skin. *JACEP.* 1977;6(6): 266–268.

40. Ashburn MA, Gauthier M, Love G, Basta S, Gaylord B, Kessler K. Iontophoretic administration of 2% lidocaine HCl and 1:100,000 epinephrine in humans. *Clin J Pain.* 1997;13(1):22–26.

41. Greenbaum SS, Bernstein EF. Comparison of iontophoresis of lidocaine with a eutectic mixture of lidocaine and prilocaine (EMLA) for topically administered local anesthesia. *J Dermatol Surg Oncol.* 1994;20(3):579–583.

42. Kim MK, Kini NM, Troshynski TJ, Hennes HM. A randomized clinical trial of dermal anesthesia by iontophoresis for peripheral intravenous catheter placement in children. *Ann Emerg Med.* 1999;33(4): 395–399.

43. Scott DB, Jebson PJ, Braid DP, Ortengren B, Frisch P. Factors affecting plasma levels of lignocaine and prilocaine. *Br J Anaesth.* 1972;44(10):1040–1049.

44. Waterbrook AL, Germann CA, Southall JC. Is epinephrine harmful when used with anesthetics for digital nerve blocks? *Ann Emerg Med.* 2007;50(4): 472–475.

45. Chandler MJ, Grammer LC, Patterson R. Provocative challenge with local anesthetics in patients with a prior history of reaction. *J Allergy Clin Immunol.* 1987;79(6):883–886.

46. Incaudo G, Schatz M, Patterson R, Rosenberg M, Yamamoto F, Hamburger RN. Administration of local anesthetics to patients with a history of prior adverse reaction. *J Allergy Clin Immunol.* 1978;61(5):339–345.

47. Adriani J, Zepernick R. Allergic reactions to local anesthetics. *South Med J.* 1981;74(6):694–699, 703.

48. Green SM, Rothrock SG, Gorchynski J. Validation of diphenhydramine as a dermal local anesthetic. *Ann Emerg Med.* 1994;23(6):1284–1289.

49. Ernst AA, Anand P, Nick T, Wassmuth S. Lidocaine versus diphenhydramine for anesthesia in the

repair of minor lacerations. *J Trauma*. 1993;34(3): 354–357.

50. Ernst AA, Marvez-Valls E, Mall G, Patterson J, Xie X, Weiss SJ. 1% lidocaine versus 0.5% diphenhydramine for local anesthesia in minor laceration repair. *Ann Emerg Med*. 1994;23(6):1328–1332.

51. Dire DJ, Hogan DE. Double-blinded comparison of diphenhydramine versus lidocaine as a local anesthetic. *Ann Emerg Med*. 1993;22(9):1419–1422.

52. Singer AJ, Hollander JE. Infiltration pain and local anesthetic effects of buffered vs plain 1% diphenhydramine. *Acad Emerg Med*. 1995;2(10):884–888.

53. Wilson L, Martin S. Benzyl alcohol with epinephrine as an alternative local anesthetic. *Ann Emerg Med*. 1999;33(5):495–499.

54. Thomas DV. Saline with benzyl alcohol prevents pain of needle insertion [letter]. *Anesth Analg*. 1984; 63(9):883.

55. Nuttall GA, Barnett MR, Smith RL II, Blue TK, Clark KR, Payton BW. Establishing intravenous access: a study of local anesthetic efficacy. *Anesth Analg*. 1993; 77(5):950–953.

56. Novak E, Stubbs SS, Sanborn EC, Eustice RM. The tolerance and safety of intravenously administered benzyl alcohol methylprednisolone sodium succinate formulations in normal human subjects. *Toxicol Appl Pharmacol*. 1972;23(1):54–61.

57. Kimura ET, Darby TD, Krause RA, Brondyk HD. Parenteral toxicity studies with benzyl alcohol. *Toxicol Appl Pharmacol*. 1971;18(1):60–68.

58. Bartfield JM, Jandreau SW, Raccio-Roback N. A randomized trial of diphenhydramine versus benzyl alcohol with epinephrine as an alternative to lidocaine local anesthesia. *Ann Emerg Med*. 1998;32(6): 650–654.

59. Bartfield JM, May-Wheeling HE, Raccio-Robak N, Lai SY. Benzyl alcohol with epinephrine as an alternative local anesthetic to lidocaine with epinephrine. *J Emerg Med* 2001;21(4):375–379.

60. Knoop K, Trott A, Syverud S. Comparison of digital versus metacarpal blocks for repair of finger injuries. *Ann Emerg Med*. 1994;23(6):1296–1300.

61. Ferrera PC, Chandler R. Anesthesia in the emergency setting: Part I. Hand and foot injuries. *Am Fam Physician*. 1994;50(3):569–573.

62. Ferrera PC, Chandler R. Anesthesia in the emergency setting: Part II. Head and neck, eye and rib injuries. *Am Fam Physician*. 1994;50(4):797–800.

63. Lynch MT, Syverud SA, Schwab RA, Jenkins JM, Edlich R. Comparison of intraoral and percutaneous approaches for infraorbital nerve block. *Acad Emerg Med*. 1994;1(6):514–519.

64. Syverud SA, Jenkins JM, Schwab RA, Lynch MT, Knoop K, Trott A. A comparative study of the percutaneous versus intraoral technique for mental nerve block. *Acad Emerg Med*. 1994;1(6):509–513.

65. Tarsia V, Singer AJ, Cassara GA, Hein MT. Percutaneous regional compared with local anaesthesia for facial lacerations: a randomised controlled trial. *Emerg Med J*. 2005;22(1):37–40.

CHAPTER 6

Procedural Sedation and Analgesia

James Miner, MD

Procedural sedation and analgesia (PSA) is commonly used to facilitate the care of wounds in the emergency department (ED).[1,2] The use of PSA allows the physician to provide analgesia, anxiolysis, and, if necessary, amnesia for the patient, and to facilitate a patient's wound repair by limiting motion during the repair of complex wounds. Analgesia and amnesia can provide the patient a more pleasant experience during wound repair. For the physician, the patient's decreased responsiveness and movement often allow the procedure to be done more quickly and achieves better results than could be achieved without sedation. This use of PSA is safe and associated with a high degree of patient satisfaction.[2–9]

Most wounds can be repaired with local anesthesia, distraction techniques, and a calm, reassuring bedside manner. Some patients, however, require PSA because of anxiety, pain, or the complexity of the wound. The term PSA describes a wide variety of depths of sedation and agents. For some patients, the principal requirement of PSA is anxiolysis, which typically does not require more than a minimal level of sedation. Other patients, such as a child with a complex facial laceration, require decreased responsiveness to limit motion during the procedure to achieve optimal results, and require carefully titrated deep sedation to maintain an adequate level of sedation without

causing oversedation and increasing the risk of adverse events.

The use of sedation is especially important in children, who have many characteristics that can make proper wound management and laceration repair challenging. Anxious young children have a hard time trying to hold still for ideal wound care, even when appropriate local analgesia has been administered, and often require PSA. Three large, prospective series describing procedural sedation in children found that procedural sedation for laceration repair represents from 18% to 58% of all sedation provided to children.[9–11] Under the right circumstances, many children can undergo wound care with only local anesthesia. This is often facilitated in children by having their parents close by to help keep them comfortable and relaxed enough to facilitate laceration repair. How a person will respond to painful stimuli and unfamiliar situations varies among individuals and situations. It is important to discuss the options that exist to facilitate laceration repair with patients in order to determine their preferences and guide their expectations.

The type of PSA that is best for a given procedure is determined by the level of sedation intended, rather than the agents used. Minimal, moderate, and deep sedation have all been described for wound care. Unlike patients who undergo sedation in other patient care settings, patients in need of acute wound care have unpredictable NPO status; may have concurrent, severe systemic disease; and usually are in pain and somewhat agitated before the procedure begins. In addition, concurrent events cannot be predicted because the injuries are not planned, which requires the procedure to adapt to a wide range of circumstances and outcomes.

INDICATIONS

Descriptions of procedural sedation are generally based on the intended depth of sedation (Table 6-1). Although sedation is generally described by its ordinal level, in reality, a spectrum exists for the depth of sedation. When a target level of sedation is chosen, plans must be made for possible excursions into deeper levels of sedation, which frequently can occur. In general, the more deeply that a patient is sedated, the higher the risk of an adverse event.[12,13] Decisions about the optimal level of sedation for patients during wound repair must take into account the patient's needs in terms of the wound care procedure, and the patient's underlying risk of an adverse event.

Minimal sedation refers to a patient who retains the ability to follow commands in an age-appropriate fashion. It is often used in procedures that require anxiolysis, but have adequate analgesia from local anesthesia, which represents a common situation in wound repair. During minimal sedation, cardiovascular and ventilatory functions are usually maintained, although patients should be monitored for inadvertent oversedation in other patient care settings, patients in need to deeper levels with oxygen saturation monitors and close supervision. Agents typically utilized for minimal sedation include nitrous oxide, alfentanil, fentanyl, midazolam, pentobarbital, and low-dose ketamine.

Moderate sedation describes patients that may have their eyes closed but respond to verbal commands, or are in a dissociative state. Unlike agents that are typically used for minimal sedation, many of the agents used for moderate sedation have been shown to be associated with amnesia of the procedure.[14] It is typically used in situations when wound complexity requires more motion control than can be achieved with minimal sedation, or the pain or anxiety caused by the procedure make amnesia an important goal of the sedation. Typically, moderate sedation patients maintain their airway and ventilatory function without support.[13,15] Inadvertent oversedation to deeper levels is common, and appropriate monitoring with direct observation of the patient's airway is important. Agents used for moderate sedation for wound care include propofol, etomidate, ketamine, methohexital, and the combination of fentanyl and midazolam.

Patients who undergo deep sedation do not respond to verbal commands but respond to pain. It is performed on patients who would benefit from a deeper level of sedation to optimally complete the wound care procedure than could be achieved with moderate sedation, such as when muscle relaxation is required. Amnesia of the procedure is similar between moderate and deep sedation, and it is not necessary to sedate patients to a deep level only to obtain

TABLE 6–1 Definition of General Anesthesia and Levels of Sedation and Analgesia[34]

	Minimal Sedation (Anxiolysis)	Moderate Sedation and Analgesia ("Conscious Sedation")	Deep Sedation and Analgesia	General Anesthesia
Responsiveness	Normal response to verbal stimulation	Purposeful response to verbal or tactile stimulation	Purposeful response following repeated or painful stimulation	Unarousable even with painful stimulus
Airway	Unaffected	No intervention required	Intervention may be required	Intervention often required
Spontaneous ventilation	Unaffected	Adequate	May be inadequate	Frequently inadequate
Cardiovascular function	Unaffected	Usually maintained	Usually maintained	May be impaired

amnesia.[13-16] Deep sedation generally is achieved in the ED with the same agents as with moderate sedation; the difference is the intended depth. Inadvertent oversedation to the level of general anesthesia (no response to pain) can occur with the use of deep sedation, and preparations must be made for airway support and management prior to starting deep sedation procedures.[13]

Generally, the deeper the level of sedation achieved and the longer the patient is sedated, the higher the risk of adverse events.[13,15,16] Patients should therefore be sedated to the lightest level of sedation necessary for their wound care, but to a depth that will allow the procedure to be completed with optimal results. If a patient only requires anxiolysis for a wound repair in which pain can otherwise be controlled locally, they should be minimally sedated. If a patient requires amnesia of a painful procedure (such as when local anesthesia will be difficult or painful to administer) they should undergo dissociative or moderate sedation. If a patient needs to be relaxed to complete a procedure, such as for a complex wound to the face or mouth, they may require deep sedation. The patient's necessity for increasing depth of sedation for his or her procedure must be balanced with the patient's pre-procedural risk of an adverse outcome to determine his or her appropriate sedation target level.

HISTORY AND COMORBIDITY

The urgency of the patient's requirement for wound repair and the patient's current medical condition must be considered in the planning of PSA. The depth and timing of the sedation can be balanced with the patient's medical condition to provide the optimal target for PSA to meet the patient's needs and minimize the risk of the procedure. A tool that can be used to assess the severity of a patient's underlying illness is the American Society of Anesthesiologists' physical status classification system (Table 6-2).[17] The risk of sedation is higher in patients with a physical status score of 3 or 4 relative to a patient with a score of 1 or 2,[18] and sedation in these patients should be undertaken with caution. Patients who are physical status class 3 and 4 are common, however, and they can be safely sedated if appropriate attention is paid to their risk and the approach to sedation. The risks of the sedatives must be appreciated and the necessary interventions to treat them must be prepared prior to starting the procedure.

A history concerning prior adverse experiences with PSA or anesthesia should be obtained in addition to the patient's current medications and allergies. The physical examination should be directed at identifying patients with a potentially difficult airway or who are at risk for cardiorespiratory instability. The airway should be examined to determine if there are abnormalities that might complicate airway management such as a short neck, micrognathia, a large tongue, trismus, tracheomalacia, laryngomalacia, morbid obesity, a history of difficult intubation, or congenital anomalies of the airway and neck.

Most PSA agents can cause vasodilatation and hypotension, and the reserve of patients with known cardiovascular disease should be assessed. Similarly, patients with decreased intravascular volume should have their fluid status optimized prior to beginning PSA to avoid hypotension from the sedative agents. Lung auscultation should be performed to assess for active pulmonary disease, especially obstructive lung disease and active upper respiratory infections that may predispose the patient to heightened airway reactivity or limit his or her reserve in the case of respiratory depression. The patient's mental status should be evaluated as well both to detect intoxication and to determine his or her baseline.

There are no routine laboratory tests necessary prior to PSA. Conditions such as airway abnormalities or infections, dehydration, fever, or hypovolemia may increase the risk of complications, and should lead to the postponement of nonurgent procedures and appropriate management prior to emergent sedations (increased monitoring, reduced level of sedation, or the use of reversible agents). The duration of the effects of the sedatives may be prolonged in infants less than 6 months of age, the elderly, and patients with hepatic or renal disease because of delayed metabolism and should be carefully evaluated during the procedure.

TABLE 6–2	**ASA Physical Status Classification**[17]
Class I	A normally healthy patient
Class II	A patient with mild systemic disease
Class III	A patient with severe systemic disease
Class IV	A patient with severe systemic disease that is a constant threat to life
Class V	A moribund patient who is not expected to survive without the procedure
Class E	Emergency procedure

PROCEDURAL URGENCY

The urgency of a patient's need for his or her wound care procedure is determined by the nature of the wound. Emergent indications for procedures include the treatment of wounds associated with vascular compromise, or intractable pain or suffering. Most wound care procedures can be delayed to some extent if necessary to mitigate procedural risk. Dirty wounds and lacerations sometimes benefit from urgent repair, depending on the degree of contamination and the location of the wound. The care of clean wounds, foreign body removal, and abscess incision and drainage can be considered semiurgent. Nonurgent indications for sedation include the removal of a chronic soft tissue foreign body, delayed primary closure of wounds, and dressing changes.

RISKS AND PRECAUTIONS

Fasting State

The complication of greatest concern for patients undergoing PSA is the development of impaired protective airway reflexes and associated aspiration pneumonia. Normally, protective airway reflexes prevent aspiration. During sedation, patients who go past the point of deep sedation to general anesthesia may lose their normal protective airway reflexes. If the patient vomits in this situation, they can aspirate gastric contents. To prevent this, elective PSA is done in patients who have an empty stomach. The amount of time required for the stomach to empty is variable depending on the patient and the most recent food eaten, and an optimal time since the most recent meal is not known.

There is insufficient evidence to support specific fasting requirements prior to procedural sedation, regardless of the target depth of sedation or the agent administered. A guideline for emergency physicians[19] has made recommendations for the proper risk stratification of patients based on their most recent oral intake. In general, the risk of aspiration from recent oral intake increases with the depth of sedation and the length of the procedure, and must be balanced with the urgency of the procedure when one is deciding whether to delay sedation because of recent oral intake.

Patients who have not had oral intake other than clear liquids for 3 hours prior to their wound repair have a low risk of aspiration at any level of sedation. For patients with recent oral intake in need of an emergent procedure, the risk of aspiration is unlikely to outweigh the risk of delaying the procedure. Because the risk of aspiration increases with the depth of sedation, it is prudent to target the lightest level of sedation feasible for the necessary procedure. For nonurgent

procedures where a time delay is unlikely to have a negative effect on the patient, patients who have eaten more than clear liquids in the prior 3 hours should have the procedure delayed until 3 hours after their most recent intake. For urgent procedures, patients who have had a small amount of oral intake, such as a light snack or a nonclear liquid, should be limited to brief (single bolus with a short-acting agent) deep sedation, and patients who have eaten a larger meal should be limited to moderate sedation for the shortest period possible. Balancing the urgency of the procedure and the nature of the oral intake with the length and depth of PSA allows for a safe approach to the timing of the start of sedation.

Patients who are intoxicated, especially with alcohol, can be especially difficult to sedate. They often have food in their stomachs and the achieved level of sedation can be difficult to predict. In urgent procedures, intoxicated patients may benefit from a delay in their sedation until the progression of their mental status (getting worse or getting better) can be ascertained through observation.

PERSONNEL

Physicians who perform PSA must be prepared to rescue patients from inadvertent oversedation and the adverse events typical of PSA. Similarly, nurses must be qualified for the role of directly monitoring PSA patients.[2,20] The necessity of two physicians to perform PSA, one for PSA administration and a second to perform the wound care procedure, has not been evaluated specifically. Many of the studies of PSA that included wound care used two physicians. A description of 1028 PSA procedures with a single physician simultaneously administering sedation and performing the procedure found adverse event rates similar to previous studies of PSA, suggesting that the use of a single physician practitioner is a safe practice.[21]

EQUIPMENT

The immediate sedation area should include all necessary age-appropriate equipment for airway management and resuscitation, including oxygen, a bag mask, suction, and oral and nasal airways. A defibrillator should be available for subjects with significant cardiovascular disease. For situations in which sedation is initiated by the intramuscular (IM), oral, nasal, inhalational, or rectal routes, intravenous (IV) access is not required. When sedation is performed without IV access, however, equipment to obtain IV access should be immediately available.

PROCEDURAL MONITORING

There are two types of monitoring used for PSA: interactive and mechanical monitoring.

Interactive Monitoring

Interactive PSA monitoring is the direct observation of the patient to assess the depth of sedation and recognize adverse events such as upper airway obstruction, impaired protective airway reflexes, hypoventilation, apnea, and vomiting. This requires continuous observation of the patient's face, mouth, and chest wall and access to the patient to address any situation that may occur.

Moderate and deep sedation require at least two medical providers; a physician and a nurse or respiratory therapist. The physician typically oversees drug administration and performs the procedure, while the nurse or respiratory therapist interactively monitors the patient. The individual dedicated to patient monitoring should have no other responsibilities that would interfere with his or her direct observation of the patient while the patient is at a moderate or deep level of sedation. Minimal sedation does not typically require dedicated interactive monitoring.

Mechanical Monitoring

Oxygenation

A patient's oxygen saturation should be monitored during PSA with pulse oximetry. Pulse oximetry is not a substitute for monitoring ventilation, as there is a variable lag time between the onset of hypoventilation or apnea and a change in oxygen saturation, especially in patients who receive supplemental oxygen.[22,23] Patients who are receiving supplemental oxygen require a ventilation monitoring modality in addition to pulse oximetry, such as interactive monitoring or a capnograph. A decline in oxygen saturation should always prompt an evaluation of respiratory rate, and adequacy of ventilation and circulation.

Ventilation

Ventilation can be monitored with capnography, the measurement of the partial pressure of carbon dioxide (CO_2) in exhaled breath, represented by the CO_2 waveform (capnogram). Changes in the capnogram shape can demonstrate changes in ventilation, and changes in end-tidal CO_2 (the maximum CO_2 concentration at the end of each tidal breath) can be used to assess the severity of these changes and the response to interventions.[24,25]

Capnography can rapidly detect apnea, upper airway obstruction, laryngospasm, bronchospasm, and respiratory failure.[24] The absence of the capnogram waveform can distinguish upper airway obstruction and laryngospasm (in the presence of chest wall motion) from apnea (in the absence of chest wall motion). Return of the waveform after airway alignment maneuvers (chin lift, jaw thrust, oral airway placement) then distinguishes upper airway obstruction from laryngospasm. Similarly, changes in the respiratory rate, depth of ventilation, and the presence of airway obstruction can be detected. In general, hypoventilation results in an increase in end tidal CO_2 as the patient retains CO_2. When there is an airway obstruction, increased airway turbulence results in the mixing of expired air with ambient air, resulting in a sudden drop in the end tidal CO_2, indicating the need for airway repositioning.

Hemodynamics

The patient's heart rate and blood pressure should be monitored during PSA. Pulse oximetry and continuous electrocardiography both provide a continuous measure of heart rate. If pulse oximetry is providing an adequate waveform, the addition of cardiac monitoring is only necessary for patients with preexisting cardiac disease.

Monitor Frequency

At a minimum, the parameters monitored during PSA should be recorded prior to the procedure, after each dose of sedative, upon completion of the procedure, at the beginning of the recovery period, and prior to discharge. During moderate and deep sedation, they should be recorded more frequently. Patients are at the highest risk of complications during the period following IV medication administration until the peak effect of the medication has been reached, and during the immediate postprocedure period when external stimuli are discontinued and the pain of the procedure has subsided, and it is common to record the vital signs at these times.

SEDATION TECHNIQUE

The approach to a patient's sedation will vary with the nature of the wound and his or her medical condition. The underlying principle to minimize risk is that the deeper the level of sedation, the longer a patient is sedated, and the greater number of doses of sedative that a patient receives, the more likely the patient is to have an adverse event.[13,26] The patient benefits from receiving the lightest level of sedation possible, but if the patient is not sufficiently sedated to facilitate the wound repair, and the procedure ends up taking longer than it would have in a more deeply sedated patient, the risk of the procedure is increased because of the length of the sedation. Finding the balance between the depth and length of the procedure is an important part of providing PSA and is essential to maximizing the safety of the procedure.

The potential adverse events of PSA must be anticipated prior to the start of the procedure. The exact depth of sedation a particular patient will reach cannot be predicted in a patient that has not received the medication before. Patients may therefore inadvertently be sedated to a deeper level than expected, and equipment must be in place to rescue a patient from oversedation to the point of general anesthesia prior to starting the sedation. Preparations should include the immediate proximity of all equipment necessary to secure a patient's airway in the case of respiratory depression. This includes supplemental oxygen, suction equipment, an oral airway, a bag-valve-mask apparatus, a laryngoscope, and an endotracheal tube.

Pre-procedure Pain Management

In patients with pain who do not obtain relief with local anesthesia prior to the sedation, the administration of 0.1 mg/kg of morphine sulfate followed by 0.05 mg/kg every 5 to 10 minutes of fentanyl 1 µg/kg followed by 0.5 µg/kg every 3 minutes until pain control is adequate prior to the start of PSA can be used to provide analgesia before and during PSA. Analgesics should be given until the patient is comfortable while at rest prior to starting the procedure. Patients whose pain cannot be controlled with analgesics at doses that do not cause an apparent decrease in their level of consciousness should be considered to have intractable pain and should undergo their wound care procedure as quickly as can safely be achieved.

The PSA procedure should begin after the last dose of analgesic has been given and has had sufficient time to reach its peak affect (2 to 5 minutes for IV morphine). Administration of combinations of sedatives such as propofol and etomidate concurrently with analgesics may increase the likelihood of adverse outcomes.[27] Many of the medications used for analgesia in the ED have half-lives that are significantly longer than the sedatives used for PSA. Unlike midazolam and fentanyl, which are classically titrated together, propofol and etomidate should be administered as sole agents after complete or near-complete analgesia has been achieved with an opioid.

The quantity of analgesics needed to make a patient comfortable before a procedure may differ drastically after the procedure than before. Once a procedure has been completed, patients can have less pain than before the procedure started. Using long-acting medications to achieve sufficient pain relief to perform a procedure without using PSA can lead to patients that are oversedated after their procedure, possibly leading to respiratory depression.

Supplemental Oxygen During PSA

The use of supplemental oxygen prior to and during PSA is a common practice. Several studies have shown that supplemental oxygen during procedural sedation can delay changes in pulse oximetry that were noted by capnography.[22] Emergency department PSA studies that have used supplemental oxygen have documented desaturation rates ranging from 5% to 7%, but similar rates have been reported in patients that did not receive supplemental oxygen.[28] It would seem that a preoxygenated patient could tolerate a longer period of apnea or hypoventilation without requiring assisted ventilation, but the oxygen does not protect the patient from the true complication of aspiration. Because supplemental oxygen may blunt or delay changes in oxygen saturation findings, it should be used in conjunction with capnography and interactive airway monitoring.

SEDATION MANAGEMENT

Once a patient has been evaluated, the appropriate sedation target level and timing have been selected, pain treatment has been initiated, and preparations have been made for possible adverse events, the procedure can begin. The patient should receive his or her initial bolus of sedative and then be closely monitored until the peak effect of the medication has been reached. If the patient has achieved the target sedation level, the wound care procedure may begin. If not, smaller repeat boluses of the sedative are given at the same time interval as the time to the onset of the peak effect of the first bolus until the appropriate sedation depth is achieved. If the patient begins to regain consciousness before wound care is completed, additional boluses of the medication can be given to extend the duration of the sedation, although this practice has been associated with an increased risk of respiratory depression and should be done cautiously.[26] Many of the sedatives used in PSA (and especially propofol) have a duration of effect dependent on the redistribution of the drug. As larger cumulative doses of the drug are given, the duration of effect will increase as redistribution occurs more slowly, making it necessary to adjust the size of the boluses and closely observe the response to each bolus before giving further medication to avoid oversedation.

Once a patient has begun to develop changes associated with oversedation, such as unresponsiveness to pain, respiratory depression, or cardiovascular compromise, it is not appropriate to sedate them further for a procedure. Patients should be monitored closely between aliquots of sedatives to determine the safety of further doses and to initiate appropriate interventions for adverse events as soon as they arise. Table 6-3 shows the general workflow of PSA procedures. Table 6-4 shows agents and doses used in PSA. Table 6-5 lists examples of agents to achieve various sedation target levels. Table 6-6 lists examples of sedation levels typical to various wound care procedures.

MINIMAL SEDATION AGENTS

Midazolam

Midazolam is a short-acting benzodiazepine that is commonly used for minimal sedation. It can be combined with an opioid such as fentanyl for moderate or deep PSA. Benzodiazepines and opioids synergistically increase respiratory depression when they are given together, and have a long duration of effect relative to most other agents used for moderate and deep PSA, making close monitoring during titration of these medications important. Midazolam causes mild cardiovascular depression, and hypotension can arise when it is given to patients who are hypovolemic. Paradoxical agitation has been reported with the use of midazolam for PSA in 1% to 15% of patients.

Midazolam can be administered through multiple routes. Oral administration leads to unreliable levels of sedation because of first-pass hepatic metabolism. The intranasal route has an irritating effect on the mucosa from the preservative benzyl alcohol that accompanies it, and can be painful and provoke anxiety. The rectal route has a variable effect and onset, but is easy to administer. Intramuscular administration also has a variable onset and duration of effect. Intravenous dosing has the most predictable onset and duration of effect.

The benzodiazepine antagonist flumazenil quickly reverses sedation and respiratory depression caused by benzodiazepines. It lowers the seizure threshold and can precipitate seizures in patients with benzodiazepine dependence, known seizure disorder, cyclic antidepressant overdose, and intracranial hypertension, and in patients on medications that also lower the seizure threshold (e.g., cyclosporin, INH, lithium, propoxyphene and TCAs). The duration of action of flumazenil is shorter than that of most benzodiazepines, and close observation should be continued for, at least, the expected duration of action of the sedative agent.

Opioids

Fentanyl

Fentanyl is a potent opioid with a short half-life. A single intravenous dose has rapid onset (<30 s), peaks in 2 to 3 minutes, and has a duration of effect of 40 minutes. It is easily titratable for use alone for minimal

TABLE 6–3	**Procedural Sedation and Analgesia (PSA) Workflow by Procedural Urgency**

Emergent procedure

- Single bolus agent targeted to minimal or moderate sedation
- Perform Procedure
- Administer local anesthetics during the sedation if possible
- Allow patient to regain baseline mental status prior to repeating dose of sedative agent
- Begin systemic analgesia therapy after sedation recovery if the patient remains in pain

Urgent, Semiurgent Procedure

- Administer analgesics if patient has pain prior to procedure, wait 20 to 30 minutes for peak effect of analgesics prior to beginning PSA
- Perform sedation, choose target sedation level based on need for relaxation (moderate and deep sedation are the same to the patient's perception)

Nonurgent procedure

- Administer analgesics if patient has pain prior to procedure, wait 20 to 30 minutes for peak effect of analgesics prior to beginning PSA
- Ensure that patient has been NPO (clear liquids only) for at least 3 hours prior to starting procedure
- Perform PSA

TABLE 6–4	Sedative Agents			
Agent	**Dose**	**Onset of Peak Effect**	**Duration of Effect**	**Typical Use**
Midazolam IV	0.05 to 0.1 mg/kg IV Repeat 0.05 mg/kg every 2 min until adequately sedated	1 to 3 min	1 hr	Minimal or moderate sedation
Midazolam IM	0.1 mg/kg IM	15 to 30 min	1 to 2 hr	Minimal sedation
Midazolam intranasal	0.2 to 0.5 mg/kg PN	2 to 5 min	1 to 2 hr	Minimal sedation
Midazolam PO/PR	0.5 to 0.75 mg/kg PO or PR	10 to 30 min	1 to 2 hr	Minimal sedation
Fentanyl IV	1 to 3 µg/kg IV, titrated up to 5 µg/kg IV	1 to 2 min	30 to 45 min	Minimal sedation
Fentanyl PN/ nebulized	3 µg/kg PN/inhaled	10 min	1 hr	Minimal sedation
Alfentanil IV	10 to 20 µg/kg IV	1 to 2 min	5 to 8 min	Minimal sedation
Nitrous oxide (inhaled)	30% to 70% inhaled with oxygen	5 min	Until discontinued	Minimal sedation
Methohexital PR	25 mg/kg PR	2 to 5 min	45 minutes	Minimal sedation
Methohexital IV	1 mg/kg IV	1 min	10 min	Moderate and/or deep sedation
Fentanyl and midazolam	1 to 2 µg/kg fentanyl plus 0.1 mg/kg midazolam	1 to 2 min	1 hr	Moderate and/or deep sedation
Etomidate	0.15 mg/kg, followed by 0.1 mg/kg every 2 min	30 to 60 seconds	5 to 10 min	Moderate and/or deep sedation
Propofol	1 to 1.5 mg/kg, followed by 0.5 mg/kg every 2 min	1 to 2 min	5 to 10 min	Moderate and/or deep sedation
Ketamine IV	1 mg/kg IV	1 to 3 min	10 to 20 min	Dissociative sedation
Ketamine IM	2 to 5 mg/kg	5 to 20 min	30 to 60 min	Dissociative sedation
Ketamine PN	6 mg/kg	15 to 30 min	30 to 60 min	Dissociative sedation
Ketamine PO	10 to 15 mg/kg PO	15 to 30 min	30 to 60 min	Dissociative sedation
Ketamine PR	10 to 15 mg/kg	15 to 30 min	30 to 60 min	Dissociative sedation

Note: IV=intravenously; IM=intramuscularly; PO=orally; PR=rectally; PN=nasally.

sedation, and can be used in combination with midazolam for moderate and deep PSA. Rigid chest syndrome, a rare complication characterized by spasm of the respiratory muscles leading to respiratory depression or apnea, is seen when large doses of fentanyl are given rapidly. In small children, it may be precipitated by flushing the IV after a dose of fentanyl is given. It is unclear if rigid chest syndrome is reversible with narcotic antagonist administration. Rapid sequence induction and pharmacologic paralysis are usually required to ventilate the patient in this situation. Slow administration of fentanyl (2 to 3 µg/kg over 5 minutes) followed by slow and careful flushing of the IV line can prevent this problem.

Alfentanil

Alfentanil is an ultra–short-acting opioid that can be used for minimal sedation. When given in doses of 10 to 20 µg/kg, it provides sedation for 5 to 8 minutes. The incidence of respiratory depression increases with the dose of alfentanil. The sedation from alfentanil is

TABLE 6–5	Examples of Agents Used for Target Sedation Levels

Minimal sedation

- Midazolam 0.1 mg/kg IV
- Fentanyl 1.5 µg/kg
- Alfentanil 10 to 15 µg/kg
- Nitrous oxide 30% to 70%

Brief moderate or deep sedation

- Methohexital 1 mg/kg
- Propofol 1 mg/kg
- Etomidate 0.15 mg/kg
- Ketamine 1.0 mg/kg IV

Extended moderate or deep sedation

- Propofol 1 mg/kg followed by 0.5 mg/kg every 3 minutes as needed
- Ketamine 1 mg/kg IV +/– midazolam 0.05 mg/kg IV

necessary stimulation to breathe, making the period initially after completing the procedure the most prone to respiratory depression if the procedure is completed before the effect of the alfentanil has begun to decrease. The duration of action of alfentanil increases with the size of the dose, and total doses greater than 20 µg/kg have not been described for PSA.

Typically, patients minimally sedated with opioids for PSA can recall the procedure, although they often do not recall it as unpleasant, even if the procedure was painful. It is not clear why this occurs, but it is likely the patient's memories are imprinted differently when formed in a high opioid state relative to memories formed while under a stressful state.

Naloxone

Opioids, including fentanyl, can be reversed with the opioid antagonist naloxone. It can be given IV, IM, subcutaneously, or down an endotracheal tube. Administration of naloxone can cause nausea, anxiety, and sympathetic stimulation and can prevent adequate analgesia subsequent to the procedure. Careful titration of small amount to provide partial reversal to reverse respiratory depression may allow adequate respiratory efforts without blocking subsequent analgesia.

very similar to that of fentanyl, except for the very short duration of action. Pain is a powerful respiratory stimulant, and the procedure provides the patient the

TABLE 6–6	Examples of Sedation Levels Typical to Specific Wound Care Procedures		
Specific Procedures	**Depth of Sedation**	**Sedation Goal**	**Example of Agent**
Minor wounds in cooperative patients	Local anesthesia only	NA	NA
Large wounds in cooperative patients	Minimal sedation	Analgesia, anxiolysis	Fentanyl, alfentanil, low-dose ketamine, nitrous oxide
Minor wounds in anxious patients	Minimal sedation	Anxiolysis	Midazolam, nitrous oxide, alfentanil
Wounds in agitated/ uncooperative patients	Moderate/deep sedation	Anxiolysis, decreased motion during procedure	Ketamine, propofol, methohexital, etomidate
Incision and drainage of simple abscess	Minimal sedation	Analgesia	Midazolam, nitrous oxide, alfentanil
Incision and drainage of complex abscess	Moderate/deep sedation	Analgesia, amnesia	Ketamine, propofol, methohexital, etomidate
Burn débridement (small)	Minimal sedation	Analgesia	Midazolam, nitrous oxide, alfentanil
Burn débridement (large)	Moderate/deep sedation	Analgesia, amnesia	Ketamine, propofol, methohexital, etomidate

Nitrous Oxide

Nitrous oxide can be administered to provide minimal sedation. It is administered with oxygen in a mixture that ranges from 30% nitrous oxide up to 70%. It provides minimal sedation that is similar in appearance to the sedation provided by opioids, but has the benefit of not requiring an IV and wearing off quickly when the gas is removed. It is associated with nausea and vomiting at higher doses, but this typically resolves when the gas is decreased or discontinued. Nitrous oxide is a folate inhibitor and is associated with birth defects when pregnant patients are exposed to it, and, therefore, must be used with a scavenger system and cannot be given to pregnant patients. Typically, the patient is placed on a mask from the scavenger system 5 minutes prior to the procedure, and started at a low level. After 5 minutes, the nitrous oxide is titrated up until the patient is adequately sedated. When the procedure is completed, the patient is placed on 100% oxygen until he or she has regained the baseline mental status.

MODERATE AND DEEP SEDATION AGENTS

Methohexital

Methohexital is a short-acting barbiturate that produces sedation within 1 minute of IV administration with a duration of effect of 3 to 5 minutes. It induces significant respiratory depression, which increases if additional boluses are given subsequent to the initial dose.[26] It is best used for brief moderate and deep sedation.

Ketamine

Ketamine is frequently used and well described for ED PSA.[29] Ketamine produces a state of dissociation that is characterized by analgesia, sedation, and amnesia. Ketamine does not have the typical dose-response continuum seen with other moderate and deep PSA agents. At doses lower than the dissociative threshold, analgesia and sedation occur. Once a certain threshold is exceeded, (approximately 1 to 1.5 mg/kg IV or 3 to 4 mg/kg IM), the characteristic dissociative state abruptly appears. This dissociation has no observable levels of depth; the only value of additional titration of ketamine is to prolong the dissociated state.

Ketamine can be given either IM or IV. The IM route allows for approximately 40 minutes of sedation, whereas the IV route has much shorter duration of 10 to 15 minutes. Intramuscular ketamine is not typically associated with respiratory depression. Respiratory depression is sometimes seen with IV dosing.[30] It can also induce hypersalivation, and anticholinergics (atropine at 0.01 mg/kg or glycopyrrolate at 0.01 mg/kg) are usually administered to counter this effect if it occurs. Adverse effects also include laryngospasm, vomiting (most often in the late recovery phase), and emergence reactions. Ketamine has minimal effects on blood pressure.

Emergence reactions are commonly seen in PSA with ketamine, and range from mild agitation to recurrent nightmares and hallucinations. There is not convincing evidence that the coadministration of midazolam can prevent this, although the use of midazolam with ketamine to blunt the emergence reactions is common. It is probably sufficient to give ketamine without midazolam, and then treat patients who develop emergence reactions with midazolam as they occur.

Etomidate

Etomidate is an nonbarbiturate sedative–hypnotic. It has a rapid onset (15 to 30 seconds), and a duration of effect of 3 to 8 minutes. It causes less cardiovascular depression that most other sedatives, but causes similar respiratory depression at a given depth of sedation. Myoclonic jerking can occur after administration in up to 20% of patients, which can interfere with the wound care procedure.[18,31] It is known to cause suppression of the adrenal-cortical axis after prolonged repeated dosing. No clinically significant adrenal suppression has been detected from the short exposures used during procedural sedation.

Propofol

Propofol is frequently used for moderate and deep PSA in the ED[20] and is associated with fewer complications than etomidate or methohexital in patients who received multiple doses.[26,31] The most serious adverse effect of propofol is respiratory depression, which can arise suddenly. Propofol can also produce hypotension, as a result of both negative inotropy and vasodilatation, but this is typically transient in euvolemic patients. Propofol is formulated in a soybean oil, glycerol, and egg lecithin emulsion, and is contraindicated in patients who are allergic to eggs or soy protein. Propofol causes pain during administration. Methods used to treat this include placing a tourniquet proximal to the IV and injecting 0.05 mg/kg of lidocaine through the IV approximately 60 seconds before injecting the propofol, mixing the propofol with lidocaine, or coadministering the short-acting narcotic alfentanil at 10 μg/kg.[32]

DISCHARGE

Adverse Events

From the patient's perspective, the absence of recall of the procedure constitutes a successful sedation. From the physician perspective, the presence and nature of any adverse events that occurred during PSA is a good measure of the outcome of the procedure, in terms of an assessment of the risk to the patient. Reported complication rates for ED PSA have ranged from 2.5% to 7.7%,[2] but the actual rate depends on what is considered an adverse event, and it has varied among research studies. Sedation to a deeper level than intended, brief hypoxia, the need for assisted ventilation, and hypotension are adverse events unlikely to have a clinically significant effect other than a brief intervention during the procedure. These types of complications are a common and expected part of the of PSA. Aspiration and endotracheal intubation are significant events with profound effects on the patient, but fortunately are very rare. Appropriate procedural monitoring and careful selection of the target sedation level minimize both the rate of occurrence of these events and their impact on the patient when they occur.

Follow Up and Patient Instructions

At the completion of the wound care procedure, patients should be monitored until they have returned to their baseline mental status. Once the patient's condition has returned to baseline, the patient can be discharged. Adverse events have been shown to be rare 25 minutes after sedative dosing.[33] The necessary duration of the observation before discharge depends on the quantity of sedatives given, the patient's response to them, the duration of the procedure, and whether or not the patient experienced any adverse events during the sedation. Patients should be encouraged to return to be evaluated if they develop respiratory problems or are unable to tolerate oral intake because of nausea and vomiting. Otherwise, follow up is determined by the needs of the wound for which they were sedated.

CONCLUSION

Procedural sedation and analgesia is an important tool for the facilitation of wound care procedures. It is generally safe, but preparation and vigilance for the possible adverse events associated with the practice are important to insure patient safety and to perform these procedures successfully.

REFERENCES

1. Clinical policy for procedural sedation and analgesia in the emergency department. American College of Emergency Physicians. *Ann Emerg Med.* 1998;31(5):663–677.
2. Godwin SA, Caro DA, Wold SJ, et al. Clinical policy: procedural sedation and analgesia in the emergency department. *Ann Emerg Med.* 2005;45(2):177–196.
3. Green SM, Krauss B. Ketamine is a safe, effective, and appropriate technique for emergency department paediatric procedural sedation. *Emerg Med J.* 2004;21(3):271–272.
4. Peña BM, Krauss B. Adverse events of procedural sedation and analgesia in a pediatric emergency department. *Ann Emerg Med.* 1999;34(4 pt 1):483–491.
5. McQueen A, Wright RO, Kido MM, Kaye E, Krauss B. Procedural sedation and analgesia outcomes in children after discharge from the emergency department: ketamine versus fentanyl/midazolam. *Ann Emerg Med.* 2009;54(2):191–197, e1–4.
6. Mensour M, Pineau R, Sahai V, Michaud J. Emergency department procedural sedation and analgesia: a Canadian Community Effectiveness and Safety Study (ACCESS). *CJEM.* 2006;8(2):94–99.
7. Misra S, Mahajan PV, Chen X, Kannikeswaran N. Safety of procedural sedation and analgesia in children less than 2 years of age in a pediatric emergency department. *Int J Emerg Med.* 2008;1(3):173–177.
8. Shavit I, Steiner IP, Idelman S, et al. Comparison of adverse events during procedural sedation between specially trained pediatric residents and pediatric emergency physicians in Israel. *Acad Emerg Med.* 2008;15(7):617–622.
9. Roback MG, Wathen JE, Bajaj L, Bothner JP. Adverse events associated with procedural sedation and analgesia in a pediatric emergency department: a comparison of common parenteral drugs. *Acad Emerg Med.* 2005;12(6):508–513.
10. Green SM, Rothrock SG, Lynch EL, et al. Intramuscular ketamine for pediatric sedation in the emergency department: safety profile in 1,022 cases. *Ann Emerg Med.* 1998;31(6):688–697.
11. Singer AJ, Thode HC Jr, Hollander JE. National trends in ED lacerations between 1992 and 2002. *Am J Emerg Med.* 2006;24(2):183–188.
12. Avramov MN, White PF. Methods for monitoring the level of sedation. *Crit Care Clin.* 1995;11(4):803–826.
13. Miner JR, Biros MH, Heegaard W, Plummer D. Bispectral electroencephalographic analysis of patients undergoing procedural sedation in the emergency department. *Acad Emerg Med.* 2003;10(6):638–643.
14. Miner JR, Bachman A, Kosman L, Teng B, Heegaard W, Biros MN. Assessment of the onset and persistence of amnesia during procedural sedation with propofol. *Acad Emerg Med.* 2005;12(6):491–496.
15. Miner JR, Huber D, Nichols S, Biros M. The effect of the assignment of a pre-sedation target level on procedural sedation using propofol. *J Emerg Med.* 2007;32(3):249–255.

16. Miner JR, Biros MN, Seigel T, Ross K. The utility of the bispectral index in procedural sedation with propofol in the emergency department. *Acad Emerg Med.* 2005;12(3):190–196.

17. American Society of Anesthesiologists. *Physical Status Classification System.* 2004. Available at: http://www.asahq.org/clinical/physicalstatus.htm. JAN 27, 2010

18. Miner JR, Martel ML, Meyer M, Reardon R, Biros MH. Procedural sedation of critically ill patients in the emergency department. *Acad Emerg Med.* 2005;12(2):124–128.

19. Green S, Roback MG, Miner J, Burton JH, Krauss B. Fasting and emergency department procedural sedation and analgesia: a consensus-based clinical practice advisory. *Ann Emerg Med.* 2007;49(4):454–461.

20. Miner JR, Burton JH. Clinical practice advisory: emergency department procedural sedation with propofol. *Ann Emerg Med.* 2007;50(2):182–187, 187.e1.

21. Sacchetti A, Senula G, Strickland J, Dubin R. Procedural sedation in the community emergency department: initial results of the ProSCED registry. *Acad Emerg Med.* 2007;14(1):41–46.

22. Deitch K, Chudnofsky CR, Dominici P. The utility of supplemental oxygen during emergency department procedural sedation with propofol: a randomized, controlled trial. *Ann Emerg Med.* 2008;52(1):1–8.

23. Deitch K, Miner J, Chudnofsky, Dominici P, Latta D. Does end tidal CO_2 monitoring during emergency department procedural sedation and analgesia with propofol decrease the incidence of hypoxic events? A randomized, controlled trial. *Ann Emerg Med.* 2010; 55(3):258–264.

24. Krauss B, Hess DR. Capnography for procedural sedation and analgesia in the emergency department. *Ann Emerg Med.* 2007;50(2):172–181.

25. Miner JR, Heegaard W, Plummer D. End-tidal carbon dioxide monitoring during procedural sedation. *Acad Emerg Med.* 2002;9(4):275–280.

26. Miner JR, Biros M, Krieg S, Johnson C, Heegaard W, Plummer D. Randomized clinical trial of propofol versus methohexital for procedural sedation during fracture and dislocation reduction in the emergency department. *Acad Emerg Med.* 2003; 10(9):931–937.

27. Messenger DW, Murray HE, Dungey PE, van Vlymen J, Sivilotti ML. Subdissociative-dose ketamine versus fentanyl for analgesia during propofol procedural sedation: a randomized clinical trial. *Acad Emerg Med.* 2008;15(10):877–886.

28. Green SM, Krauss B. Propofol in emergency medicine: pushing the sedation frontier. *Ann Emerg Med.* 2003;42(6):792–797.

29. Green SM, Krauss B. Clinical practice guideline for emergency department ketamine dissociative sedation in children. *Ann Emerg Med.* 2004;44(5):460–471.

30. Chudnofsky CR, Weber JE, Stoyanoff PJ, et al. A combination of midazolam and ketamine for procedural sedation and analgesia in adult emergency department patients. *Acad Emerg Med.* 2000;7(3):228–235.

31. Miner JR, Danahy M, Moch A, Biros M. Randomized clinical trial of etomidate versus propofol for procedural sedation in the emergency department. *Ann Emerg Med.* 2007;49(1):15–22.

32. Nathanson MH, Gajraj NM, Russell JA. Prevention of pain on injection of propofol: a comparison of lidocaine with alfentanil. *Anesth Analg.* 1996;82(3): 469–471.

33. Newman DH, Azer MM, Pitetti RD, Singh S. When is a patient safe for discharge after procedural sedation? The timing of adverse effect events in 1367 pediatric procedural sedations. *Ann Emerg Med.* 2003;42(5):627–635.

34. American Society of Anesthesiologists Task Force on Sedation and Analgesia by Nonanesthesiologists. Practice guidelines for sedation and analgesia by non-anesthesiologists. *Anesthesiology.* 2002;96(4): 1004–1017.

CHAPTER 7

Wound Closure Devices

Judd E. Hollander, MD, Adam J. Singer, MD

Most lacerations will heal without sequelae but a minority will develop wound infections, and unsightly or dysfunctional scars. The goals of wound management are simple: avoid infection and achieve a functional and aesthetically pleasing scar.[1] These goals may be accomplished by reducing tissue contamination, débriding devitalized tissue, restoring perfusion in poorly perfused wounds, and achieving a well-approximated skin closure.

Various wound closure devices have been used for several millennia. The earliest record of sutures dates back nearly 4,500 years,[2,3] while "biological" staples in the form of insect jaws have also been used by ancient civilizations.[4] The advantages and disadvantages of the currently available wound closure methods are presented in Table 7-1. Preferred methods of wound closure based on the type of wound are presented in Table 7-2. This chapter will present a general overview of the various wound closure methods, which will be discussed in more detail in the following chapters.

TIMING OF WOUND CLOSURE

Most lacerations can be closed primarily. Primary closure results in more rapid healing and less patient discomfort than secondary closure. The time interval from injury to closure of a laceration is directly related to the risk of subsequent infec-tion, but the length of this "golden period" is highly variable.[5–7] In one study of 300 hand and forearm lacerations, Morgan and colleagues[5] found that lacerations closed within 4 hours had a 7% infection rate, compared to 21% for those closed more than 4 hours after injury. On the other hand, Baker and Lanuti,[6] in a study of 2834 pediatric patients, found that the infection rate for lacerations closed more than 6 hours after the time of injury was no greater than the rate for lacerations closed within 6 hours. The most widely quoted study comes from Jamaica, where the authors used healing (defined as epithelialization without infection) as the main outcome.[7] This study of 204 lacerations found that facial lacerations healed well regardless of the time to closure. In contrast, lacerations of the trunk or extremity had lower rates of healing if they were closed more than 19 hours from the time of injury (63% to 75%) than if they were closed earlier (75% to 91%). The subgroups were small, however, ranging from eight to 44 patients.[7]

On the basis of these studies, it seems most prudent to consider each individual laceration separately. Before closing a wound, consider time from injury until presentation, etiology, location, degree of contamination, host risk factors, and the importance of cosmetic appearance. Then decide whether to perform primary wound closure. For example, a 20-hour-old laceration on the face of a healthy 4-year-old child, which has a low

TABLE 7–1	Comparative Merits of Common Wound Closure Techniques	
Technique	Advantages	Disadvantages
Suture	Long history of use Meticulous closure Greatest tensile strength Lowest dehiscence rate	Slowest application Requires anesthesia, removal Greatest tissue reactivity Highest cost
Staples	Faster application Low tissue reactivity Lower cost Low risk of needle-stick	Less meticulous closure May interfere with certain imaging techniques (computed tomography, magnetic resonance imaging)
Tissue adhesives	Faster application Patient comfort Resistant to bacterial growth No removal or risk of needle stick Lower cost	Lower tensile strength than sutures Dehiscence over high tension areas (e.g., joints) Not useful on hands Cannot bathe or swim
Surgical tapes	Faster application Least reactive Lowest infection rates Patient comfort Lower cost No risk of needle-stick	Often fall off Lower tensile strength than sutures Highest rate of dehiscence Require use of toxic adjuncts Cannot be used in areas of hair Cannot get wet

likelihood of infection, may be closed primarily, whereas a deep laceration in the foot of a diabetic patient will be at increased risk of infection and may be best off if it is not closed primarily. Thus, the timing during which wound closure is safe needs to be individualized.[1] Wounds that are not closed primarily because of a high risk of infection should be considered for delayed primary closure after 3 to 5 days. After 3 to 5 days of open wound management, the risk of infection substantially decreases.

METHODS OF WOUND CLOSURE

The ideal wound closure technique would allow a meticulous wound closure, would be easy and rapid to apply, would be painless, would have a low infection rate, would cause no risk to the health care provider, would be inexpensive, and would result in minimal scarring. Sutures are the most commonly employed wound closure technique.[8] Tissue adhesives can be

TABLE 7–2	Selection of Wound Closure Method	
Type of Wound	Preferred Closure Method	Alternative Closure Method
Scalp laceration	Staples	Sutures (particularly with deep, bloody wounds)
Nongaping, superficial facial laceration	Tissue adhesives	Sutures
Gaping or complex facial laceration	Sutures	
High-tension lacerations	Sutures	Tissue adhesives with immobilization
Hand and foot lacerations	Sutures	No good alternatives
Avulsion lacerations with fragile skin or tenuous blood supply	Tissue adhesives	Surgical tapes
Long linear lacerations	Staples	Tissue adhesives

used rather than sutures in one quarter to one third of laceration repairs and many surgical incisions.[9] Other alternatives include staples and surgical tapes.

Sutures

Sutures are the time-honored and most reliable method of wound closure. They produce a meticulous wound closure with the greatest tensile strength and lowest likelihood of dehiscence. Even the most complex laceration can be well approximated by suturing. Nonabsorbable sutures retain most of their tensile strength for more than 60 days, are relatively nonreactive, and are appropriate for closure of the outermost layer of the laceration or for repair of tendons.[10–12] The need for removal of nonabsorbable sutures is a disadvantage, as it requires patient revisit and the associated work-life disruptions.

Absorbable sutures are usually used to close structures deeper than the epidermis. Rapidly dissolving absorbable sutures are sometimes used to close the outer layers of the skin, especially in children or in patients with poor follow up because they do not require removal. Most absorbable sutures increase the duration of time that the wound retains 50% of its tensile strength up to 1 month. Some synthetic absorbable sutures retain their tensile strength for as long as 2 months, making them useful in areas with high dynamic and static tensions.

Deep sutures can be used to relieve skin tension, and should be used to decrease dead space and hematoma formation. They may improve cosmetic outcome. Many advise the use of deep sutures to reduce scar width (especially on the face), but little evidence supports this recommendation. In fact, a study comparing closure of laminectomy incisions with and without deep sutures failed to demonstrate any differences in scar width.[13] A study in nongaping facial lacerations found that cosmetic outcome and scar width were similar with single- or double-layer closure.[14] Animal studies suggest that deep sutures should be avoided in highly contaminated wounds, where they increase the risk of infection.[15,16] Although the use of absorbable sutures is generally reserved for the subcuticular tissues, rapidly dissolving forms can be used to close the skin of children to avoid the discomfort associated with suture removal.[17,18]

Suture closure does have several disadvantages. Local anesthesia is generally needed to decrease the pain of the suturing. Suture placement is the most time-consuming wound closure option. Sutures produce more tissue reactivity and inflammation than any of the other options. The placement of sutures poses a small but real risk of blood and body fluid exposure through skin puncture of the health care provider. If not removed in a timely manner, sutures may leave unsightly hatch marks on either side of the wound. The cost and inconvenience of suturing and suture removal may make other wound closure options more attractive for some lacerations.

Staples

Staples are the most rapid method of closure, and are especially well suited for scalp wounds.[19,20] They are associated with a lower rate of foreign body reaction and infection.[19,21,22] Staples also reduce the risk of needle-sticks to the health care provider. Brickman and Lambert[22] used staples in 75 patients with 87 lacerations to the scalp, trunk, and extremities. No patient developed an infection and only one patient had a dehiscence. Ritchie and Rocke[19] performed a randomized controlled trial comparing sutures to staples for scalp lacerations. They found that lacerations healed equally well, with low infection rates (<2%) in both groups. In general, staples are considered particularly useful for scalp,[19,23] trunk, and extremity wounds,[1] and when saving time is essential, such as in mass casualties and in victims of multiple trauma.[1] However, they do not allow as meticulous a closure as sutures and they are slightly more painful to remove.[20] In animal models, staples are associated with lower rates of bacterial growth and lower infection rates than sutures.[21] In clinical series, these differences may be statistically significant but have limited clinical significance.[23]

Staple removal requires a special device. These devices are readily available in emergency departments (EDs) but are not stocked in all primary care offices. The removal of staples is more painful that the removal of sutures.

Adhesive Tapes

Adhesive tapes are associated with the lowest rate of infection but tend to slough off with any tension. Advantages of adhesive tapes to the patient and health care provider include rapid application, little or no patient discomfort, low cost, and no risk of needle-stick. They are associated with minimal tissue reactivity and they may be left on for long periods without resulting in suture hatch marks.

Surgical tapes are even less reactive than staples,[21] but they require the use of adhesive adjuncts (for example, tincture of benzoin), which increase local induration and wound infection.[24] Adhesive adjuncts are toxic to wounds and care should be taken so that they do not enter the wound. Adhesive tapes have the lowest tensile strength of wound closure devices and will not maintain the integrity of wound closure in areas subject to tension.[25] Adhesive tape may cause a shearing force on the epidermis resulting in blister formation.

They are seldom recommended for primary wound closure in the ED,[1] but are often used after suture removal to decrease tension on the wound until they fall off. The reasons for very low use rates are high rates of dislodgement and dehiscence, the inability to use them in hair-bearing areas, and the need to keep them dry. Their use is typically reserved for linear lacerations under minimal tension.

Postoperative care of wounds closed with adhesive tapes requires limited movement of the area. The area also should be kept as dry as possible because moisture will result in rapid tape dislodgement and subsequent wound dehiscence.

Tissue Adhesives

Tissue adhesives provide cost-effective, needle-free, rapid closure of easily approximated wound edges, with long-term cosmesis comparable to 5-0 and 6-0 sutures. Tissue adhesives can be used for lacerations and incisions that have easily apposed wound edges. They may produce a mild burning sensation but in general they are less painful than sutures or staples. The cyanoacrylates also provide some resistance to bacterial growth and function as a microbial barrier.[26] The reduced need for local anesthesia before wound closure and for return visits for removal makes them a more cost-effective wound closure device than sutures or staples.[27] The risk of needle-stick to the health care provider also is eliminated.

Observational studies of children with small scalp, face, or limb lacerations treated with a butyl-2-cyanoacrylate (Histoacryl Blue, B. Braun, Melsungen, Germany) found low infection rates (<2%) and dehiscence rates (0.6%–1.8%). Histoacryl Blue results in similar long-term cosmetic outcomes as 5-0 or 6-0 sutures when used for repair of small facial lacerations.[28] Several clinical studies have compared the use of 2-octylcyanoacrylate to 5-0 and 6-0 sutures.[29-32] In all studies, the 3-month cosmetic outcomes, short-term infection rates, and wound dehiscence rates were all similar when the use of 2-octylcyanoacrylate was compared with skin closure with sutures. The time required to close the wound was more than 50% shorter in the group treated with 2-octylcyanoacrylate. One study found that the use of octylcyanoacrylate for skin closure following elective facial plastic surgical procedures produced better long-term results than sutures.[33]

Tissue adhesives are a needle-free alternative to sutures and staples for the closure of many lacerations and surgical incisions as well as skin tears. They produce an excellent cosmetic appearance, comparable to sutures. The 2-octylcyanoacrylates can be used in locations that would otherwise be closed with 5-0 or 6-0 nonabsorbable sutures. These adhesives can be used in areas of higher tension only if subcutaneous or subcuticular absorbable sutures are placed to relieve tension on the skin. The butylcyanoacrylates have less tensile strength than 5-0 sutures and only approximately one third the tensile strength of the octylcyanoacrylates.[1] Their use is restricted to very small low-tension lacerations.

Tissue adhesives have some disadvantages and limitations. They cannot be used in complex lacerations that cannot be manually approximated. They are not as strong as larger (4-0) sutures. The 2-octylcyanoacrylates can be used in areas of higher tension only if subcutaneous or subcuticular absorbable sutures are also used to relieve tension on the skin edges. They should not be used over areas subject to great tension or repetitive movement, such as over joints or hands[34] unless the repaired wound is splinted and covered by a dressing. Increasing rates and amounts of polymerization may be associated with increased heat sensation by the patient. For optimal results, they should be applied to a bloodless field. If oozing of blood continues, sutures or staples might provide a better alternative.

Butylcyanoacrylates should not get wet for at least 48 hours. It is acceptable to shower and wash when using octylcyanoacrylates, but lacerations and incisions should not receive prolonged exposure to water, such as in swimming. When tissue adhesives are used for laceration or surgical incision closure, topical ointments and creams should not be applied. They will loosen the tissue adhesives and may result in dehiscence.

REFERENCES

1. Singer AJ, Hollander JE, Quinn JV. Evaluation and management of traumatic lacerations. *N Engl J Med.* 1997;337(16):1142–1148.
2. Majno G. *The Healing Hand. Man and Wound in the Ancient World.* Cambridge, MA: Harvard University Press; 1975.
3. Forrest RD. Early history of wound treatment. *J R Soc Med.* 1982;75(3):198–205.
4. Wheeler WM. *Ants, Their Structure and Behavior.* New York, NY: Columbia University Press; 1960.

5. Morgan WJ, Hutchison D, Johnson HM. The delayed treatment of wounds of the hand and forearm under antibiotic cover. *Br J Surg.* 1980;67(2):140–141.

6. Baker MD, Lanuti M. The management and outcome of lacerations in urban children. *Ann Emerg Med.* 1990;19(9):1001–1005.

7. Berk WA, Osbourne DD, Taylor DD. Evaluation of the "golden period" for wound repair: 204 cases from a Third World emergency department. *Ann Emerg Med.* 1988;17(5):496–500.

8. Hollander JE, Singer AJ, Valentine S, Henry MC. Wound registry: development and validation. *Ann Emerg Med.* 1995;25(5):675–685.

9. Singer AJ, Hollander JE. Tissue adhesives for laceration closure [letter]. *JAMA.* 1997;278(9):703–704.

10. Markovchick V. Suture materials and mechanical after care. *Emerg Med Clin North Am.* 1992;10(4):673–689.

11. Swanson NA, Tromovitch TA. Suture materials, 1980s: properties, uses, and abuses. *Int J Dermatol.* 1982;21(7):373–378.

12. Ratner D, Nelson BR, Johnson TM. Basic suture materials and suturing techniques. *Semin Dermatol.* 1994;13(1):20–26.

13. Winn HR, Jane JA, Rodeheaver G, Edgerton MT, Edlich RF. Influence of subcuticular sutures on scar formation. *Am J Surg.* 1977;133(2):257–259.

14. Singer AJ, Gulla J, Hein M, Marchini S, Chale S, Arora BP. Single-layer versus double-layer closure of facial lacerations: a randomized control trial. *Plast Reconstr Surg.* 2005;116(2):363–368.

15. Mehta PH, Dunn KA, Bradfield JF, Austin PE. Contaminated wounds: infection rates with subcutaneous sutures. *Ann Emerg Med.* 1996;27(1):43–48.

16. De Holl D, Rodeheaver G, Edgerton MT, Edlich RF. Potentiation of infection by suture closure of dead space. *Am J Surg.* 1974;127(6):716–720.

17. Start NJ, Armstrong AM, Robson WJ. The use of chromic catgut in the primary closure of scalp wounds in children. *Arch Emerg Med.* 1989;6(3):216–219.

18. Tandon SC, Kelly J, Turtle M, Irwin ST. Irradiated polyglactin 910: a new synthetic absorbable suture. *J R Coll Surg Edinb.* 1995;40(3):185–187.

19. Ritchie AJ, Rocke LG. Staples versus sutures in the closure of scalp wounds: a prospective, double-blind, randomized trial. *Injury.* 1989;20(4):217–218.

20. George TK, Simpson DC. Skin wound closure with staples in the accident and emergency department. *J R Coll Surg Edinburgh.* 1985;30(1):54–56.

21. Johnson A, Rodeheaver GT, Durand LS, Edgerton MT, Edlich RF. Automatic disposable stapling devices for wound closure. *Ann Emerg Med.* 1981;10(12):631–635.

22. Brickman KR, Lambert RW. Evaluation of skin stapling for wound closure in the emergency department. *Ann Emerg Med.* 1989;18(10):1122–1125.

23. Hollander JE, Giarrusso E, Cassara G, Valentine S, Singer AJ. Comparison of staples and sutures for closure of scalp lacerations [abstract]. *Acad Emerg Med.* 1997;4:460–461.

24. Panek PH, Prusak MP, Bolt D, Edlich RF. Potentiation of wound infection by adhesive adjuncts. *Am Surg.* 1972;38(6):343–345.

25. Rothnie NG, Taylor GW. Sutureless skin closure. A clinical trial. *Br Med J.* 1963;26(2);1027–1030.

26. Quinn JV, Ramotar K, Osmond MH. Antimicrobial effects of a new tissue adhesive. [abstract] *Acad Emerg Med.* 1996;3:536–537.

27. Osmond MH, Klassen TP, Quinn JV. Economic comparison of a tissue adhesive and suturing in the repair of pediatric facial lacerations. *J Pediatr.* 1995;126(6):892–895.

28. Quinn JV, Drzewiecki A, Li MM, et al. A randomized, controlled trial comparing a tissue adhesive with suturing in the repair of pediatric facial lacerations. *Ann Emerg Med.* 1993;22(7):1130–1135.

29. Quinn J, Wells G, Sutcliffe T, et al. A randomized trial comparing octylcyanoacrylate tissue adhesive and sutures in the management of lacerations. *JAMA.* 1997;277(19):1527–1530.

30. Quinn J, Wells G, Sutcliffe T, et al. Tissue adhesive versus suture wound repair at 1 year: randomized clinical trial correlating early, 3-month, and 1-year cosmetic outcome. *Ann Emerg Med.* 1998;32(6):645–649.

31. Singer AJ, Hollander JE, Valentine SM, Turque TW, McCuskey CF, Quinn JV. Prospective randomized controlled trial of tissue adhesive (2-octylcyanoacrylate) vs standard wound closure techniques for laceration repair. Stony Brook Octylcyanoacrylate Study Group. *Acad Emerg Med.* 1998;5(2):94–99.

32. Bruns TB, Robinson BS, Smith RJ, et al. A new tissue adhesive for laceration repair in children. *J Pediatr.* 1998;132(6):1067–1070.

33. Toriumi DM, O'Grady K, Desai D, Bagal A. Use of octyl-2-cyanoacrylate for skin closure in facial plastic surgery. *Plast Reconstr Surg.* 1998;102(6):2209–2219.

34. Saxena AK, Willital GH. Octylcyanoacrylate tissue adhesive in the repair of pediatric extremity lacerations. *Am Surg.* 1999;65(5):470–472.

CHAPTER 8

Wound Dressings

Rose Moran-Kelly, RN, MSN, APRN, FNP-BC,
Mary Farren, RN, MSN, CWOCN, and Adam J. Singer, MD

Historically the wound dressing has served to cover and protect the wound. The wound was kept dry and a scab was allowed to form to protect the underlying skin. It was not until 1962 that Winter's work with young domestic pigs demonstrated that reepithelialization was increased by 50% when wounds were kept moist and not allowed to form scabs as they do when exposed to air.[1] One year later Hinman and Maibach reached the same conclusion based on their studies with humans.[2] They found that histologically, with wounds exposed to the air, the epithelium had to grow at right angles to the surface to find a place of cleavage to proliferate under the eschar. Occluded wounds do not allow eschar formation so that the epithelium grows directly across the surface. Though Winter's seminal study of moist wound healing has been questioned[3] the theory of moist wound healing is widely accepted.

There had been concern that moisture under a dressing would increase the risk of infection, but this has been disproven in subsequent studies. In fact, wounds treated with occlusive dressings are less likely than those covered by traditional dressings to become infected.[4] Theoretically it would seem that keeping gauze moist would achieve the same results as using a new generation of moisture-retentive dressing. The newer dressings provide additional benefits including properties that interact within the wound environment to reduce bacterial burden, maintain moisture balance, and promote chemical or autolytic débridement in addition to providing a barrier to protect the wound from contamination by from urine, feces, and incontinence and other external contaminants.[5–7]

Though the use of a petrolatum dressing was found not to increase the incidence of infection for sterile wounds,[8] evidence supports the common practice of using topical antibiotics for acute contaminated wounds to prevent infection,[9] promote moist wound healing, and decrease pain caused by dressing adherence.[10] In a study by Dire et al. comparing wounds treated with triple antibiotic ointment (neomycin, bacitracin zinc, and polymyxin), silver sulfadiazine, and petrolatum, infection rates were significantly lower for wounds treated with topical antibiotics.[9] The triple antibiotic ointment uses the neomycin to improve the antibacterial spectrum of antibiotics such as bacitracin and polymixin but one must be aware of potential sensitivity to neomycin and the potential though rare risk of ototoxicity especially in those with renal disease.[11] Hood et al. compared triple antibiotic ointment and mupirocin and found similar rates of wound infection and adverse events.[12] Mupirocin is more expensive than the triple antibiotic ointment so the mupirocin should be reserved for suspected staphylococcal and streptococcal infections. Systemic antibiotics should only be considered for those who are at a higher risk for infection such as patients with age extremes, diabetes mellitus, or corticosteroid use.

ACUTE WOUNDS

The vast majority of simple, uncomplicated wounds treated in the emergency department (ED) or office setting can be cared for with a topical antibiotic, a nonstick adherent pad (e.g., Telfa) or petrolatum-impregnated mesh (e.g., Adaptic) covered with a secondary gauze dressing for absorption of small amounts of exudate and protection against minor trauma, attached to the patient by tape and cotton gauze or conforming dressing. Splints and crutches should be used to prevent increased tension over joints and reduced weight-bearing as indicated.

Modern Dressings (Advanced Wound Products)

Advanced wound products can enhance wound management by reducing the need for frequent dressing changes by addressing the characteristics of the wound bed and impediments to the healing trajectory.

There is considerable information in the literature describing the attributes of the ideal dressing.[13,14] These include:

- The ability to absorb and contain exudate without leakage or "strike through"
- Lack of particulate matter left in the wound by the dressing
- Thermal insulation
- Permeability to water and bacteria
- Suitability for use with different skin closures (sutures, staples)
- Avoidance of wound trauma on dressing removal
- Frequency with which the dressing needs to be changed
- Provision of pain relief
- Cosmesis and comfort
- Effect on formation of scar tissue

Although there are multiple studies that report decreased pain with use of some of the advanced dressings[15-17] and less pain with low-adherent dressings[18] as well as fewer dressing changes,[19] there was no difference in healing rates[20] in many studies. None have strong evidence to support their preference over another with the possible exception of dressings used for burns. There is some literature that reports that the use of silver-coated dressings may decrease healing time, reduce the number of dressing changes, and reduce the rate of cellulitis.[21,22] The current use of silver sulfadiazine for burns for the full duration of treatment should also be reconsidered as there is no evidence to support its use.[22]

Additionally, the use of negative pressure wound therapy (NPWT) has become increasingly popular but research to date is inconclusive regarding whether such dressings lead to improved healing.[23] There are specific indications and contraindications to the use of these devices that practitioners must be educated about prior to selection of this treatment for a specific wound. If one is discharging a patient to the community, referral to a home health agency should be initiated prior to the patient's leaving the ED and caregiver and patient must have basic knowledge about the NPWT.

Many are concerned with the perceived increased costs of advanced dressings because the dressings are individually more expensive. There have been multiple studies that show cost savings when healing times are decreased and fewer dressing changes are needed.[24] Moreover, the fact that traditional saline-moistened wet-to-dry dressings require moistening every 3 hours and, therefore, more frequent changes, suggests that one should take into consideration the cost of nursing time and additional supplies. As our population ages the demand for scarce financial and nursing resources will increase, and these resources will be strained.

There are more than 350 brands of moisture-retentive dressings produced by 50 manufacturers.[25] Many of them serve primary and secondary requirements of the wound. It is increasingly complex to select from among the available products. It is recommended that health care professionals acquaint themselves with the classes of products available and become familiar with one or two products in each category. Dressing choice can be matched to address the specific characteristics of a particular wound. It is helpful to standardize the selection of wound care products, and most institutions have product formularies from which to choose. Table 8-1 may help with selection of the appropriate wound care product for a specific type of acute wound.

Chronic Wounds

In the ED and office setting many patients will present with wounds that are not healing or chronic wounds. As patients are discharged earlier from the hospital after surgical procedures the risk of complications will rise. As the population ages there is an increased incidence of chronic wounds and health care providers need to be familiar with acute and chronic wound diagnoses and treatment. An estimated 938,000 patients are admitted each year with the diagnosis of chronic wound.[26] In 2006 there was noted to be an 80% increase in admissions since 1993 for the diagnosis of

TABLE 8-1 | Dressings for Acute Wounds

Therapy	Examples	Advantages	Disadvantages	Uses
Topical antimicrobial agents				
Silver sulfadiazine	Silvadene	Wide antimicrobial coverage, painless	Requires frequent dressing changes, delays reepithelialization, stains tissue, may cause allergic reaction, may cause transient leukopenia	Deep burns, weeping burns, heavily contaminated or infected burns
Mafenide acetate	Sulfamylon	Wide antimicrobial coverage, penetrates eschar	Painful, may cause metabolic acidosis, may delay reepithelialization	Deep burns with eschar
Bacitracin		Painless, inexpensive, does not cause staining	Narrower antimicrobial coverage, requires frequent dressing changes, may cause allergic reaction	Facial burns, small burns, abrasions, lacerations, bites
Mupirocin	Bactroban	Painless, good coverage of gram-positive organisms	Expensive, requires frequent dressing changes	Facial burns, abrasions, bites
Triple antibiotic		Wide antimicrobial coverage, inexpensive, painless	Requires frequent dressing changes	Facial burns, small burns, abrasions, lacerations, bites

(Continued)

TABLE 8–1	Dressings for Acute Wounds (Continued)			
Therapy	**Examples**	**Advantages**	**Disadvantages**	**Uses**
Nonabsorptive dressings				
Impregnated nonadherent	Xeroform, Adaptic, Vaseline gauze	Painless, inexpensive	No antimicrobial activity, messy	Superficial burns and abrasions, lacerations
Nonabsorptive polyurethane film	OpSite, Tegaderm	Reduces pain, transparent	Promotes maceration	Minor abrasions, dry superficial burns
Silver-impregnated dressings	Acticoat, Actisorb, Aquacell	Wide antimicrobial coverage, reduces pain	Expensive, needs to be kept moist	Burns
Silicone	Mepitel	Painless, allows seepage of exudates into secondary dressing	Expensive	Burns, deep abrasions
Absorptive dressings				
Hydrocolloids	DuoDERM, Tegasorb	Reduce pain	Malodorous, opaque	Weeping burns, deep abrasions, skin tears
Hydrogels	Aquasorb, Vigilon, Curagel, FlexiGel, Nu-Gel	Rehydrate dry wounds		Weeping burns, deep abrasions, crusted surface exudate
Alginates		Absorb exudate	Require frequent dressing changes, nonadhesive, has been less extensively studied than other dressings	Weeping burns

Source: Singer AJ, Dagum AB. Current management of acute cutaneous wounds. *N Engl J Med.* 2008;359(10):1037.

pressure ulcer.[27] Any wound that does not improve or is getting worse is a cause for concern. In a study, Golinko et al. observed in patients presenting to the ED that despite a lack of systemic signs of infection, many of the patients studied grew antibiotic-resistant organisms and had histological signs of necrosis, ulceration, or osteomyelitis. They further noted that undermining is frequently missed on exam, is a sign of serious infection, and requires prompt surgical débridement.[28] These patients should be seriously considered for admission to prevent a deterioration of their condition that will ultimately lead to their return to the ED.

Table 8-2 may help to guide selection of dressing for use with acute and chronic wounds. The assessment of the wound bed characteristics and level of exudate drive the product choice. The amount of wound exudate is the critical factor in determining the product selection. The shaded boxes indicate the preferred product.

DRESSING CATEGORIES

Gauzes

Plain dry gauze is one of the earliest dressings to be used in modern medicine. Although gauze can absorb exudate it tends to dry and adhere to the wound bed causing pain and further trauma when removed. Plain gauze also is not an effective microbial barrier. There is now an antimicrobial gauze that is available in packing strips and in pad versions. Gauze may also be impregnated with various substances, such as petrolatum, that are less drying; however, impregnated gauze has little ability to absorb exudate. Saline-impregnated gauze maintains a moist wound environment but must be kept wet to be effective and avoid wound dessication. There are also hypertonic saline gauze dressings that absorb exudate and cleanse the wound.

Films

Films are transparent adhesive dressings generally made of polyurethane that are semiocclusive allowing water vapor and oxygen transmission while preventing liquid transmission. Although they are useful in relatively dry wounds, films cannot absorb exudate. As a result, films should not be used on wounds with moderate or heavy exudate. Films also may strip the fragile neoepidermis upon removal. Because they are transparent they allow visual examination of the wound without requiring their removal. Films are beneficial over secondary dressings as a barrier to contamination from urine and feces.

Hydrocolloids

Hydrocolloids can be either semiocclusive or occlusive (depending on manufacturer) adhesive dressings composed of various combinations of gelatin and pectin with little moisture transmission. Unlike films, hydrocolloids have the ability to absorb exudate and are most appropriate for wounds with small to moderate exudate. With heavy exudate hydrocolloids can become malodorous and may cause maceration of the surrounding skin. The hydrocolloids are comfortable and may be left in place for relatively long periods.

Hydrogels

The hydrogels are glycerin- or water-based dressings that help maintain a moist wound environment. Because they do not absorb exudate they are best used in dry wounds or those with minimal exudate. Hydrogels may be used in patients with contraindication to sharp surgical débridement because they promote autolytic debridement and sloughing of necrotic tissue. Hydrogels require a secondary dressing.

Foams

The foams are generally made of polyvinyl alcohol or polyurethane. They are moderately absorbent, semiocclusive dressings that are most appropriate for wounds with moderate to large exudate. The foams also protect the wound from heat loss and shearing forces. Some foams contain an outer layer of film that prevents leakage of exudate and provides an additional microbial barrier. Foam dressings are usually changed three times per week if exudate is managed. There are thin foam dressings designed for wounds with small exudate. Foams are also used as secondary dressings for wounds with depths that require packing with alginates.

Alginates

Alginates are derived from seaweed and have a high capacity to absorb exudate. Their use is generally limited to wounds with heavy exudate. On application to a moist wound the alginates form a gelatinous mass that helps maintain a moist wound environment. Alginates also have hemostatic properties making them appropriate for hemorrhagic wounds. Alginates should not be used on dry wounds. Because they may cause maceration of the peri-wound skin, the alginates should be trimmed to fit the size of the wound. There are apparent differences between

TABLE 8–2 | Guideline to Selection of Wound Dressings

VNSNY WOUND TREATMENT GUIDELINE

* Blue box with asterisk indicates appropriate treatment

Product Type — Refer To VNSNY Wound Care Formulary For Specific Products By Name	Granular — Objective: Keep Moist — Exudate S	M/L	Depth — Objective: Fill Space — Exudate S	M/L	Tunneling/Undermining — Objective: Fill Space — Exudate S	M/L	Necrotic Tissue: Slough — Objective: Debride — Exudate S	M/L	Necrotic Tissue: Eschar — Objective: Debride — Exudate S	M/L	Infected/Critically colonized — Objective: Reduce Bioburden — Exudate S	M/L
Hydrogel Wound Gel / Gauze — Maintains moisture balance to facilitate either granulation or autolytic debridement — Available as an antimicrobial	*		*		*		* <25% slough		* <25% eschar			
Hydrocolloid Wafer — Maintains moisture balance to facilitate either granulation or autolytic debridement — Available as an antimicrobial	*						* <25% slough		*			
Hydrocolloid/Hydrophilic paste — Fills depth & maintains moisture balance to facilitate granulation or autolytic debridement	*		*				* <25% slough					
Calcium Alginate or Hydrofiber — Absorbs exudate to maintain moisture balance — Available as an antimicrobial		*		*		*		* <25% slough				
Foam — Absorbs exudate to maintain moisture balance — Available as an antimicrobial		*						* <25% slough				
Antimicrobial — (Silver, Cadexomer Iodine, AMDs) — Available in gels, foams, alginates, hydrofiber, gauze pads/packing strips and collagen dsgs											*	*
Debriding Agents:									100% eschar should first be crosshatched by MD			
Enzymatic: Collagenase/Santyl — Needs MD prescription. — Cannot be used with silver products							*					
Cadexomer Iodine: Iodosorb/Iodoflex — Debrides slough, antimicrobial, absorbs exudate						*		*				*
Hypertonic Saline Gauze — Cleanses debrides slough, absorbs exudate						*		*				*
Hypertonic Saline Gel: Hypergel — Softens dry eschar to promote debridement. — Not to be used on intact skin							*		*	*		
Negative Pressure Wound TX	*		*	*		*	*				* Must tx infection	* Must tx infection

the various alginates on the market. There are also silver-impregnated alginates that provide absorption and antimicrobial activity.

Antimicrobial-Impregnated Dressings

A large number of silver-coated dressings (e.g., gauzes, gels, foams, hydrocolloids, alginates) that slowly release silver ions are now available on the market. Silver ions are effective against a large number of organisms with very low resistance rates. Silver-impregnated dressings may be used to prevent bacterial contamination or more commonly to reduce the bacterial bioburden in contaminated wounds. Silver should not be used in combination with enzymatic débridement. Cadexomer iodine product comes in both a paste and a pad. This antimicrobial product absorbs exudate and helps to débride slough. It is contraindicated for patients with thyroid disease or iodine sensitivity, and in nursing mothers.

FURTHER EVIDENCE AND GUIDELINES FOR SELECTING WOUND DRESSINGS

A recent systematic review was conducted that assessed dressings for acute and chronic wounds.[29] Although there were no level A studies, 14 level B and 79 level C studies were reviewed. The authors concluded that there was good (level B) evidence that the hydrocolloid dressings were better than saline gauze or paraffin gauze for chronic wounds. They further concluded that alginates, used either singly or in sequential treatment, are better than other modern dressings in reducing wound area, perhaps because they débride necrotic tissue. There was no difference between hydrocolloids and foam dressings in terms of healing. In the case of acute wounds, only one study reported a difference in healing rates between hydrofiber dressings and paraffin gauze or wet-to-dry gauze dressings. Hyaluronic acid and silver-coated dressings delayed healing compared with glycerine impregnated dressings or foam dressings, respectively. A subsequent consensus panel recommended the use of hydrogels for the débriding stage, foam or low-adherence dressings for the granulation stage, and hydrocolloids or low-adherence dressings for the reepithelialization phase of chronic wounds.[30] For fragile skin, low-adherence dressings were favored, and alginates were favored for hemorrhagic wounds. Alginates were also preferred for malodorous wounds.

REFERENCES

1. Winter GD. Formation of the scab and the rate of epithelization of superficial wounds in the skin of the young domestic pig. *Nature.* 1962;193:293–294.
2. Hinman CD, Maibach H. Effect of air exposure and occlusion on experimental human skin wounds. *Nature.* 1963;200:377–378.
3. Jones J. Winter's concept of moist wound healing: a review of the evidence and impact on clinical practice. *J Wound Care.* 2005;14(6):273–276.
4. Hutchinson JJ, McGuckin M. Occlusive dressings: a microbiologic and clinical review. *Am J Infect Control.* 1990;18(4):257–268.
5. Hansson C. Interactive wound dressings. A practical guide to their use in older patients. *Drugs Aging.* 1997;11(4):271–284.
6. Cho CY, Lo JS. Dressing the part. Dermatologic Clinics 1998;16(1):25–46.
7. Thomas S. The role of dressings in the treatment of moisture-related skin damage. 2008. Available at: http://www.worldwidewounds.com/2008/march/Thomas/Maceration-and-the-role-of-dressings.html. Accessed May 4, 2009.
8. Smack P, Harrington AC, Dunn C, et al. Infection and allergy incidence in ambulatory surgery patients using white petrolatum vs bacitracin ointment. A randomized controlled trial. *JAMA.* 1996;276(12):972–977.
9. Dire DJ, Coppola M, Dwyer DA, Lorette JJ, Karr JL. A prospective evaluation of topical antibiotics for preventing infections in uncomplicated soft-tissue wounds repaired in the ED. *Acad Emerg Med.* 1995;2(1):4–10.
10. Meaume S, Téot L, Lazareth I, Martini J, Bohbot S. The importance of pain reduction through dressing selection in routine wound management; the MAPP study. *J Wound Care.* 2004;13(10):409–413.
11. Johnson CA. Hearing loss following the application of topical neomycin. *J Burn Care Rehabil.* 1988;9(2):162–164.
12. Hood R, Shermock KM, Emerman C. A prospective, randomized pilot evaluation of topical triple antibiotic versus mupirocin for the prevention of uncomplicated soft tissue wound infection. *Am J Emerg Med.* 2004;22(1):1–3.
13. Sharp KA, McLaws ML. Wound dressings for surgical sites. *Cochrane Database Syst Rev.* 2001;(2):CD003091.
14. Zhai H. The effect of occlusion and semi-occlusion on experimental skin wound healing: a re-evaluation. *Wounds.* 2007;19(10):270–276.
15. Hedman LA. Effect of a hydrocolloid dressing on the pain level from abrasions on the feet during intensive marching. *Mil Med.* 1988;153(4):188–190.
16. Hermans MH, Hermans RP. Duoderm, an alternative dressing for smaller burns. *Burns Incl Therm Inj.* 1986;12(3):214–219.
17. Vermeulen H, Ubbink DT, de Vos R, Legemate DA, Semin-Goossens A. Dressings and topical agents for surgical wounds healing by secondary intention. *Cochrane Database Syst Rev.* 2004;(2):CD003554.

18. Briggs M, Closs SJ. Patients' perceptions of the impact of treatments and products on their experience of leg ulcer pain. *J Wound Care.* 2006;15(8):333–337.

19. Holm C, Petersen JS, Grønboek F, Gottrup F. Effects of occlusive and conventional gauze dressings on incisional healing after abdominal operations. *Eur J Surg.* 1998;164(3):179–183.

20. Palfreyman SJ, Nelson EA, Lochiel R, Michaels JA. Dressings for healing venous leg ulcers. *Cochrane Database Syst Rev.* 2006;(3):CD001103.

21. Fong J, Wood F, Fowler B. A silver coated dressing reduces the incidence of early burn wound cellulitis and associated costs of inpatient treatment: comparative patient care audits. *Burns.* 2005;31(5):562–567.

22. Wasiak J, Cleland H, Campbell F. Dressings for superficial and partial thickness burns. *Cochrane Database Syst Rev.* 2008;(4):CD002106.

23. Ubbink DT, Westerbos SJ, Nelson EA, Vermeulen H. A systematic review of topical negative pressure therapy for acute and chronic wounds. *Br J Surg.* 2008; 95(6):685–692.

24. Jones AM, San Miguel L. Are modern wound dressings a clinical and cost-effective alternative to the use of gauze? *J Wound Care.* 2006;15(2):65–69.

25. Ovington LG. Hanging wet-to-dry dressings out to dry. *Adv Skin Wound Care.* 2002;15(2):79–84.

26. Agency for Healthcare Research and Quality. Healthcare Cost and Utilization Project. Available at: http://www.hcupnet.ahrq.gov. Accessed July 2, 2009.

27. Russo CA, Steiner C, Spector W. Hospitalizations related to pressure ulcers, 2006. HCUP Statistical Brief 64. Rockville, MD: Agency for Healthcare Research and Quality. Available at: http://www.hcup-us.ahrq.gov/reports/statbriefs/sb64.pdf. Accessed July 2, 2009.

28. Golinko. MS, Clark S, Rennert R, Flattau A, Boulton JM, Brem H. Wound emergencies: the importance of assessment, documentation and early treatment using a wound electronic medical record. *Ostomy Wound Manage.* 2009;55(5):54–61.

29. Chaby G, Senet P, Vaneau M, et al. Dressings for acute and chronic wounds: a systematic review. *Arch Dermatol.* 2007;143(10):1297–1304.

30. Vaneau M, Chaby G, Guillot B, et al. Consensus panel recommendations for chronic and acute wound dressings. *Arch Dermatol.* 2007;143(10):1291–1294.

Antibiotics in Wound Management and Necrotizing Infections

Gregory J. Moran, MD, and Hans R. House, MD

Although virtually all wounds are contaminated with bacteria to some extent, only a small fraction will develop an infectious complication. Estimates of the incidence of infection of traumatic wounds vary tremendously, depending upon the method of study and the population examined, but most studies have found an incidence of 4.5% to 6.3%.[1] The best way to prevent wound infections is thorough wound cleansing and appropriate closure technique. Despite good wound care, some infections will still occur. Antibiotics have an important role in the management of wound infections, and may have a role in prophylaxis of certain high-risk wounds.

This chapter will discuss the optimal use of antibiotics in the management of wounds and wound infections. The use of antibiotics for animal bites, plantar puncture wounds, and abscesses is discussed in Chapters 15, 17, and 18, respectively.

PRINCIPLES OF ANTIBIOTIC USE FOR WOUNDS AND WOUND INFECTIONS

Effectiveness

Activity against the likely pathogens is the most important consideration in choosing an antibiotic; other important factors include cost, convenience, and adverse effects. Because bacterial cultures require at least 1 to 2 days, initial treatment in the emergency department (ED) or office setting is almost never guided by culture results. A reasonable determination of the likely pathogens can be made, however, by considering the mechanism, the circumstances of the wound, the location on the body, and host factors.

The antimicrobial spectrum of a particular agent is determined by in vitro studies. This may not necessarily correlate with clinical effectiveness, as simple in vitro sensitivities do not take into account the complex interactions of tissue fluids, fibrin coagulum, contaminated skin, the interaction of bacterial species, and the immune response. Most antibiotics in common use, including penicillins, cephalosporins, trimethoprim/sulfamethoxazole, macrolides, aminoglycosides, and fluoroquinolones, will achieve adequate levels in skin and soft tissues. Many antibiotics do not penetrate well into fluid collections and abscesses, so it is important that these infections be drained adequately. Aminoglycosides have especially poor penetration into abscesses, and their activity is inhibited by the low pH environment.

Practical Issues

Practical issues such as cost and dosing convenience must also be considered. Selecting a broad-spectrum antibiotic is usually not the best solution, as they are typically more expensive and may be more likely to select resistant organisms or cause adverse effects by disrupting normal flora.

Antibiotics with more frequent dosing are clearly associated with lower compliance rates. Some drugs commonly used for wound infections, including cephalexin, cephradine, dicloxacillin, clindamycin, and erythromycin, have inconvenient four-times-daily dosing. Some physicians will prescribe cephalexin 500 mg three times daily instead of 250 mg four times daily to simplify the regimen. Cefadroxil is a first-generation cephalosporin with two-times-daily dosing. Amoxicillin–clavulanate has traditionally been given three times daily, but the 875-/125-mg dose can be given twice daily and appears to have fewer gastrointestinal side effects. Although some fluoroquinolones with once-daily dosing are approved for treating infections of skin and soft tissue, they generally are not considered first-line agents because of higher cost and because other agents are available that have greater activity against skin pathogens.

In pediatric patients, the palatability and dosing convenience of a drug can be very important in determining the success of a clinical regimen.[2] Dicloxacillin and erythromycin have been noted to have a bitter taste that may interfere with compliance.[3]

Adverse Reactions

Adverse reactions to antibiotics must also be considered. Fortunately, the β-lactam antibiotics preferred for most wound infections have a low incidence of adverse reactions, although some β-lactam antibiotics have more adverse effects than others. Diarrhea, for example, is reported by 9% of patients taking amoxicillin–clavulanate, but is only rarely reported among users of cephalexin. Some drugs within a class carry a milder adverse effect profile than others. Although erythromycin causes gastrointestinal distress in approximately 20% to 25% of patients, azithromycin and clarithromycin have a much lower incidence of gastrointestinal adverse effects as well as less-frequent dosing.

EMPIRIC ANTIBIOTIC THERAPY FOR WOUND INFECTIONS

Gram-positive organisms such as *Streptococcus pyogenes* and *Staphylococcus aureus* are responsible for the large majority of wound infections. These are ubiquitous organisms that may be found in the normal flora of the skin, and will be introduced into any injury that causes a break in the integrity of the epidermis. Pathogens isolated from traumatic wounds have been found to be primarily the resident flora of the skin. Although recent bacteriological surveys of traumatic wound infections are limited (most data in the literature focus on surgical wound infections), the few studies published confirm the predominance of these two pathogens. *S aureus* has been found in about half of traumatic wounds, one third yielded *S pyogenes*, and 10% to 15% grew both organisms.[4] Gram-negative rods, enterococci, and anaerobes appeared in only about 10% of wound cultures. Although *Escherichia coli* has been found in as many as 25% of wound infections,[5] most studies have found a low incidence of gram-negative pathogens in uncomplicated infections.[6]

Since the year 2000, community-associated methicillin-resistant *S aureus* (CA-MRSA) has emerged as the predominant cause of skin and soft tissue infections in the United States.[7] CA-MRSA is relatively more common as a cause of skin abscesses, but is also a frequent cause of wound infections. Certain types of wounds (e.g., "turf burn" abrasions in football players) may be at higher risk of CA-MRSA infection, but there are no clinical or epidemiologic features that can reliably exclude a CA-MRSA etiology.[8] In areas with CA-MRSA it is reasonable to include activity against this organism when one is choosing empiric therapy.[9] Newer rapid tests that use technology such as polymerase chain reaction or fluorescent in-situ hybridization may be able to reliably identify or exclude MRSA in wound infections for the purposes of empiric treatment.

Most patients with simple wound infections can be safely treated as outpatients with oral agents. First-generation cephalosporins, such as cephalexin (250 to 500 mg every 6 hours), or antistaphylococcal penicillins, such as dicloxacillin (500 mg every 6 hours), have been the most commonly used therapy for most simple wound infections.

Because CA-MRSA has now become a common etiology of wound infections in many areas, β-lactam antibiotics alone may not be adequate. Oral antimicrobials with in vitro activity against most CA-MRSA isolates include trimethoprim–sulfamethoxazole, clindamycin, doxycycline, rifampin, and linezolid.[10] Most MRSA isolates are resistant to macrolides and quinolones. Because trimethoprim–sulfamethoxazole may not have good activity against streptococci, it can be combined with cephalexin when reliable streptococcal activity is desired in addition to MRSA activity.

Clindamycin has good activity as monotherapy against both CA-MRSA and streptococci, though it is relatively more expensive and has more frequent adverse effects such as diarrhea. Some macrolide-resistant strains of MRSA have what has been termed "inducible" clindamycin resistance. There have been case reports of treatment failures or recurrences associated with clindamycin therapy for these strains, but it appears that most patients will recover with clindamycin therapy.

Doxycycline is active against about 85% of CA-MRSA strains as well as most streptococci. Rifampin quickly selects for resistant isolates so it should not be used alone. There are no data showing that outcomes are improved by adding rifampin to other agents, but it has a theoretical advantage of possibly preventing recurrence by improved decolonization with combination therapy.

Occasionally, intravenous administration of antibiotics in an inpatient setting is indicated. Relative indications for admission include signs of systemic toxicity or underlying immunodeficiency states such as poorly controlled diabetes, renal failure, and chronic steroid use. Patients should also be considered for admission if they suffer a severe infection in a specific vital area such as the face, orbit, hand, perineum, or lower extremity—any region that would result in disastrous morbidity if the infection continued to spread. Intravenous therapy may also be warranted in suspected mixed flora or gram-negative infections. For most simple wound infections in which gram-positive organisms (including CA-MRSA) are the more likely etiology, clindamycin 900 mg IV every 6 hours will cover the likely pathogens, including about 85% to 90% of CA-MRSA strains. Vancomycin 15 mg/kg IV every 12 hours is an alternative that is active against virtually all CA-MRSA, as well as streptococci. Linezolid and daptomycin are also active against MRSA and other gram-positive skin pathogens, but higher cost usually precludes their use as first-line agents.

If culture results or a rapid test show methicillin-susceptible *S aureus*, the antibiotic can be switched to cefazolin (1 g every 8 hours), oxacillin (2 g every 4 hours), or nafcillin (2 g every 4 hours). If streptococci are found, then penicillin G 2 million units every 4 hours (or by continuous infusion) is an alternative to the other β-lactam regimens. Vancomycin would also be appropriate for persons with prosthetic heart valves, synthetic vascular implants, or orthopedic hardware underlying the infection because coagulase-negative staphylococci can cause prosthesis infection. A number of newer agents may soon be available, including new cephalosporins such as ceftobiprole and ceftaroline that are active against MRSA.

Infections in patients with underlying diseases such as poorly controlled diabetes may call for more broad-spectrum antibiotics. Serious or recurrent infections are more likely to be polymicrobial, with gram-negative and anaerobic organisms as well as *S aureus* and streptococcus. Agents such as amoxicillin–clavulanate (which lacks activity against CA-MRSA) or a combination of clindamycin plus a fluoroquinolone would be appropriate.

Although most bacteria involved in wound infections originate from the patient's own body, exogenous pathogens may be introduced from the environment where the injury occurred, and may require specific treatment in some circumstances. *Clostridium perfringens* or *Clostridium tetani* are associated with soil contamination, particularly in puncture wounds or those associated with crush injury. Wounds contaminated with animal or human feces (e.g., barnyard puncture wounds) are more likely to be infected with gram-negative enteric organisms and anaerobes.

Wounds with a history of marine or freshwater exposure are at risk for involvement of certain unique organisms. Marine exposures may be associated with infection from *Vibrio* species, especially in patients with underlying liver disease.[11] *Vibrio* skin infections tend to cause hemorrhagic, bullous lesions, and should be treated with ceftazidime with or without doxycycline, or ciprofloxacin. *Mycobacterium marinum* may also be found with saltwater exposures. *Aeromonas hydrophilia* or *Pseudomonas aeruginosa* may be seen in wounds exposed to fresh water. For serious infections resulting from freshwater exposures, consider adding an antipseudomonal aminoglycoside or fluoroquinolone to agents traditionally used to treat gram-positive organisms. Agents such as imipenem, meropenem, ticarcillin–clavulanate, or piperacillin–tazobactam could be used instead. Wounds that result from the handling of fish are at risk for the unusual pathogen *Erysipelothrix rhusiopathiae*. This organism responds to penicillin or ampicillin, and fluoroquinolones may be used in the penicillin-allergic patient.[12] The recommended choices for empiric antibiotic treatment of wound infections are presented in Table 9-1.

NECROTIZING INFECTIONS

The most severe skin infections are deep, necrotizing soft tissue infections. These may initially be subtle in presentation, but they pose a significant threat to life and limb if not treated expediently. The tissue involvement is usually extensive and quickly spreading, but the classic signs of swelling, warmth, and erythema may not be present. The hallmark findings are crepitus on physical exam or tissue gas seen on radiographs,

TABLE 9–1 Empiric Antibiotics for Wound Infections

Clinical Situation	First-line Agent	Alternative Therapy	Comment
Uncomplicated cellulitis	1st generation cephalosporin (or antistaphylococcal penicillin) plus trimethoprim–sulfamethoxazole	Clindamycin	CA-MRSA now a common cause of wound infections in most areas
Patient with underlying immunodeficiency	Amoxicillin–clavulanate plus trimethoprim–sulfamethoxazole	Clindamycin plus a fluoroquinolone	Consider prophylaxis, especially in contaminated wounds
Patient with prosthetic heart valve or orthopedic implant	Consider adding vancomycin to standard regimen		Give prophylaxis when manipulating abscesses
Barnyard injuries, fecal contamination	Amoxicillin–clavulanate or 2nd-generation cephalosporin	Fluoroquinolone plus clindamycin or metronidazole	Prophylaxis should be strongly considered
Salt water exposure	3rd-generation cephalosporin +/– doxycycline	Fluoroquinolone	*Vibrio* may cause hemorrhagic, bullous lesions
Freshwater exposure	Antipseudomonal aminoglycoside or antipseudomonal penicillin	Fluoroquinolone	*Aeromonas* or *Pseudomonas* may be involved
Abscesses, infections associated with IV drug use	Clindamycin	Trimethoprim–sulfamethoxazole	Antibiotics usually not necessary; incision and drainage essential
Necrotizing fasciitis	Ampicillin–sulbactam plus clindamycin +/– vancomycin	Ertapenem plus clindamycin +/– vancomycin	Clindamycin active against most CA-MRSA, but consider adding vancomycin if CA-MRSA likely
Bite wounds	Amoxicillin–clavulanate or cefoxitin/cefotetan	Azithromycin or ciprofloxacin plus clindamycin	Consider prophylaxis for high-risk: deep puncture, crush, hand
Open fracture	1st generation cephalosporin or antistaphylococcal penicillin	Vancomycin	Add gentamicin for prophylaxis of severe open fractures
Plantar puncture wound osteomyelitis	Ceftazidime	Ciprofloxacin	

CA-MRSA=community-associated methicillin-resistant *Staphylococcus aureus*.

but these are late findings. Necrotizing infections may present initially with severe pain and tenderness out of proportion to physical findings. Systemic toxicity may be severe as the infection progresses.

Necrotizing infections are typically polymicrobial and should be treated aggressively; broad-spectrum antimicrobials such as a β-lactamase inhibitor combination plus vancomycin plus clindamycin would be appropriate.[10] The nomenclature of necrotizing infections is somewhat inconsistent and can be confusing. The terms necrotizing fasciitis, monomicrobial necrotizing cellulitis, and Meleney's synergistic gangrene are used to describe various types of necrotizing infections. As mentioned, most are polymicrobial, occurring in patients with underlying chronic disease such as diabetes or renal failure. Organisms include S aureus, streptococci, enteric gram-negative rods, and a variety of anaerobic organisms. Necrotizing infections can follow traumatic wounds, abdominal surgery, cutaneous ulcers, perirectal infections, and intravenous drug use. Fournier's gangrene is a variant of polymicrobial necrotizing fasciitis that occurs in the perineum.

Group A streptococcus (GAS), popularly known as "flesh-eating bacteria," can cause a rapidly progressing necrotizing infection in previously healthy individuals, sometimes following trivial trauma. This infection predominantly involves the subcutaneous tissue and fascia, with early sparing of the skin and only very late involvement of the muscle. Initially, the skin is painful but appears only mildly erythematous, and the area of involvement is not distinctly demarcated. As vessel thrombosis within the subdermal tissues occurs, the surface becomes mottled, edematous, or frankly necrotic, and blebs appear. After incision, thin, reddish-brown pus ("dishwater pus") may be released and the skin may be found to be undermined.[13] Group A streptococcus infections also may be associated with toxic shock syndrome. CA-MRSA has also been reported to cause necrotizing infections, though they may not be as rapidly progressive as GAS infections.[14]

Gas gangrene, or clostridial myonecrosis, results from a deep injury to skeletal muscle and leads to ischemia and tissue necrosis. Tissue gas can be found within muscle groups on radiograph. Toxins liberated by clostridial species infecting the wound can lead to profound systemic disease and mortality. A less severe form, known as clostridial cellulitis, has no muscle involvement and a more gradual onset.

Regardless of the specific syndrome involved, every necrotizing infection should be recognized as a life-threatening emergency. Immediate surgical consultation and broad-spectrum antibiotics must be initiated. Appropriate empiric antibiotic combinations would include a β-lactamase inhibitor drug (e.g., ampicillin–sulbactam) or carbapenem (e.g., ertapenem) plus clindamycin; vancomycin can be added if MRSA is considered likely. For GAS infections, animal data suggest that a regimen including clindamycin may be superior to penicillin.[13] This superiority is believed to be attributable to reduced efficacy of penicillin when large numbers of organisms are present, and the ability of clindamycin to limit toxin production by inhibiting protein synthesis.

PROPHYLAXIS FOR WOUND INFECTIONS

Topical Antibiotics

Although topical antibiotics such as mupirocin can be used successfully to treat minor wound infections, the primary use of topical antibiotics is for prevention of infection in fresh wounds.[15] Topical ointments containing bacitracin, neomycin, or polymyxin are routinely used by many physicians for fresh wounds: a survey of US emergency physicians found that 71% use a topical antibiotic on simple lacerations.[16] Despite the frequent use of topical antibiotics, there are surprisingly few studies that assess the efficacy of topical antibiotics on the suture line after closure. Animal studies have shown that topical antimicrobials inside the wound prior to closure may reduce infection in contaminated wounds.[17] One double-blind, randomized human trial found a 5% infection rate with antibiotic ointment, compared to an unexpectedly high 17.6% with petrolatum control.[18] Other studies have found no significant reduction in infection rates with topical antibiotics.[19] Because the risk of infection is higher for crush injuries than for sharp lacerations, some practitioners use topical antibiotics only for stellate wounds with abraded skin edges, but this suggestion is not based on comparative trial data.

Systemic Antibiotic Prophylaxis

Antibiotic prophylaxis is not necessary for uncomplicated wounds in immunocompetent individuals. Although it is tempting to give prophylactic antibiotics to prevent wound infections, it is important to note the limitations of this strategy. In many situations prophylactic antibiotics will not reduce the overall rate of infection, but may skew the bacteriology toward more unusual or resistant pathogens. To date, no randomized trials have demonstrated a benefit of antibiotic prophylaxis for simple wounds in immunocompetent patients.[20–24] A meta-analysis of randomized trials has also confirmed the lack of benefit for simple wounds.[25] Despite these data, it is still unclear whether there is a subset of high-risk wounds for which prophylactic antibiotics may be beneficial. Although it is known that certain types of wounds are more likely to develop infection, there is a paucity of good studies of prophylaxis for uninfected high-risk wounds. It is reasonable

TABLE 9–2	**Considerations for Prophylactic Systemic Antibiotics for Wounds**

Immunocompromised host

- Poorly controlled diabetes mellitus
- Systemic corticosteroids or other immuno-suppressants
- Renal failure
- Lymphedema
- AIDS

High-risk anatomical sites

- Oral lacerations
- Exposed tendon, bone, or joint

High-risk wounds

- Large amount of crushed or devitalized tissue
- Heavily contaminated wounds, possible retained foreign body
- Puncture wounds
- Bites
- Significant delay before presentation

to give prophylaxis for some high-risk wounds. Situations in which prophylaxis is sometimes recommended include an immunosuppressed host; an open fracture; a wound involving a joint, tendon, or cartilage; a grossly contaminated, high-risk bite wound (puncture, crush, extremity); oral wounds; or significant delay before presentation (Table 9-2).

Immune impairment

Prospective outcome studies have found an increased infection rate in patients with immune impairment.[26,27] Diabetes mellitus, malnutrition, renal failure, HIV infection, steroid use, chemotherapy treatment, extremes of age, and obesity have all been associated with more infectious complications. Patients with cardiac lesions at high risk for endocarditis should receive prophylactic antibiotics as recommended by the American Heart Association when undergoing procedures likely to induce transient bacteremia, such as the incision and drainage of a large abscess.[28] However, repair of a wound that is not grossly infected does not require antibiotic prophylaxis.

Anatomical Site

The anatomical site of the wound may influence the risk of infection. Foot wounds appear to become infected more often than those involving other parts of the body, and injuries to the head and neck have the lowest rates of complication.[26] This disparity is often attributed to differences in regional blood flow, but greater contamination (both from environmental sources and endogenous flora) of lower extremity injuries is also important. Although most minor oral wounds probably do not require prophylaxis, there may be a benefit of oral penicillin prophylaxis for more severe wounds, in particular through-and-through wounds.[29] Although hand wounds are often classified as high-risk, studies have failed to demonstrate a benefit of antibiotic prophylaxis for simple hand wounds.[30,31]

Most experts recommend prophylactic antibiotics for wounds in which tendons are lacerated or exposed. Although no randomized studies have been done in this group, it is reasonable to give prophylaxis for these high-risk injuries. Prospective studies have not been done to validate antibiotic prophylaxis for wounds involving the cartilage of the ear or nose, but this also seems reasonable. Open fractures or wounds into joint spaces typically require débridement and irrigation in the operating room in conjunction with parenteral antibiotics. Minor open fractures of distal fingers appear to have a low risk of infection,[32,33] but prophylaxis should be considered for higher-risk patients.

Wound Mechanism and Contamination

The mechanism causing the wound may or may not influence the infection rate. Although some studies have found that crush injuries are higher risk,[34] presumably because of more devitalized tissue, which is impaired in its ability to resist bacterial growth, other prospective studies suggest that sharp and blunt mechanisms have similar rates of infection. The presence of collected blood within a wound acts as a growth medium and has been shown to increase risk of infection.[35] Wounds contaminated with more than 10^5 organisms per gram are at greater risk of infection, although there are no practical means to make this determination at the time of repair. Antibiotic prophylaxis should be considered for wounds that are grossly contaminated and cannot be adequately cleaned. One of the most important local factors promoting infection is the presence of foreign bodies, including dirt, glass, metal, wood, bits of rubber or clothing, and even subcutaneous sutures.[36] Soft-tissue gunshot wounds appear to be at low risk for infection and should not require antibiotic prophylaxis.

Delayed presentation

Much has been written about the "golden period" of time after injury in which a wound can be safely closed, and opinions differ as to when the increased risk of infection becomes significant. Although some studies have found that delayed closure does seem to influence the infection rate, several studies have shown that delayed closure does not seem to be a significant factor, at least up to 18 hours after injury.[37] Some experts recommend antibiotic prophylaxis for wounds with significantly delayed presentation, often in conjunction with delayed primary closure.

Deciding on prophylaxis

Although the available literature does not support the routine use of prophylactic antibiotics in all simple wounds, and prophylaxis is poorly studied in high-risk subsets, it is reasonable to use prophylaxis in select settings. It is impossible to make generic recommendations that can account for the multiple factors present in any individual patient, so clinicians must use their own judgment. Prophylaxis should be *considered* in the situations shown in Table 9-2, especially if multiple factors are present.

Choice of agents for prophylaxis

The specific antibiotics used for prophylaxis are similar to those used for treatment of established infections. In most settings, a first-generation cephalosporin, antistaphylococcal penicillin (e.g., dicloxacillin), or macrolide would be appropriate. Penicillin would be an appropriate choice for intraoral wounds because of the activity against most common oral pathogens. Amoxicillin–clavulanate is the preferred prophylactic agent for high-risk bite wounds (because of its activity against *Pasteurella* sp. for animal bites and *Eikenella corrodens* for human bites)[38,39] and for grossly contaminated, devitalized wounds in immunocompromised patients.

Although many experts recommend a dose of parenteral antibiotics at the time of repair to quickly obtain high levels in the tissues, parenteral antibiotics have not been shown to be any more effective than oral antibiotics for wound repair.[20–23] For open fractures or joints, a parenteral antistaphylococcal agent should be given, and an aminoglycoside should be added for severe open fractures.[40] It is not necessary to give a prolonged course of antibiotics for wound prophylaxis; a 3- to 5-day course is adequate to reduce infection during the highest-risk period.

Although CA-MRSA has emerged as the most common cause of skin infections, it is not necessary to include activity against CA-MRSA for most wound prophylaxis. The antimicrobial spectrum of prophylactic antibiotics should be selected based on the bacterial flora that are likely to exist on the skin at the time of injury and other bacteria that may be introduced through wound contamination (e.g., bite wounds, marine exposure, barnyard injuries). Carriage rates for MRSA among the general population remain low, and there are no studies supporting the use of antibiotic prophylaxis for wounds directed against this pathogen. Nevertheless, prophylactic regimens with activity against CA-MRSA would be logical for patients at high risk for CA-MRSA colonization, such as those with a history of CA-MRSA infection or with a close household contact with a known carrier of CA-MRSA.

SUMMARY

Despite good wound care, some infections will continue to occur. The choice of antibiotic for prevention and treatment of wound infections is guided by the spectrum of likely pathogens, which can be surmised by considering the mechanism, the circumstances of the wound, location on the body, and host factors. Other factors such as cost, dosing convenience, and adverse effects must also be considered. For most simple wound infections, activity against common gram-positive organisms such as *S aureus* (including CA-MRSA) and *S pyogenes* is important. Appropriate agents would include a first-generation cephalosporin (or dicloxacillin) in combination with trimethoprim–sulfamethoxazole, or clindamycin alone. More broad-spectrum activity may be appropriate for more serious wound infections such as animal or human bites, wounds exposed to freshwater or other contaminants, or necrotizing infections.

Although the routine use of prophylactic antibiotics is not supported by the available literature, certain high-risk wounds may benefit from antibiotics at the initial presentation. Situations for which prophylaxis should be considered include patients with significant immunocompromise; wounds involving bones, joints, tendons, or cartilage; grossly contaminated wounds that cannot be adequately cleaned; high-risk bite wounds (e.g., puncture wounds, crushed or devitalized tissue, hand involvement); high-risk intraoral wounds; or wounds with a significant delay before presentation. Prophylactic antibiotics for puncture wounds to the foot are controversial.

PEARLS

- The best way to prevent wound infections is thorough wound cleansing and appropriate closure technique.

- Activity against the likely pathogens is the most important consideration in choosing an antibiotic; other important factors include cost, convenience, and adverse effects.
- Gram-positive organisms such as *S pyogenes* and *S aureus* (including CA-MRSA) are responsible for the large majority of wound infections.
- Appropriate choices for empiric treatment for most wound infections would include a first-generation cephalosporin such as cephalexin or antistaphylococcal penicillin such as dicloxacillin, plus an agent such as trimethoprim–sulfamethoxazole for CA-MRSA activity. Clindamycin could be used alone as an alternative.
- Necrotizing infections may present initially with severe pain and tenderness out of proportion to physical findings.
- Necrotizing infections are typically polymicrobial and should be treated aggressively; broad-spectrum antimicrobials such as a β-lactamase inhibitor combination plus clindamycin would be appropriate.
- Antibiotic prophylaxis is not necessary for uncomplicated wounds in immunocompetent individuals.
- Situations in which antimicrobial prophylaxis is sometimes recommended for wounds include an immunosuppressed host; an open fracture; a wound involving a joint, tendon, or cartilage; a grossly contaminated, high-risk bite wound (puncture, crush, extremity); oral wounds; or significant delay before presentation.

References

1. Hollander JE, Singer AJ, Valentine S, Henry MC. Wound registry: development and validation. *Ann Emerg Med.* 1995;25(5):675–685.
2. Bauchner H, Klein JO. Parental issues in selection of antimicrobial agents for infants and children. *Clin Pediatr.* 1997;36(4):201–205.
3. Steele RW, Estrada B, Begue RE, Mirza A, Travillion DA, Thomas MP. A double-blind taste comparison of pediatric antibiotic suspensions. *Clin Pediatr (Phila).* 1997;36(4):193–199.
4. Kontiainen S, Rinne E. Bacteria isolated from skin and soft tissue lesions. *Eur J Clin Microbiol.* 1987; 6(4):420–422.
5. Brook I, Frazier EH. Aerobic and anaerobic microbiology of infection after trauma. *Am J Emerg Med.* 1998;16:585–591.
6. Moet GJ, Jones RN, Biedenbach DJ, Stilwell MG, Fritsche TR. Contemporary causes of skin and soft tissue infections in North America, Latin America, and Europe: report from the SENTRY Antimicrobial Surveillance Program (1998–2004). *Diagn Microbiol Infect Dis.* 2007;57(1):7–13.
7. Moran GJ, Krishnadasan A, Gorwitz RJ, et al. Methicillin-resistant *S. aureus* infections among patients in the emergency department. *New Engl J Med.* 2006;355(7):666–674.
8. Miller LG, Perdreau-Remington F, Bayer AS, et al. Clinical and epidemiologic characteristics cannot distinguish community-associated methicillin-resistant Staphylococcus aureus infection from methicillin-susceptible S. aureus infection: a prospective investigation. *Clin Infect Dis.* 2007;44(4): 471–482.
9. Moran GJ, Talan DA. Methicillin-resistant *Staphylococcus aureus*: is it in your community and should it change practice? *Ann Emerg Med.* 2005;45(3): 321–322.
10. Abrahamian FM, Talan DA, Moran GJ. Management of skin and soft tissue infections in the emergency department. *Infect Dis Clin North Am.* 2008;22(1): 89–116, vi.
11. Dechet AM, Yu PA, Koram N, Painter J. Nonfoodborne Vibrio infections: an important cause of morbidity and mortality in the United States, 1997–2006. *Clin Infect Dis.* 2008;46(7):970–976.
12. Eron LJ. Targeting lurking pathogens in acute traumatic and chronic wounds. *J Emerg Med.* 1999;17(1): 189–195.
13. Bisno AL, Stevens DL. Streptococcal infections of skin and soft tissues. *N Engl J Med.* 1996;334(4): 240–245.
14. Miller LG, Perdreau-Remington F, Rieg G, et al. Necrotizing fasciitis caused by community-associated methicillin-resistant Staphylococcus aureus in Los Angeles. *N Engl J Med.* 2005;352(14):1445–1453.
15. Moran GJ, Talan DA, Abrahamian FM. Antimicrobial prophylaxis for wounds and procedures in the emergency department. *Infect Dis Clin North Am.* 2008;22(1):117–143.
16. Howell JM, Chisholm CD. Outpatient wound preparation and care: a national survey. *Ann Emerg Med.* 1992;21:976–981.
17. Edlich RF, Smith QT, Edgerton MT. Resistance of the surgical wound to antimicrobial prophylaxis and its mechanisms of development. *Am J Surg.* 1973: 126(5):583–591.
18. Dire DJ, Coppola M, Dwyer DA, Lorette JJ, Karr JL. Prospective evaluation of topical antibiotics for preventing infections in uncomplicated soft-tissue wounds repaired in the ED. *Acad Emerg Med.* 1995; 2(1):4–10.
19. Caro D, Reynolds KW, De Smith J. An investigation to evaluate a topical antibiotic in the prevention of wound sepsis in a casualty department. *Br J Clin Pract.* 1967;21(12):605–607.
20. Hutton PA, Jones BM, Law DJ. Depot penicillin as prophylaxis in accidental wounds. *Br J Surg.* 1978; 65(8):549–550.
21. Thirlby RC, Blair AJ III, Thal ER. The value of prophylactic antibiotics for simple lacerations. *Surg Gynecol Obstet.* 1983;156(2):212–216.
22. Edlich RF, Kenny JG, Morgan RF, Nichter LS, Friedman HI, Rodeheaver GT. Antimicrobial treatment of minor soft tissue lacerations: a critical review. *Emerg Med Clin North Am.* 1986;4(3):561–580.

23. Day TK. Controlled trial of prophylactic antibiotics in minor wounds requiring suture. *Lancet.* 1975; 2(7946):1174–1176.

24. Baker MD, Lanuti M. The management and outcome of lacerations in urban children. *Ann Emerg Med.* 1990;19(9):1001–1005.

25. Cummings P, Del Beccaro MA. Antibiotics to prevent infection of simple wounds: a meta-analysis of randomized studies. *Am J Emerg Med.* 1995;13(4): 396–400.

26. Singer AJ, Hollander JE, Quinn JV. Evaluation and management of traumatic lacerations. *N Engl J Med.* 1997;337(16):1142–1148.

27. Cruse PJ, Foord R. A five-year prospective study of 23,649 surgical wounds. *Arch Surg.* 1973;107(2): 206–210.

28. Wilson W, Taubert KA, Gewitz M, et al. Prevention of infective endocarditis: guidelines from the American Heart Association: a guideline from the American Heart Association Rheumatic Fever, Endocarditis, and Kawasaki Disease Committee, Council on Cardiovascular Disease in the Young, and the Council on Clinical Cardiology, Council on Cardiovascular Surgery and Anesthesia, and the Quality of Care and Outcomes Research Interdisciplinary Working Group. *Circulation.* 2007;116(15): 1736–1754.

29. Mark DG, Granquist EJ. Are prophylactic oral antibiotics indicated for the treatment of intraoral wounds? *Ann Emerg Med.* 2008;52(4):368–372.

30. Zehtabchi S. Evidence-based emergency medicine/critically appraised topic. The role of antibiotic prophylaxis for prevention of infection in patients with simple hand lacerations. *Ann Emerg Med.* 2007;49(5):682–689, 689.e1.

31. Moran GJ, Talan DA. Hand infections. *Emerg Med Clin North Am.* 1993;11(3):601–619.

32. Suprock MD, Hood JM, Lubahn JD. Role of antibiotics in open fractures of the finger. *J Hand Surg Am.* 1990;15(5):761–764.

33. Zook EG, Guy R, Russell RC. A study of nail bed injuries: causes, treatment, and prognosis. *J Hand Surg.* 1984;9(2):247–252.

34. Cardany CR, Rodeheaver GT, Thacker J, Edgerton MT, Edlich RF. The crush injury: a high risk wound. *JACEP.* 1976;5(12):965–970.

35. Krizek TJ, Davis JH. The role of the red cell in subcutaneous infection. *J Trauma* 1965;5:85–95.

36. Mehta PH, Dunn KA, Bradfield JF, Austin PE. Contaminated wounds: infection rates with subcutaneous sutures. *Ann Emerg Med.* 1996;27(1): 43–48.

37. Berk WA, Welch RD, Bock BF. Controversial issues in clinical management of the simple wound. *Ann Emerg Med.* 1992;21(1):72–80.

38. Talan DA, Citron DM, Abrahamian FM, Moran GJ, Goldstein EJ. Bacteriologic analysis of infected dog and cat bites. Emergency Medicine Animal Bite Infection Study Group. *N Engl J Med.* 1999;340(2): 85–92.

39. Talan DA, Abrahamian FM, Moran GJ, et al. Clinical presentation and bacteriologic analysis of infected human bites in patients presenting to emergency departments. *Clin Infect Dis.* 2003;37(11) 1481–1489.

40. Hauser CJ, Adams CA, Eachempati SR; Council of the Surgical Infection Society. Surgical Infection Society guideline: prophylactic antibiotic use in open fractures: an evidence-based guideline. *Surg Infect (Larchmt).* 2006;7(4):379–405.

CHAPTER 10

Adhesive Tapes for Closure of Acute Wounds and Surgical Incisions

Robert M. Blumm, MA, PA-C, DFAAPA

What is the best type of closure or the best technique for closing wounds? The answer is straightforward: the one that meets the need of the hour. Our interest in wounds can be dated back to our ancestor, *Australopithecus africanus*, who needed to deal with wounds as violence and war appeared in his culture.[1] Historically, man has utilized his intelligence and the materials that were known to him to close or protect wounds. Our very early ancestors used mud packs, hemp, leaves, and grass to "dress" a wound. When a person sustained a significant wound such as a gaping abdominal wound, spikes were inserted at the wound margins and tied together by attaching hides, leather, or cloth to the lateral surfaces and pulling them together.[2] This is the genesis of the Montgomery Binder, a binder that was used predominantly in the 1960s; however, it is still utilized for certain wounds in the first decade of the 21st century. The history of wound healing is filled with information that has caused modern man to adapt and to transform.[3] We are always evolving and lessons from the past will always be a part of the mosaic of what we like to consider "modern medicine." All techniques, even that of utilization of tapes, has a forerunner in human history.[4]

Primitive man was known to sew wounds together with pieces of tendon or hair, bind wounds with tapes, or use various alternative medicine types of packs to seal wounds. Bleeding was controlled with hot pokers that seared the tissue as well as the bleeder. To achieve hemostasis, suturing was a contribution of the Romans, Egyptians, and Indians. Students of history discovered that suture techniques were a double-edged sword as they often caused infection and delayed wound healing. The first use of adhesive and gum tapes dates back 4000 years. Twenty-first century clinicians continue to refine sutures and needles but the search for the Holy Grail, a perfect closure device, continues.[3]

Although sutures are considered the "gold standard" for wound closure,[5] they sometimes produce a less favorable result than staples, tapes, and adhesives.[6,7] Surgical tapes are easy to use, do not leave suture marks, are not associated with any risk of a needle stick, and are very gentle on the skin. Because no foreign body is left inside the wound, they also have a lower risk of infection than do sutures. However, tapes cannot be utilized on mucosal surfaces or over hairy and oily skin.

INDICATIONS FOR ADHESIVE TAPES

Adhesive tapes are multifunctional as they can be used as a closure device, as reinforcement after suture closure, and as a postoperative adjunct that lends support to the healing wound and simultaneously reduces tension on the suture line. Because of their tendency to easily dislodge, adhesive tapes are often used in conjunction with an adhesive adjunct such as tincture of benzoin or Mastisol.[6] Because these adjuncts are toxic to the wound, care should be taken to avoid their entering the wound.

Adhesive tapes were designed to be used under many circumstances, from closing a superficial laceration to closing wounds after intracuticular closure. Tapes are highly functional and are among the least expensive and most cost-effective closure devices in use today.[7,8] A survey of the surgical tape marketplace in 2002 demonstrated that there were a dozen types of paper, plastic, silk, elastic, cloth, and waterproof tapes.[9] Thus, the clinician has a wide range from which to choose based mostly on personal preference.

A study evaluated nonwoven microporous tapes, a nonwoven microporous reinforced tape, a gauze tape, and a polyurethane tape.[10,11] This study assessed their breaking strength, degree of elongation under pressure, adhesion to the skin, air and vapor transmission, and bacterial growth under the tape. The investigators concluded that the nonwoven microporous tape (unnamed in the study) performed the best because of an adhesive that aggressively adhered to the underlying skin, resisted breakage during clinical use, and elongated enough to prevent the formation of blisters. It was also found that its microporous structure permits rapid air transmission in vitro and results in an environment that prevents bacterial growth.[11,12]

COMPLICATIONS AND POTENTIAL ADVERSE EFFECTS

All closure methods have both positives and negatives or drawbacks. Many of today's tapes are hypoallergenic, breathable, and latex-free, which helps to prevent some of the negative sequelae such as contact dermatitis. The astute clinician will note dermatitis if they see the cardinal signs of edema, erythema, blisters, pustules, or exudates. One study included 100 patients treated with an adhesive tape who were monitored for cutaneous reactions.[12] Twelve patients were diagnosed with irritant (mechanical) dermatitis, one with allergic contact dermatitis from tincture of benzoin, and one demonstrated a positive patch test to thiuram mix, rubber accelerators formerly present in adhesive tapes. Thus, local irritation from the adhesive tapes is a major disadvantage with their use, and a history of prior reactions to adhesive tapes should be obtained before using tape. The formation of blisters is often thought to be the consequence of a shearing force on the skin's surface that separates the epidermis from the underlying dermis.

ADVANTAGES AND DISADVANTAGES

Perhaps one of the greatest advantages of tape compared with sutures and staples is that tapes are noninvasive and create no fistulous track for the promotion and spread of bacteria through a wound.[8,10,13] Multiple studies comparing tapes and sutures have found that the adhesive tapes are very safe to use and have low rates of infection.[12,14,15] The learning curve for tape application is also easier than that for other wound closure modalities. Cross-hatch marks, common sequelae of wounds under tension or sutures left in place beyond the recommended time, are literally impossible after tape application. Not unlike with skin adhesives, there is no anesthesia required for a superficial laceration that requires no other suture closure. There is also no need to purchase additional disposable trays for the removal of tapes and there is no threat to the health care provider who removes the tapes. Tape closure allows for an even distribution of tension over the entire wound and then a parallel layer locks the first layer of tapes.

Avulsions of the thin onionlike skin or parchment-type skin on elderly patients (or those patients on long-term corticosteroids) present a particularly difficult problem for the clinician. The skin over the bony prominences of some of these patients cannot be sutured because of the quality of epidermis and the lack of dermis. Application of adhesive tapes to the adjacent proximal and distal aspects of the avulsed skin followed by 4-0 nylon through the adhesive tape permits the proper tension and allows proper healing time to facilitate a closure (Figure 10-1). The use of antimicrobial strips to reduce the risk of infection may be particularly useful in these patients who are often

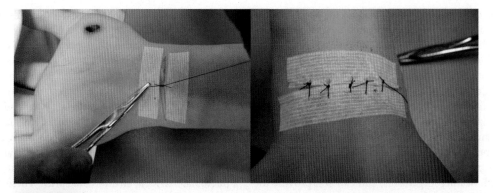

FIGURE 10-1

Closing parchmentlike fragile skin with tapes and sutures. Strips of adhesive tape are placed on either side of the wound and sutures are then passed through the skin and overlying tape to prevent tearing of the skin.

immunocompromised because of the steroids or poor organ perfusion.

COMPARISON WITH TOPICAL SKIN ADHESIVES

Great debate exists between advocates of adhesive tape closure and tissue adhesives. Patients want good cosmetic results but also desire to return to almost full activity without the need of additional office visits for suture and staple removal.[16] Adhesive tapes help to bring about a meticulous apposition of the surgical wound edges, and create a flat wound without step-off. They improve efficiency and may reduce hypertrophic scarring and infection—particularly when a prosthetic device is being inserted into the body.[17] A study in the Royal Hospital for Sick Children in the United Kingdom came to the conclusion that both tissue adhesives and adhesive strips are excellent "no needle" alternatives for the closure of appropriate low-tension lacerations in children and both techniques are equal in efficacy, parental acceptability, and cosmetic outcome. The choice in this study was reduced to economics and operator preference.[18] Another study conducted at a children's hospital compared the cosmetic outcomes of simple, low-tension facial lacerations closed with tape or a topical skin adhesive and concluded that the outcomes were similar. They added that closure of the wounds with adhesive tape may represent a low-cost alternative in this type of wound.[19] Some clinicians will argue that the potential time required for closure of a long wound with topical skin adhesives is somewhat prohibitive as is the potential for irritation of internal tissues and the inability to readjust the apposition of the closure once the wound

is dry.[16] In defense of topical skin adhesives, other clinicians have been comfortable with the tissue adhesive technique and have commented that it speeds up the closure process. Wound closure may be a significant portion of a procedure and time saving reduces anesthesia and decreases operating room costs.[16,20] In some cases use of topical skin adhesive is discretional; in others the adhesive is preferred because of the location of the wound (e.g., groin). One can use an adhesive in moist areas of the body such as after a thigh lift and the patient can shower immediately whereas this is not possible with the adhesive tapes. In many cases where tape or adhesives are used, meticulous subcutaneous or deep dermal closure is necessary. This suggests that, in many cases, setting up the deep closure properly can produce an equally good effect utilizing either technique.[16,17]

COMPARISON OF ADHESIVE TAPES TO THE "GOLD STANDARD"

There is no question that sutures can close dead spaces, set up the deeper layers of closure such as fascia, and remove tension from the wound edges, which remains the largest reason for wound dehiscence and for hypertrophic scarring.[1,15] When used appropriately, sutures set up wound edges and offer many techniques that can remove excessive tension such as mattress sutures and and half-buried sutures that are capable of bringing points of wounds together providing superb safety and excellent cosmesis. A half-buried mattress is the personal favorite of many plastic surgeons who place the starting suture in a pigmented area such as the areola and suture to the dermis on the other side, returning to the pigmented area. This technique has only one entry and exit point. Perhaps there needs to be the thought process of a "marriage" between both methods of closure.

Certainly, it has been proven that a running subcuticular or intracuticular closure with either absorbable or nonabsorbable sutures creates a clean line and good strength until the suture absorbs or is pulled out.[17] The addition of an antimicrobial-impregnated tape seals the wound, prevents the growth of microorganisms, and can still provide the patient with the ability to shower 2 days postoperatively. The tapes then are adding to the support of the wound and can be easily removed to perform a wound check and reapplied to add strength to the wound closure. This has been proven in studies utilizing staples and adhesive tapes. There was a final outcome of greater inflammatory reaction in wounds where the staples were in place for 7 days versus staple removal at 3 days with application of adhesive tapes, which demonstrated far less inflammation and better results. The long-term follow-up demonstrated no puncture marks on the side of wounds where tapes were applied early in the healing process.

A randomized, controlled trial comparing the long-term cosmetic outcomes of traumatic pediatric lacerations repaired with absorbable plain gut versus nonabsorbable nylon sutures[15] supports the assertion that an adhesive closure tape combined with a suture that would self-dissolve within 3 days is superior to a nonabsorbable suture such as nylon.[20] This technique seems to be acceptable in clean wounds where the chance of infection is low and the need for critically accurate wound levels is essential to the overall cosmetic result. Once again, the adhesive closures need to be removed accurately and reapplied for additional wound support for another 5 days.

ADJUNCT INNOVATIONS UTILIZING ADHESIVE TAPES AND VARIOUS NEW SYSTEMS

3M Health Care (St. Paul, MN) has created a wound closure system that provides the cosmetic benefits of tape with the added barrier protection of a polyurethane foam dressing to provide a package with all of the sterile essentials. This innovation has its place in laparoscopic procedures performed in an operating room as the port sites are between 5 mm and 15 mm in length and usually require 1 or 2 deep sutures to

prevent herniation and then 1 or 2 external sutures, staples, or a subcuticular closure. This new system provides the clinician with a precut adhesive tape and a transparent dressing that allows for showering while resisting infection. Long-term prepping agents provide an extended antimicrobial barrier and this presents the surgical team with a faster and safer closure method than traditional sutures. This is also a great adjunct in the acute care setting as many of our closures are less than 2 cm and these strips and the transparent dressing allow for good apposition and a microbial barrier at an affordable price. These dressings may be worn for up to 7 days without requiring a change and then can be resupported for an additional 5 days by the application of another strip. The limitations of this system are areas of high moisture, hairy areas, and areas exposed to constant drainage such as the lip.

Steri-Strip S Surgical Skin Closure (3M Health Care, St. Paul, MN) is another of the enhancements made to this family of products. This system allows for quick closure of skin lacerations or incisions with good cosmetic results. The unique, interlaced design facilitates alignment of skin edges, disperses tension more evenly over the wound and provides both the clinician and the patient with a sense of security (Figure 10-2). Unlike all of the other adhesive tape devices, S Surgical

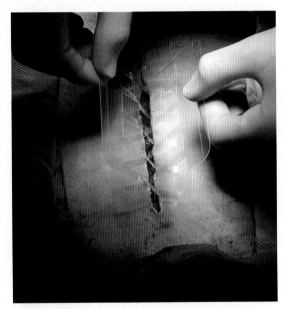

FIGURE 10-2

Steri-Strip S Surgical Skin Closure: The interlacing strips are placed on either side of the wound and pulled together across the wound to approximate the wound edges.

Skin Closures are part of a system that requires some minimal instruction and a "hands-on" experience to facilitate a smooth and correct application. These tapes will stay in place for 2 weeks or longer even after showering. The area of the laceration or incision needs no adjunctive care and can be readily observed with the clear filament strips intact. This system has application in emergency departments, acute care clinics, surgicenters, and operating rooms. Utilization of this device is for low-tension lacerations or incisions, an adjunct to suture closures in higher tension wounds, and, like all adhesive tapes, for reinforcement of a wound after early suture or staple removal. This new product has been marketed to the dermatological services because of the lack of deep invasion in their usual excisions and the smaller wound surfaces.[21] A small pilot study in the operating room supports the efficacy of this product.

Elastic and Blend adhesive closures (3M Health Care, St. Paul, MN) are also newcomers on the block and are considered to be a 21st century continued improvement over all tapes of the past. Obviously, aesthetics are important to many of our patients and a tape that considers normal flesh tones causes assimilation of the normal characteristics of the skin. These tapes are less obvious and are not likened to "a stamp on an envelope." Integration of a tape or dressing into a patient's lifestyle is considered a positive innovation to both patient and clinician. When one is considering lifestyle, it is important to realize that function is one of the main considerations when repairing a wound. Lacerations are the result of accidents and, therefore, we cannot preplan the location or direction of the wound. Elastic closure strips have entered the market and offer the clinician a tape that can be used over the joints of fingers, elbows, knees, and the shoulder. These tapes "stretch" with the flexion and extension of the extremity, allowing a more versatile closure and reducing the shearing of skin that can sometimes occur because of incorrect application of tapes. This newcomer is slowly becoming known to both orthopedic and podiatric surgeons and their use will likely increase in these specialty groups who deal with high-tension wounds over the extremities.

COST OF ADHESIVE TAPE CLOSURES VERSUS SUTURES AND TOPICAL SKIN ADHESIVES

A recent study that included 28 articles attempted to compare the cost of tapes, sutures, and topical adhe-

sives. In this study the investigators used a health economic model to estimate variables such as dehiscence, infection, time, and cost of materials. This study found that for low-tension wounds, all three closure devices had approximately the same cosmetic outcome and that adhesive tapes were the lowest-cost option both in purchase price and when the rates of infection or dehiscence and application time were considered (see Table 10-1)

APPLICATION AND REMOVAL OF ADHESIVE TAPES

The approach to utilizing adhesive closure tapes or strips requires the same judicious care of the wound to remove foreign bodies, properly cleanse and irrigate, and to utilize a sterile field in closure. The wound requires the same documentation and examination as a wound that is to be sutured or stapled. The wound is then prepped with the appropriate solution presently being utilized at the treating institution. It is important that the wound edges and an area 2 or 3 inches from the wound on both sides be dry. As in all closures, hemostasis must be achieved. There are numerous tapes that can be used in closure and some function better when an adjunct is used to enhance adhesiveness. Both tincture of benzoin and Mastisol are presently used for this purpose. Follow the instructions of these products for drying time as this creates the appropriate tackiness to facilitate a better adhesion of the strip to the wound and the surrounding area. An area is considered dry when it has become tacky. Tackiness is dependent on the amount of solution used. According to some, Mastisol is seven times more effective than tincture of benzoin.[6]

Tapes can be opened and cut to the size that is most appropriate for the wound. Gloves should be utilized for application but they need not be sterile.[22,23] The perforated backing is removed from the tapes and, with the practioner using forceps or gloved fingers, the tape is then removed. With the technique of "halving" or bisecting the wound as used in suture repair, the tape is applied to the skin on one side of the wound at the midpoint (Figure 10-3). The opposite side of the wound is then gently pushed toward the side with the tape to approximate the wound edges and the strip is applied in a fashion of "place and pat" (Figure 10-3). At no time should tension be placed on one side of the wound and used to pull the wound edges together. This improper technique causes friction and tension and ultimately can cause shearing of the epidermis on removal, which can result in blister formation and may leave a hyper- or hypopigmented

TABLE 10–1	Advantages and Disadvantages of Adhesive Tapes

Advantages	Disadvantages
Far less expensive than alternatives	Cannot be used on mucosa or hair
Short learning curve	Cannot be used on wet or oily skin
No risk to clinician from sharps	May require adjunct such as tincture of benzoin or Mastisol
No suture set required	Cannot close incisions requiring "deep sutures"
No local anesthesia required	Should never be placed circumferentially around a digit
No suture or staple removal	Requires hemostasis prior to application
Various new wound-specific tapes	Can be removed by noncompliant patient
Wound Closure System allowing showers Steri-Strips S Skin Closure Sytem 3M Healthcare, Minneapolis, MN	May cause shearing of epidermis and blister formation
No separate removal sterile trays	
Skin color blended	
Elastic for joints	
Does not compromise blood supply	
Rapid application	
Ability to cover with a polyurethane film, a common practice among clinicians	
Least compromising to host defenses	
Longest shelf life for emergency preparedness kits	

scar. With the use of "halfing" throughout the closure, tapes should be approximately 2 mm to 5 mm from each other. As an additional support and to prevent shearing or blistering, additional tapes can be placed at the end of each row of strips, parallel to the others (Figure 10-4). Depending on the type, length, and width of the wound, size selection should be at the discretion of the clinician. Strips come in different widths and it is reasonable to believe that an ophthalmologist would use a narrower width than an orthopedist.

Ongoing care and removal of the adhesive tapes is quite easy and can readily be done by other office or hospital personnel such as nurses and technicians.

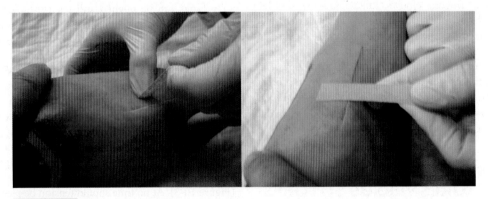

FIGURE 10-3

The first tape is placed across the center of the wound bisecting it into halves (upper). The wound edges are approximated by applying the tape to one side of the wound and "pushing" the other side toward the first (lower). Pulling of the tape and skin across the wound should not be performed to avoid shearing of the skin and subsequent blister formation.

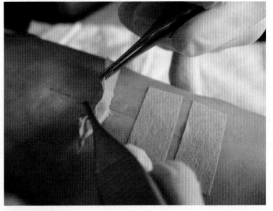

FIGURE 10-5

Removal of tape strips.

CONCLUSIONS

There have been studies of sutured and sutureless wounds, clinical comparisons of both, and studies that have focused on contaminated wounds as well as on specialty patients such as plastic surgery and pediatrics. There is ample evidence that supports use of tapes after removal of sutures and staples and we have seen studies and reports on the comparison of adhesives versus tapes. It is undisputed in this age of hepatitis and HIV infection that we need to be aware of the potential for contamination or injury to health care professionals that are involved in the closure of acute wounds and during surgical procedures. Evidence supports that there is no one perfect method of wound closure and that decisions related to closure are made based upon exposure, tradition, experience, location, and presence or absence of infection, as well as modalities such as cost. Evidence also supports that closure with wound tapes certainly has its place in our armamentarium and that it needs to be rediscovered by this new generation of physicians, physician assistants, nurse practitioners, and other providers of wound care. It is essential, as we look to the future, that we keep our eyes on the past and capture all the available methods that have proven the test of time.

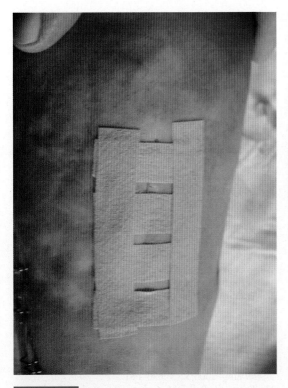

FIGURE 10-4

Further tape strips are then placed across the wounds with a distance of 2 mm to 3 mm between the strips to completely appose the wound edges. Additional tape strips are then placed parallel to the wound to reinforce the original tape strips to avoid their premature dislodgement.

A nice rule of thumb is that the tapes should remain at least as long as other accepted modalities such as suture.[13] In most cases the strips are removed as they begin to lift from the skin. If there is premature lifting at the edges, this can be cut carefully with a scissor to prevent early removal. The strip should remain dry initially and no antibiotic ointments should be applied to it. If the patient desires to shower the injured area, a plastic wrap can be applied to make the area watertight or a polyurethane dressing may be applied at the time of closure. Removal should proceed in an orderly manner, gently lifting one side until it is adjacent to the laceration and then doing likewise on the other. A gentle upward removal in the direction of the wound is then utilized, which will prevent the wound margins from being traumatized (Figure 10-5). A second set of adhesive strips can be applied for an additional week to further support the wound. Gentle cleansing of the area with alcohol or an antibacterial soap can facilitate preparation and the area should then be completely dry prior to reapplication.

REFERENCES

1. Quinn JV. *Tissue Adhesives in Wound Care*. ED1. Hamilton, Ontario: BC Decker Inc; 1998.
2. Sipos P, Győry H, Hagymási K, Ondrejka P, Blázovics A. Special wound healing methods used in ancient Egypt and in the mythological background. *World J Surg*. 2004;28(2):211–216.

3. Majno G. *The Healing Hand. Man and Wound in the Ancient World.* Cambridge, MA: Harvard University Press; 1975.

4. Van Gulik TM. The dry suture, forerunner of surgical adhesive tape. *Neth J Surg.* 1988;40(2): 55–56.

5. Edlich, Rodehover, Thacker, Edgarton. *A Manual for Wound Closure.* 2nd ed. Minnesota Mining and Manufacturing Company, St. Paul, MN: 1980.

6. Mikhail GR, Selak L, Salo S. Reinforcement of surgical adhesive strips. *J Dermatol Surg Oncol.* 1986; 12(9):904–905, 908.

7. Liew SW, Haw CS. The use of taped skin closure in orthopedic wounds. *Aust N Z J Surg.* 1993;63(2): 131–133.

8. Pepicello J, Yavorek H. Five year experience with tape closure of abdominal wounds. *Surg Gynecol Obstet.* 1989;169(4):310–314.

9. Surgical tape (Market Choices). *RN.* June 2002. Available at: http://www.findarticles.com/cf_O/M3235/6_65/87469046/print.jhtml. Accessed July 2009.

10. Rodehaver GT, McLane M, West L, Edlich RF. Evaluation of surgical tapes for wound closures. *J Surg Res.* 1985;39(3):251–257.

11. Hirshman HP, Schurman DJ, Kajiyama G. Penetration of Staphylococcus aureus into sutured wounds. *J Orthop Res.* 1984;2(3):269–271.

12. Marks JG Jr, Rainey MA. Cutaneous reactions to surgical preparations and dressings. *Contact Dermatitis.* 1984;10(1):1–5.

13. Singer AJ, "Chapter 7, Adhesive Tapes," in Singer AJ, Hollander JE. *Lacerations and Acute Wounds, An Evidence Based Guide.* Philadelphia, PA: FA Davis Co; 2003;7:64–71.

14. Edlich RF, et al. Technique of closure: contaminated wounds. *JACEP.* 1974;3:375–381.

15. Conolly BW, Hunt TK, Zederfeldt B, Cafferata TH, Dunphy JE. Clinical comparison of surgical wounds closed by sutures and adhesive tapes. *Am J Surg.* 1969;17(3):318–322.

16. Lenanski MJ. Achieving closure. *Cosmetic Surgery Times.* July 2007.

17. Karounis H, Gouin S, Eisman H, Chalut D, Pelletier H, Williams B. A randomized, controlled trial comparing long-term cosmetic outcomes of traumatic pediatric lacerations repaired with absorbable plain gut versus nonabsorbable nylon sutures. *Acad Emerg Med.* 2004;11(7):730–735.

18. Coulthard P, Worthington H, Esposito M, Waes OJ. Tissue adhesives for closure of surgical incisions. *Cochrane Database Syst Rev.* 2004;(2):CD004287.

19. Zempsky WT, Parrotti D, Grem C, Nichols J. Randomized controlled comparison of cosmetic outcomes of simple facial lacerations closed with Steri Strip Skin Closures or Dermabond tissue adhesive. *Pediatr Emerg Care.* 2004;20(8):519–524.

20. Farion K, Osmond MH, Hartling L, et al. Tissue adhesives for traumatic lacerations in children and adults. *Cochran Database Syst Rev.* 2002;(3):CD003326.

21. Traub AC, Quattlebaum FW. Cutaneous wound closure: early staple removal and replacement by skin tapes. *Contemp Surg.* 1981;18:93–101.

22. Kuo F, Lee D, Rogers GS. Prospective, randomized, blinded study of a new wound closure film versus cutaneous suture for surgical wound closure. *Dermatol Surg.* 2006;32(5):676–681.

23. Tokars JI, Bell DM, Culver DH, et al. Percutaneous injuries during surgical procedures. *JAMA.* 1992; 267(21):2899–2904.

24. Henry K, Campbell S. Needlestick/sharps injuries and HIV exposure among health care workers. National estimates based on survey of US hospitals. *Minn Med.* 1995;78(11):41–44.

25. *3M Steri Strip Adhesive Skin Closures, Second Edition, 3 M Medical Division, Minnesota Mining and Manufacturing Company, 1980:* St. Paul, MN: 8–10.

CHAPTER 11

Surgical Staples

Adam J. Singer, MD, and Mary Jo McBride, PA

The first stapler dates back to 18th century France. It is believed that the first stapling devices were made for King Louis XV of France and that each staple was inscribed with the royal court insignia. The first surgical stapler was invented by Victor Fischer, who was a well-known designer of surgical devices.[1] The first surgical staple was designed at the request of the Hungarian surgeon Humer Hultl who requested Fischer to design a "mechanical stitching device, which would shorten the duration of an operation as much as possible. . .". This stapling device was completed in 1908 and first used clinically in 1909. Since then, many different stapling devices have been invented. However, the modern surgical stapling devices are derivatives of inventers from the Soviet Union in the 1950s. The use of "biological" staples has been attributed to the ancient Hindu civilization where insect mandibles were used to approximate wounds.[2]

The major advantage of the stapler over sutures is the speed in which wounds can be closed. Staples are also less irritating to wounds than sutures. However, the use of staples is mostly limited to linear lacerations and incisions because it does not allow fine adjustment of the wound edges.

CLINICAL EVIDENCE

Within the emergency department, stapling has been studied mostly for the closure of scalp lacerations. Khan et al. conducted a randomized trial comparing the cosmetic outcome of pediatric scalp lacerations closed with staples or sutures in 42 children.[3] Procedure time was significantly shorter in the stapling group (P=.001) and the mean visual analog cosmetic scores at 12 months (+/–4 months) were 96.3 (+/–8.1) for the suturing group and 97.0 (+/–7.0) for the stapling group (P=.17). Kanegaye et al. conducted a similar study in 88 children with scalp lacerations and found that stapling was twice as fast as sutures and 40% cheaper with similar short-term outcomes.[4] Two systematic reviews of pediatric and adult scalp lacerations also concluded that stapling is faster and cheaper than sutures yet is as effective.[5,6] Another noncomparative study evaluated the use of stapling in 76 emergency department (ED) patients with 87 lacerations of the scalp, trunk, and extremities. In the authors' experience, stapling was faster and less expensive than suturing.[7]

In the context of the operating room, several studies have compared incision closure with staples and sutures. Eldrup et al. conducted a randomized trial comparing suturing and stapling in 137 patients with elective abdominal and breast surgery.[8] The median duration of wound closure with the stapler was 80 seconds versus a median of 242 seconds with suturing. Although infection rates were similar, postoperative pain was more common after stapling. Another study of 48 patients undergoing laparotomy randomized patients to closure with skin staples or subcuticular sutures.[9] In this study the mean time saved by stapling was 77 seconds. However, wound pain and requirements for analgesia were significantly lower in the sutured group. A study of 162 patients undergoing coronary artery bypass grafting compared subcuticular sutures and surgical clips for sternal and leg repair.[10] Closure with subcuticular sutures resulted in fewer wound infections and similar cosmetic outcomes compared with surgical clips.

A recent addition to the armamentarium of wound closure devices has been the dermal stapler that introduces absorbable staples within the dermis.[11] A clinical trial of 11 patients with bilateral breast reconstruction randomized one side to be closed with dermal absorbable sutures while the other side was closed with dermal absorbable staples. Wound closure was significantly faster with the stapling device and early (1-month) but not late (6-month) cosmetic outcome was improved.

Staples have also been evaluated for securing central venous catheters. A randomized trial compared sutures and staples in human cadavers and found that a greater force was needed to cause the catheter hub to break free from the skin when staples were used to secure the catheter on the chest versus when sutures were used.[12]

CHOOSING A STAPLING DEVICE

There are several commercially available stapling devices available to clinicians. A study conducted nearly 30 years ago compared the mechanical properties of three commercially available stapling devices (Proximate™, Ethicon Inc, Somerville, NJ; Premium™, US Surgical, Norwalk, CT; and Precise™, 3M Center, St. Paul, MN) and found that, of the three, the Premium stapler had the best handling characteristics.[13] Ultimately the choice of the stapler should be based on availability and clinician preference.

ADVANTAGES AND DISADVANTAGES OF STAPLES

The major advantage of staples is their speed and ability to shorten the time required to close the skin. Time savings is most significant for longer lacerations and incisions. Depending on the number of staples in the device and the length of the wound, staples are generally more cost-effective than sutures.[4,14] For example, a study of 141 patients randomized to closure with sutures or staples found that the cost of wound repair was less with staples ($7.84) than with sutures ($21.00).[14]

Another potential advantage of staples is their ability to evert the wound's edges, which may be associated with superior wound cosmesis compared with non-everted or inverted wound edges. This may be especially helpful in older patients with lax skin. However, there is little if any evidence to support this claim. Staples are also less reactive than sutures in non-contaminated skin incisions in a pig model.[15] When evaluated in a contaminated animal wound model, staples were also more resistant to abscess formation than were sutures.[16]

A major disadvantage of stapling is the difficulty in achieving a meticulous wound closure, especially with nonlinear or jagged wounds. Stapling may sometimes cause overlapping of the wound edges that may delay healing. Staple removal has also been shown to be more painful than suture removal.[17] Generally patients are less satisfied with staples than they are other wound closure devices. For example, a survey of 724 adults found that, if given a choice, only 3% would choose to have their wounds closed with staples.[18] Another study of patients undergoing hip and knee surgery found that there was a higher incidence of inflammation, discomfort on removal, and spreading of the healing scar associated with staples.[19] Staples are especially uncomfortable when used over uneven surfaces such as the groin. A retrospective review of 45 skin flap operations found that partial necrosis or delayed healing of the flap was more common in staples than in sutured wounds (62% vs 21%) possibly because of crimping of the skin edges by the staples resulting in tension across the flap.[20]

INDICATIONS AND CONTRAINDICATIONS

Staples are most appropriate for closing long, linear nonfacial surgical incisions and lacerations. They are commonly used to close scalp wounds; however, they should not be used alone when hemostasis is problematic and when there is a large tear in the galea aponeurotica that requires closure separately. Although there are no absolute contraindications (except for infected or heavily contaminated wounds) staples probably should not be used for irregular or stellate lacerations or for facial wounds.

STAPLING METHOD

Before pressing on the trigger of the stapler it is important for the practitioner to line up the wound edges with the center indicator of the stapler (Figure 11-1).

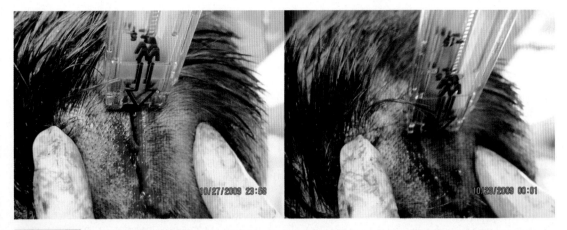

FIGURE 11-1

Alignment of stapling device: Proper alignment is shown with arrow indicator over the center of the wound (left). Improper alignment of stapling device is shown on the right.

In this way the arms of the staple enter the skin on both sides of the wound at the same distance from the wound edge. With long wounds the first staple should be placed in the center thus dividing the wound into several more manageable segments. If the staple is improperly placed, overlapping of the wound edges can occur. If overlapping occurs, the staple should be removed and replaced by a new staple (Figure 11-2). Stapling can sometimes be facilitated by having an assistant approximate and evert the wound edges with fine forceps. Excessive pressure on the skin should be avoided. After the practitioner places the staple, slight backward pulling on the stapler allows disengagement of the stapling instrument from the staple.

POSTOPERATIVE CARE FOR THE STAPLED WOUND

Staples may be covered with a topical antibiotic and a nonadherent dressing. The stapled wound should be cleaned daily with warm water and soap. Particular care should be taken when one is combing or brushing the hair in the area of a stapled scalp laceration to avoid premature dislodgement. Timing of staple removal parallels that for sutured wounds (see Chapter 23).

The staples are removed with a specialized staple remover. The bottom double prongs are gently inserted between the staple and the skin (Figure 11-3). The lever of the staple remover is then slowly depressed to slowly lower the single prong. This results in

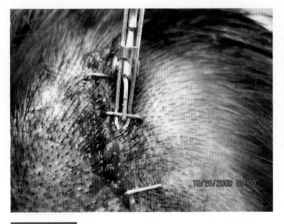

FIGURE 11-2

Improper alignment of the stapling device may result in overlapping of wound edges noted in the bottom two staples. The upper staple is properly placed. If improperly placed, the staple should be removed as demonstrated.

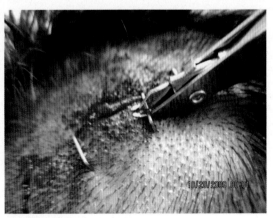

FIGURE 11-3

Removing a staple by placing the lower two limbs of the staple remover between the horizontal portion of the staple and the underlying skin is shown.

bending of the arms of the staple and its removal from the skin. After removal, the staples should be discarded using a sharp instrument container.

REFERENCES

1. Robicsek F. Development of the surgical stapling device. *Thorac Cardiovasc Surg.* 1993;41(4):207–215.
2. Chamas PJ, Cragel MD. The use of skin stapling in podiatric surgery: a review and update. *J Foot Ankle Surg.* 1993;32(5):536–538.
3. Khan AN, Dayan PS, Miller S, Rosen M, Rubin DH. Cosmetic outcome of scalp wound closure with staples in pediatric emergency department: a prospective randomized trial. *Pediatr Emerg Care.* 2002; 18(3):171–173.
4. Kanegaye JT, Vance CW, Chan L, Schonfeld N. Comparison of skin stapling devices and standard sutures for pediatric scalp lacerations: a randomized study of cost and time benefits. *J Pediatr.* 1997;130(5):808–813.
5. Hogg K, Carley S. Towards evidence based emergency medicine: best BETs from the Manchester Royal Infirmary. Staples or sutures in children with scalp lacerations. *Emerg Med J.* 2002;19(4):328–329.
6. Hogg K. Towards evidence based emergency medicine: best BETs from the Manchester Royal Infirmary. Staples or sutures for repair of scalp lacerations in adults. *Emerg Med J.* 2002;19(4):327–328.
7. Brickman KR, Lambert RW. Evaluation of skin stapling for wound closure in the emergency department. *Ann Emerg Med.* 1989;18(10):1122–1125.
8. Eldrup J, Wied U, Andersen B. Randomised trial comparing Proximate stapler with conventional skin closure. *Acta Chir Scand.* 1981;147(7);501–502.
9. Ranaboldo CJ, Rowe-Jones DC. Closure of laparotomy wounds: skin staples versus sutures. *Br J Surg.* 1992;79(11):1172–1173.
10. Chughtai T, Chen LQ, Salasidis G, Nguyen D, Tchervenkov C, Morin JF. Clips versus suture technique: is there a difference? *Can J Cardiol.* 2000; 16(11):1403–1407.
11. Cross KJ, Teo EH, Wong SL, et al. The absorbable dermal staple device: a faster, more cost-effective method for incisional closure. 2009;124(1):156–162.
12. Hightower D, March J, Ausband S, Brown LH. Comparison of staples vs suturing for securing central venous catheters. *Acad Emerg Med.* 1996;3(12); 1103–1105.
13. Johnson A, Rodeheaver GT, Durand LS, Edgerton MT, Edlich RF. Automatic disposable stapling devices for wound closure. *Ann Emerg Med.* 1981; 10(12):631–635.
14. Orlinsky M, Goldberg RM, Chan L, Puertos A, Slajer HL. Cost analysis of stapling versus suturing for skin closure. 1995;13(1):77–81.
15. Roth JH, Windle BH. Staple versus suture closure of skin incisions in a pig model. *Can J Surg.* 1988;31(1): 19–20.
16. Stillman AM, Marino CA, Seligman SJ. Skin staples in potentially contaminated wounds. *Arch Surg.* 1984;119(7):821–822.
17. George TK, Simpson DC. Skin wound closure with staples in the accident and emergency department. *J R Coll Surg Edinb.* 1985;30(1):54–56.
18. Singer AJ, Mack C, Thode HC Jr, Hemachandra S, Shofer FS, Hollander JE. Patient priorities with traumatic lacerations. *Am J Emerg Med.* 2000;18(6): 683–686.
19. Stockley I, Elson RA. Skin closure using staples and nylon sutures: a comparison of results. *Ann R Coll Surg Engl.* 1987;69(2):76–78.
20. Coupland RM. Sutures versus staples in skin flap operations. *Ann R Coll Surg Engl.* 1986;68(1):2–4.

Topical Skin Adhesives

Adam J. Singer, MD

A tissue adhesive is defined as a substance used to cause adherence of one tissue to another tissue or a biological tissue to nontissue surfaces, such as prostheses. A topical skin adhesive (TSA) is an adhesive or glue used to close wounds in the skin, as an alternative to sutures, staples, or adhesive tapes. Currently, only the cyanoacrylates are strong enough to function as a TSA. None of the currently available TSAs are biodegradable and their use is limited to topical use as a bridge to hold the apposed wound edges together. Biodegradable cyanoacrylates for internal use (e.g., to reinforce blood vessel anastomoses) are currently under investigation.[1]

The cyanoacrylates were first developed by a chemist, Ardis, in 1949.[2] The first clinical report in which a cyanoacrylate was used for skin closure was by Coover et al. in 1959.[3] The initial short-chain cyanoacrylates were found to have histocytoxicity, especially when implanted in pharmacological doses in the retroperitoneum of rabbits.[4] However, with topical use, there is little if any systemic absorption. Furthermore, later, longer-chain cyanoacrylates were not found to have the same degree of tissue toxicity.[5] The first cyanoacrylates that were widely used were the butylcyanoacrylates. However, because of their relatively low strength and brittle nature, their use was limited mostly to simple, short, low-tension lacerations and surgical incisions.

With the development of the longer-chain octylcyanoacrylate, which is stronger and more flexible than the butylcyanoacrylates, the use of topical skin adhesives greatly expanded. In fact, with octylcyanoacrylate, there are no length or body location limitations as long as the tension on the wound is low or relieved with tension-relieving deep dermal sutures. Most recently, several blends of butyl- and octylcyanoacrylate have become commercially available. However, data concerning their use are limited.

THE CHEMISTRY AND STRUCTURE OF THE CYANOACRYLATE ADHESIVES

The cyanoacrylates are formed from the condensation of cyanoacetate and formaldehyde.[4] The resulting cyanoacrylic ester polymer is then broken down to single monomers. Additional substances, such as stabilizers and plasticizers may then be added to enhance the clinical characteristics of the adhesives. The cyanoacrylate monomers are marketed in a liquid form. On contact with the moist wound or blood they polymerize forming long chains or polymers consisting of several hundred molecules that are plasticlike materials strong enough to hold the wound edges together. The polymerization process is exothermic and therefore is associated with the release of varying degrees of

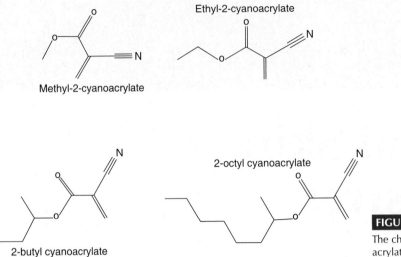

FIGURE 12-1

The chemical structure of the cyanoacrylate topical skin adhesives.

heat. The various cyanoacrylates share a similar basic structure but differ in terms of the length or number of carbons in the side chain (Figure 12-1). As the side chain becomes longer, the adhesive becomes stronger and more flexible.

CLINICAL STUDIES SUPPORTING THE USE OF THE CYANOACRYLATE TOPICAL SKIN ADHESIVES

Butylcyanoacrylate

One of the largest and earliest series concerning the use of TSA for wound closure was reported by Mizrahi et al.[6] In this retrospective study, more than 1500 traumatic pediatric lacerations were closed with a butylcyanoacrylate (Histoacryl Blue) with very low rates of infection (n=28) and dehiscences (n=10).[6] Similar studies were also reported for surgical incisions in the operating room setting including general surgery, ophthalmology, dentistry, and plastic surgery.[7–12] The first prospective randomized trial comparing sutures with a butylcyanoacrylate TSA was reported by Quinn et al. in 81 children with facial lacerations.[13] The TSA (Histoacryl Blue) was found to be faster and less painful than sutures and the cosmetic outcome was comparable to that with sutures.[13] The use of other butylcyanoacrylates, such as Indermil, has also been reported.[14–15]

Octylcyanoacrylate

In 1997, Quinn et al. reported the first randomized controlled trial comparing an octylcyanoacrylate (Dermabond) and sutures in 136 emergency department (ED) patients with traumatic lacerations.[16] He found that laceration repair with octylcyanoacrylate was faster and less painful than with sutures and that infection and dehiscence rates were similar. Both the 3-month[16] and 1-year[17] cosmetic outcomes were also similar between groups. The largest trial to date was a multicenter randomized controlled trial that included more than 800 patients and 900 wounds (lacerations and surgical incisions) closed in the ED and the operating room.[18] Patients were randomized to octylcyanoacrylate (Dermabond) or the standard closure device (mostly sutures). Closure with the TSA was faster than with sutures and the rates of dehiscence and infection were similar. Importantly, the percentage of patients with an optimal scar 3 months later was similar in both groups. These findings have been echoed in multiple similar clinical studies conducted in the following fields: neurosurgery, general surgery, plastic surgery, cardiothoracic surgery, obstetrics and gynecology, orthopedics, interventional radiology, otolaryngology, ophthalmology, pediatric surgery, and urology.[19–26] Octylcyanoacrylate has also been used successfully to close skin tears in the elderly.[27]

There have also been two systematic reviews performed by the Cochrane Collaboration groups for surgical incisions[28] and traumatic lacerations.[29] For surgical incisions, there were no significant differences for dehiscences, infection, and patient satisfaction with the cosmetic results between sutured and glued wounds.[28] However, based on the assessments of the surgeon, the glued wounds had a better cosmetic result. With regard to lacerations, a similar review found that glued and sutured lacerations had similar cosmetic outcomes and infection rates.[29] However, glue was associated with less pain and shorter closure times than sutures but was also associated with a slight increase in the rate of wound dehiscence (number needed to harm=25; 95% confidence interval=14 to 100),[29] emphasizing the need to limit the use of TSA to low-tension wounds.

Whereas most studies using a butylcyanoacrylate have been limited to short (<4 cm to 8 cm) wounds, studies with the octylcyanoacrylate (Dermabond) have not been limited to short wounds only. A study by Blondeel et al. specifically compared outcomes of 219 long surgical incisions (mean length = 16 cm; range = 4 cm to 69 cm) closed with high-viscosity Dermabond versus other commercially available devices.[30] In this study, cosmetic outcome and dehiscence rates were similar; however, infection rates were lower for the TSA. Because of small sample size, the difference in infection rates was not statistically different (3% vs 7%; P=.10).[30] Several larger subsequent studies have demonstrated lower infection rates after closure of sternotomy incisions (2.1 vs 4.9%; P<.001)[31] and body contouring incisions (0.9% vs 3.5%; P<.001).[32]

COMPARISON OF BUTYLCYANOACRYLATE AND OCTYLCYANOACRYLATE

Several animal studies have compared the wound bursting strength and flexibility of incisions closed with various butylcyanoacrylates, Dermabond, and Steri-Strips.[33–36] In all studies, the bursting strength of Dermabond was greater than that of any of the butylcyanoacrylates (including Indermil, Histoacryl Blue, and LiquiBand). Both the octylcyanoacrylates and the butylcyanoacrylates tested were stronger than Steri-Strips.[35] In one study, the flexibility and strength of Dermabond was stronger than that of the tested butylcyanoacrylates even after 48 hours of application.[36] As they are relatively brittle, the butylcyano-acrylates crack and form an irregular wound coating limiting their ability to function as a microbial barrier.[34] In contrast, the more flexible octylcyanoacrylate (Dermabond) creates a thick, uniform wound coating that allows it to continue to function as a microbial barrier for several days.

Few clinical studies have directly compared the various TSAs. A study by Osmond et al. compared outcomes of short, simple, low-tension facial lacerations in 94 children randomized to Histoacryl Blue or Dermabond.[37] In this highly select group of low-tension wounds, all outcomes (pain, duration of skin closure, infection, dehiscence, cosmesis) were similar between the two cyanoacrylates. In two subsequent studies, similar low-tension facial lacerations were closed with equally good results with either octyl-cyanoacrylate or Steri-Strips.[38,39] In contrast, Steiner and Mogilner compared the outcomes of lower abdominal and inguinal pediatric incisions closed with Histoacryl Blue or Dermabond and found significantly lower dehiscence rates in wounds closed with Dermabond (2.4% vs 9.4%; P<.01).[40]

ADVANTAGES OF TOPICAL SKIN ADHESIVES

All of the cyanoacrylate adhesives have several major advantages over other standard wound closure devices. Because they are noninvasive and do not cause pain on application, the TSA may be used without any anesthesia. Although this is not an issue in the operating room, in the ED or outpatient setting this is of major benefit, especially in children. Furthermore, gluing wounds is faster than suturing, especially with longer incisions and lacerations. As the cyanoacrylates slough off spontaneously within 5 to 10 days, there is no need to remove them. In addition to functioning as a secure wound closure device (Dermabond is equivalent to a running subcuticular 4-0 Monocryl suture),[41] the adhesives form a microbial barrier[42] and a moist wound healing environment that optimizes healing.[43,44] Although TSA applicators are more costly than sutures or staples, a formal cost analysis has demonstrated that TSAs are more cost-effective than other devices, because they eliminate the need for suture kits, suture removal kits, bandages, and topical agents.[45]

DISADVANTAGES OF TOPICAL SKIN ADHESIVES

When TSAs are used alone on high-tension wounds, there is an increased risk of wound dehiscence.[29] Because of limited moisture resistance, TSA may also slough off prematurely when subjected to recurrent and frequent scrubbing or soaking.[46] The use of TSAs has also been associated with foreign body reactions, allergic contact dermatitis, matting of the eyelashes, and even skin necrosis of the fingertip after application of Super Glue.[47–50] A summary of the indications and contraindications for using TSAs[51] are presented in Table 12-1.

OPTIMIZING THE USE OF TOPICAL SKIN ADHESIVES

As with any wound, a careful history and physical examination should be performed and wound prepa-

TABLE 12–1	Indications and Contraindications to Topical Skin Adhesives	

Indications	Contraindications
■ Easily approximated lacerations and incisions	■ Infection
■ Closure of flaps	■ Heavy contamination
■ Lacerated fragile skin	■ Mucosal surfaces
■ Attachment of grafts	■ Hair-bearing area
■ Nail bed repair	■ High-tension areas
■ Soft-tissue fingertip amputations	■ High-friction areas
	■ Allergy to cyanoacrylates, formaldehyde

ration should follow the principles discussed in greater detail elsewhere. The actual technique of gluing wounds is simple and straightforward; however, there are several potential pitfalls that can easily be avoided with proper use (Table 12-2). Several studies have demonstrated that mastery of TSA follows a rapid learning curve.[52,53] In contrast, attainment of adequate proficiency with suturing usually takes several years.[54]

Before one applies a TSA, it is essential to achieve adequate hemostasis. Hemostasis may require prolonged pressure or application of a topical vaso-constrictive agent such as epinephrine. A common mistake with the use of TSAs is application of too much glue. This should be avoided for several reasons.

First, when too much glue is applied it tends to run off risking spillage into critical areas such as the eyelashes. Second, polymerization of the cyanoacrylates is an exothermic reaction that releases heat. When a thick coat of glue is applied or when there is pooling of the adhesive this may result in a burning sensation. Because of their greater reactivity, butylcyanoacry-lates, in particular, should only be applied as a thin layer. Finally, when too much glue is applied, the gloves of the practitioner may adhere to the wound.

To avoid excessive application and runoff, only a thin layer of glue should be expressed and the wound should always be positioned in a horizontal plane. When glue is used above the eye, the patient should be

TABLE 12–2	Potential Pitfalls and Solutions With Application of Topical Skin Adhesives (TSAs)

Pitfall	Solution
Matting of eyelashes	Position wound horizontal
	Express small amount of adhesive
	Cover eyelashes with ointment and moist gauze
Getting the practitioner's gloves glued to the wound	Express small amount of adhesive
	If glue comes into contact with finger, remove hand from the wound edges while reinforcing wound closure with other hand prior to glue drying
Premature wound dehiscence	Only use TSA in easily approximated low-tension wound
	With high-tension wounds only use TSA after placement of deep dermal sutures and/or immobilization of the wound
Wound infection	Obtain extensive history for potential foreign body and high-risk wound
	Explore and prep wounds appropriately prior to closure
Poor wound edge apposition	Use surgical tape or assistant in hard-to-approximate wounds
	Consider applying traction on both ends of the wound to improve wound approximation
	Consider using deep sutures to approximate wound edges prior to TSA
	Avoid TSA if wound edges cannot be adequately approximated

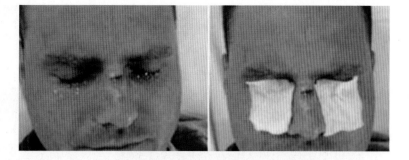

FIGURE 12-2
Avoiding runoff near the eyes: A topical ointment is applied to the eyelashes (left) and the eyes are covered with moist gauze (right).

placed in the Trendelenburg position. When the glue is used below the eye, the patient should be placed in the anti-Trendelenburg position. In addition, when one is working around the eyes, the eyelashes may be covered with an ointment (such as bacitracin) and moist gauze to avoid adherence of any stray glue (Figure 12-2). To avoid inadvertent seepage of the glue between the wound edges, complete apposition of the wound edges

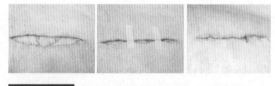

FIGURE 12-3
Use of adhesive tape to facilitate closure of long wound: The wound (left) is approximated with two adhesive tapes (middle) and then the topical adhesive is applied over the taped wound approximating its edges (right).

should be achieved prior to applying any TSA. With long or complex wounds, wound edge apposition may be facilitated by placing several surgical tapes along the wound (Figure 12-3) or by having an assistant hold the wound edges together while the glue is applied and dries. At times, it is easier to appose the wound edges by applying lateral traction on the ends of the wound parallel to the wound itself (Figure 12-4).

When one is using a butylcyanoacrylate, the glue is applied as thin beads (Figure 12-5) or a single thin layer. When one is using the octylcyanoacrylate Dermabond, the glue is applied as a continuous thin layer, like applying paint with a brush (Figure 12-5). With some formulations, a second layer is applied after the first layer dries. To avoid separation of the wound edges, direct pressure of the applicator on the wound should be avoided. An example of a wound closed with Dermabond is presented in Figure 12-6.

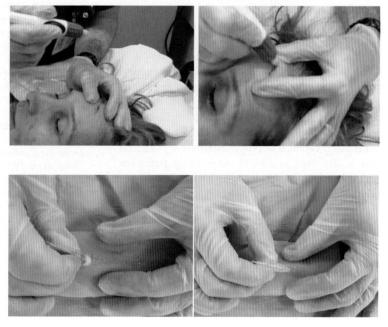

FIGURE 12-4
When apposition of the wound edges is suboptimal (left), lateral traction on both ends of the wound may result in improved wound edge approximation (right).

FIGURE 12-5
Application of topical skin adhesive: The octylcyanoacrylate (Dermabond, Ethicon Inc, Somerville, NJ) is painted on in a continuous manner (left). The butylcyanoacrylate (Indermil, Syneture, Norwalk, CT) is applied in discrete spots like welding (right).

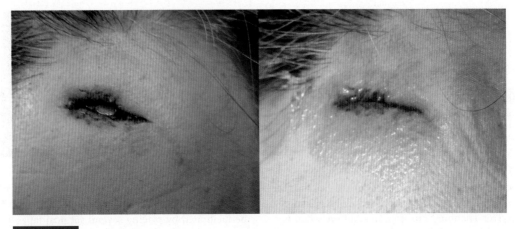

FIGURE 12-6

Forehead laceration closed with octylcyanoacrylate: before (left) and after (right) closure.

AFTERCARE OF WOUNDS CLOSED WITH TOPICAL SKIN ADHESIVES

When wounds are closed with a TSA, no additional dressings are required. However, some patients prefer covering their glued wounds. In this case, care should be taken to apply a nonadhesive dressing (such as Telfa) only after the glue is completely dry. With small wounds, a regular adhesive bandage may be used; however, application of the adhesive strip over the glue should be avoided. Because the TSAs will slough off as the stratum corneum or outer layer of the skin renews itself, there is no need to remove them. With the butyl-cyanoacrylates, the wound should be kept dry for at least 48 hours. With the octylcyanoacrylates the patient may shower immediately after application. With all TSAs, scrubbing and soaking of the wound should be avoided. To avoid premature sloughing, patients should be instructed not to apply any topical ointments or creams. If the adhesives need to be removed for any reason, a topical ointment may be applied to hasten sloughing. The burn cream silver sulfadiazine contains isopropyl myristate, a plasticizer that is also used in several eye-makeup removers. Therefore, this agent may also be used to hasten removal of the cyanoacrylates.

REFERENCES

1. Lumsden AB, Heyman ER; Closure Medical Surgical Sealant Study Group. Prospective randomized study evaluating an absorbable cyanoacrylate for use in vascular reconstructions. *J Vasc Surg.* 2006;44(5): 1002–1009.
2. Ardis AE, inventor. US patents 2467926 and 2467927. 1949.
3. Coover HW, Joyner FB, Shearer NH, Wicker TH. Chemistry and performance of cyanoacrylate adhesives. *J Soc Plast Eng.* 1959;15:413–417.
4. Mattamal GJ. History and background. In: Quinn JV, ed. *Tissue Adhesives in Clinical Medicine.* 2nd ed. Hamilton, Ontario: BC Decker Inc; 2005:15–26.
5. Leonard E. The N-alkylalphacyanoacrylate tissue adhesives. *Ann NY Acad Sci.* 1968;146(1):203–213.
6. Mizrahi S, Bickel A, Ben-Layish E. Use of tissue adhesive in the repair of lacerations in children. *J Pediatr Surg.* 1988;23(4):312–313.
7. Dalvi A, Faria M, Pinto A. Non-suture closure of wound using cyanoacrylate. *J Postgrad Med.* 1986; 32(2):97–100.
8. Farouk R, Drew PJ, Qureshi AC, Roberts AC, Duthie GS, Monson JR. Preliminary experience with butyl-2-cyanoacrylate adhesive in tension-free inguinal hernia repair. *Br J Surg.* 1996;83(8): 1100.
9. Amiel GE, Sukhotnik I, Kawar B, Siplovich L. Use of N-butyl-2-cyanoacrylate in elective surgical incisions—longterm outcomes. *J Am Coll Surg.* 1999; 189(1):21–25.
10. Spitznas M, Lossagk H, Vogel M, Meyer-Schwickerath G. Retinal surgery using cyanoacrylate as a routine procedure. *Albrecht Von Graefes Arch Klin Exp Ophthalmol.* 1973;187(2):89–101.
11. Bhaskar SN, Frisch J. Use of cyanoacrylate adhesives in dentistry. *J Am Dent Assoc.* 1968;77(4):831–837.
12. Kamer FM, Joseph JH. Histoacryl. Its use in aesthetic facial plastic surgery. *Arch Otolaryngol Head Neck Surg.* 1989;115(2):193–197.
13. Quinn JV, Drzewiecki A, Li MM, et al. A randomized, controlled trial comparing a tissue adhesive with suturing in the repair of pediatric facial lacerations. *Ann Emerg Med.* 1993;22(7):1130–1135.
14. Schonauer F, Pereira J, La Rusca I, Harris J, Cullen K. Use of Indermil tissue adhesive for closure

of superficial skin lacerations in children. *Minerva Chir.* 2001;56(4):427–429.

15. Greenhill GA, O'Regan B. Incidence of hypertrophic and keloid scars after N-butyl 2-cyanoacrylate tissue adhesive had been used to close parotidectomy wounds: a prospective study of 100 consecutive patients. *Br J Oral Maxillofac Surg.* 2009;47(4):290–293.

16. Quinn J, Wells G, Sutcliffe T, et al. A randomized trial comparing octylcyanoacrylate tissue adhesive and sutures in the management of lacerations. *JAMA.* 1997;277(19):1527–1530.

17. Quinn J, Weels G, Sutcliffe T, et al. Tissue adhesive versus suture wound repair at 1 year: randomized clinical trial correlating early, 3-month and 1-year cosmetic outcome. *Ann Emerg Med.* 1998;32(6):645–649.

18. Singer AJ, Quinn JV, Clark RE, Hollander JE. Closure of lacerations and incisions with octylcyanoacrylate: a multi-center randomized clinical trial. *Surgery.* 2002;131(3):270–276.

19. Collin TW, Blyth K, Hodgkinson PD. Cleft lip repair without suture removal. *J Plast Reconstr Aesthet Surg.* 2009;62(9):1161–1165.

20. Nipshagen MD, Hage JJ, Beekman WH. Use of 2-octyl-cyanoacrylate skin adhesive (Dermabond) for wound closure following reduction mammaplasty: a prospective, randomized intervention study. *Plast Reconstr Surg.* 2008;122(1):10–18.

21. Hancock NJ, Samuel AW. Use of Dermabond tissue adhesive in hand surgery. *J Wound Care.* 2007;16(10):441–443.

22. Laccourreye O, Cauchois R, Sharkawy EL, et al. Octylcyanoacrylate (Dermabond) for skin closure at the time of head and neck surgery: a longitudinal prospective study [in French]. *Ann Chir.* 2005;130(10):624–630.

23. Pachulski R, Sabbour H, Gupta R, Adkins D, Mirza H, Cone J. Cardiac device wound closure with 2-octyl cyanoacrylate. *J Interv Cardiol.* 2005;18(3):185–187.

24. Sofer M, Greenstein A, Chen J, Nadu A, Kaver I, Matzkin H. Immediate closure of nephrostomy tube wounds using a tissue adhesive: a novel approach following percutaneous endourological procedures. *J Urol.* 2003;169(6):2034–2036.

25. Cho J, Harrop J, Veznadaroglu E, Andrews DW. Concomitant use of computer image guidance, linear or sigmoid incisions after minimal shave, and liquid wound dressing with 2-octyl cyanoacrylate for tumor craniotomy or craniectomy: analysis of 225 consecutive surgical cases with antecedent historical control at one institution. *Neurosurgery.* 2003;52(4):832–841.

26. Yam A, Tan SH, Tan AB. A novel method of rapid nail bed repair using 2-octyl cyanoacrylate (Dermabond). *Plast Reconstr Surg.* 2008;121(3):148e–149e.

27. Milne C, Corbett LQ. A new option in the treatment of skin tears for the institutionalized resident: formulated 2-octylcyanoacrylate topical bandage. *Geriatr Nurs.* 2005;26(5):321–325.

28. Coulthard P, Worthington H, Esposito M, van der Elst M, van Waes OJ. Tissue adhesives for closure of surgical incisions. *Cochrane Database Syst Rev.* 2004;(2):CD004287.

29. Farion K, Osmond MH, Hartling L, et al. Tissue adhesives for traumatic lacerations in children and adults. *Cochrane Database Syst Rev.* 2001;(3):CD003326.

30. Blondeel PN, Murphy JW, Debrosse D, et al. Closure of long surgical incisions with a new formulation of 2-octylcyanpacrylate tissue adhesive versus commercially available methods. *Am J Surg.* 2004;188(3):307–313.

31. Souza E C, Fitaroni RB, Januzelli DM, Macruz HM, Camacho JC, Souza MR. Use of 2-octyl cyanoacrylate for skin closure of sternal incisions in cardiac surgery: observations of microbial barrier effects. *Curr Med Res Opin.* 2008;24(1):151–155.

32. Silvestri A, Brandi C, Grimaldi L, et al. Octyl-2-cyanoacrylate adhesive for skin closure and prevention of infection in plastic surgery. *Aesthetic Plast Surg.* 2006;30(6):695–699.

33. Perry LC. An evaluation of acute incisional strength with TraumaSeal surgical tissue adhesive wound closure. Leonia, NJ: Dimensional Analysis Systems Inc; 1995.

34. Singer AJ, Zimmerman T, Rooney J, Cameau P, Rudomen G, McClain SA. Comparison of wound bursting strength and surface characteristics of FDA approved tissue adhesives for skin closure. *J Adhesion Sci Technol.* 2004;18:19–27.

35. Taira BR, Singer AJ, Rooney J, Steinhauff NT, Zimmerman T. An in-vivo study of the wound-bursting strengths of octylcyanoacrylate, butyl-cyanoacrylate and surgical tape in rats. *J Emerg Med.* 2009; [Epub ahead of print].

36. Singer AJ, Perry LC, Allen RL Jr. In-vivo study of wound bursting strength and compliance of topical skin adhesives. *Acad Emerg Med.* 2008;15(12):1290–1294.

37. Osmond MH, Quinn JV, Sutcliffe T, Jarmuske M, Klassen TP. A randomized, clinical trial comparing butylcyanoacrylate with octylcyanoacrylate in the management of selected pediatric facial lacerations. *Acad Emerg Med.* 1999;6(3):171–177.

38. Mattick A, Clegg G, Beattie T, Ahmad T. A randomized, controlled trial comparing a tissue adhesive (2-octylcyanoacrylate) with adhesive strips (Steristrips) for paediatric laceration repair. *Emerg Med J.* 2002;19(5):405–407.

39. Zempsky WT, Parrotti D, Grem C, Nichols J. Randomized controlled comparison of cosmetic outcomes of simple facial lacerations closed with Steri Strip skin closures and Dermabond tissue adhesive. *Ped Emerg Care.* 2004;20(8):519–524.

40. Steiner Z, Mogilner J. Histoacryl vs Dermabond cyanoacrylate glue for closing small operative wounds [in Hebrew]. *Harefuah.* 2000;139(11–12):409–411, 496.

41. Shapiro AJ, Dinsmore RC, North JH Jr. Tensile strength of wound closure with cyanoacrylate glue. *Am Surg.* 2001;67(11):1113–1115.

42. Mertz PM, Davis SC, Cazzaniga AL, Drousou A, Eaglstein WH. Barrier and antibacterial properties of

2-octyl cyanoacrylate-derived wound treatment films. *J Cutan Med Surg.* 2003;7(1):1–6.

43. Winter GD. Formation of the scab and the rate of epithelisation of superficial wounds in the skin of the young domestic pig. *Nature.* 1962;193:293–294.

44. Hinman CD, Maibach H. Effect of air exposure and occlusion on experimental human skin wounds. *Nature.* 1963;200:377–378.

45. Osmond MH, Klassen TP, Quinn JV. Economic comparison of a tissue adhesive and suturing in the repair of pediatric facial lacerations. *J Pediatr.* 1995;126(6):892–895.

46. Carleo C, Singer AJ, Thode HC Jr. Effect of frequent water immersion on the rate of tissue adhesive sloughing: a randomized study. *CJEM.* 2005;7(6):391–395.

47. Edmonson MB. Foreign body reactions to Dermabond. *Am J Emerg Med.* 2001;19(3):240–241.

48. Hivnor CM, Hudkins ML. Allergic contact dermatitis after postsurgical repair with 2-octylcyanoacrylate. *Arch Dermatol.* 2008;144(6):814–815.

49. Rouvelas H, Saffra N, Rosen M. Inadvertent tarsorrhaphy secondary to Dermabond. *Pediatr Emerg Care.* 2000;16(5):346.

50. Wang AA, Martin CH. Full-thickness skin necrosis of the fingertip after application of superglue. *J Hand Surg Am.* 2003;28(4):696–698.

51. Singer AJ, Quinn JV, Hollander JE. The cyanoacrylate topical skin adhesives. *Am J Emerg Med.* 2008;26(4):490–496.

52. Hollander JE, Singer AJ. Application of tissue adhesives: rapid attainment of proficiency. Stony Brook Octylcyanoacrylate Study Group. *Acad Emerg Med.* 1998;5(10):1012–1017.

53. Lin M, Coates WC, Lewis RJ. Tissue adhesive skills study: the physician learning curve. *Pediatr Emerg Care.* 2004;20(4):219–223.

54. Singer AJ, Hollander JE, Valentine SM, Thode HC Jr, Henry MC. Association of training level and short-term cosmetic appearance of repaired lacerations. *Acad Emerg Med.* 1996;3(4):378–383.

Selecting Sutures and Needles for Wound Closure

Judd E. Hollander, MD, and Adam J. Singer, MD

There are several different techniques for performing a cosmetically appealing repair of lacerated or surgically incised tissue. In each individual situation, the optimal closure technique should be based upon consideration of the biological properties of the materials to be used, the anatomical configuration of the injury, and the biomechanical properties of the wound. This chapter will summarize the various suture materials and needles available for closure of traumatic lacerations and surgical incisions. The characteristics of particular suture materials are summarized in Tables 13-1 and 13-2.

CONSIDERATIONS IN SUTURE SELECTION

In general, the techniques of suture closure of skin can be divided into two types: percutaneous sutures and dermal (deep dermal or subcuticular) sutures. The choice of suture materials depends upon whether the wound closure occurs in one or more layers. The practitioner must take into account the number of layers of closure, amount of static and dynamic tension on the wound edges, depth of suture placement, anticipated amount of edema, and the anticipated timing of suture removal in selecting the most appropriate suture(s) for each particular wound.

Infection

All sutures potentially impair the local tissue defenses that prevent infection. Needle insertion itself causes a small inflammatory response. Sutures also penetrate the intact skin, thereby providing a means for bacteria to descend to the depth of the wound. The suture material serves as a nidus for bacterial colonization and biofilm formation. Bacterial biofilms consist of a complex micro-environment of single- or mixed-species bacteria attached to each other or attached to surfaces, being encased within extracellular polymeric substances.[1] The presence of a biofilm around the suture helps protect the bacteria from the innate immune system and exogenously administered antibiotics. Thus, the presence of the suture material within the wound increases the likelihood of infection. The likelihood of infection is related to both the amount of suture within the tissue and the particular suture material used. Additionally, sutures that are tied too tightly and strangulate tissue can impair host defenses, further increasing the risk of infection.[2]

TABLE 13–1	Nonabsorbable Suture Characteristics				
Suture	Structure	Raw Material	In-Vivo Tensile Strength Retention	Tissue Reactivity	Common Emergency Department Uses
Silk	Braided	Organic protein called fibroin	Degradation of fiber results in loss of strength over many months	Significant inflammatory reaction	Intraoral mucosal surfaces for comfort
Nylon (Ethilon, Dermalon)	Monofilament	Polyamide polymer	Hydrolysis results in loss of strength over years	Minimal	Soft tissue and skin reapproximation
Polypropylene (Prolene, Surgipro)	Monofilament	Polypropylene polymer	No degradation or weakening	Least	Soft tissue and skin reapproximation
Polyester (Mersilene, Ticron)	Braided and monofilament	Poly (ethylene terephthalate)	No degradation or weakening	Minimal	Tendon repair using undyed (white) color
Polybutester (Novafil)	Monofilament	Poly (butylene) and poly (tetramethylene ether) glycol terephthalate	No degradation or weakening	Minimal	Soft tissue approximation, easy handling, and knot security

TABLE 13-2	Absorbable Suture Characteristics					
Suture	Types	Material	In-Vivo Tensile Strength Retention	Absorption Rate	Tissue Reactivity	Common Emergency Department Uses
Surgical gut	Plain	Collagen derived from bovine/ovine intestine	Retains 50% tensile strength for 5 to 7 days	Absorbed by proteolytic processes in weeks	Moderate	Rarely for intraoral
Chromic gut	Chromium coating	Collagen derived from bovine or ovine intestine	Retains 50% tensile strength for 10 to 14 days	Absorbed by proteolytic processes in weeks	Moderate	Rarely for subcutaneous closures and intraoral
Polyglycolic acid (Dexon)	Braided	Polymer of glycolic acid	Retains 65% tensile strength at 2 weeks, 35% at 3 weeks	Completely absorbed by slow hydrolysis by 60 to 90 days	Minimal	Approximation of deep soft tissue structures (i.e., dermis), for ligation
Polyglactin 910 (Vicryl; Vicryl Plus Antibacterial)	Braided	Copolymer of lactide and glycolide with polyglactin 370 and calcium stearate	Retains 75% tensile strength at 2 weeks, 50% at 3 weeks	Completely absorbed by slow hydrolysis by 56 to 70 days	Minimal	Approximation of deep soft tissue structures (i.e., dermis), for ligation
Poliglecaprone 25 (Monocryl; Monocryl Plus Antibacterial)	Monofilament	Copolymer of glycolide and ε-caprolactone	Retains 50% to 70% tensile strength at 1 week, 20% to 40% at 2 weeks	Completely absorbed by hydrolysis by 91 to 119 days	Slight	Approximation of deep soft tissue structures (i.e., dermis), for ligation

TABLE 13–2	Absorbable Suture Characteristics					
Suture	**Types**	**Material**	**In-Vivo Tensile Strength Retention**	**Absorption Rate**	**Tissue Reactivity**	**Common Emergency Department Uses**
Polyglactin 910 (Vicryl Rapide)	Braided	Copolymer of glycolide and lactide coated with polyglactin 370 and calcium stearate	Retains 50% tensile strength for 5 days, 0% by 10 to 14 days	Absorbed by hydrolysis, usually complete by 42 days	Minimal to moderate	Skin approximation when absorbable sutures used
Polyglactin 910 (Lactomer)	Braided	Copolymer of glycolide and lactide coated with caprolactone and glycolide	Retains 40% tensile strength for 3 weeks	Absorbed by hydrolysis, usually complete by 56 to 70 days	Minimal	Subcutaneous soft tissue approximation
Polydioxanone (PDS II; PDS Plus Antibacterial)	Monofilament	Polyester polymer	Retains 40% tensile strength for 4 weeks; 35% for 6 weeks	Minimal until 90 days, complete by 6 months	Slight	Subcutaneous soft tissue approximation where more prolonged strength is needed
Glycomer 631	Monofilament	Terpolymer of glycolide, trimethylene carbonate, and dioxanone	Retains 70% tensile strength 28 days, 13% at 56 days.	Completely hydrolyzed by 90 to 110 days	Slight	Subcutaneous soft tissue approximation where more prolonged strength is needed
Polyglyconate (Maxon)	Monofilament	Polyglyconate polymer	Retains 70% tensile strength at 28 days; 13% at 56 days.	Completely hydrolyzed by 90 to 110 days	Slight	Subcutaneous soft tissue approximation where more prolonged strength is needed

Monofilament nylon, polypropylene, or polybutester sutures are excellent for percutaneous closure of skin wounds because these suture materials exert the least damage to the wounds' defenses.[3]

Synthetic absorbable sutures elicit the least inflammatory response of the absorbable sutures. Plain and chromic gut elicit a greater inflammatory response. Of the nonabsorbable sutures, nylon, polypropylene, polybutester, and polytetrafluoroethylene sutures are the least reactive.[2] Sutures made of natural fibers potentiate infection more than any other nonabsorbable sutures; this correlates with the tissue's reaction to these sutures in clean wounds.[3] On the basis of clinical experience and supportive experimental studies, silk and cotton sutures should not be used in wounds that have gross bacterial contamination.[5] These materials should not be used for most wound closures: they have increased inflammatory properties, and do not appear to have significantly improved handling characteristics than the less reactive monofilament nylon and polypropylene sutures. As a result, there is little if any clinical role for these natural fiber sutures in wound closure. The physical configuration of sutures is also related to the likelihood of developing infection. Monofilament sutures have lower infection rates than multifilament sutures.[4]

In general, practitioners should use the narrowest diameter suture (5-0 or 6-0) with sufficient strength to maintain wound closure, because larger diameter sutures are associated with greater impairment of tissue defenses.

Over the past few years, a number of "smart" sutures that are coated with an antibacterial agent have become available. Examples of antibacterial sutures that are coated with the antibacterial agent triclosan include Vicryl Plus, Monocryl Plus, and PDS Plus. Other than the presence of an antibacterial coating these antibacterial sutures perform very similarly to their non-antibacterial counterparts.[5] In vitro data demonstrate the antibacterial effects of these coated sutures against a wide variety of bacteria that cause wound infections including methicillin-resistant *Staphylococcus aureus* (MRSA).[6] Recent animal and human studies also suggest a significant reduction in wound infection rates when these antibacterial agents are used.[6-9] Retrospective studies have shown a significant reduction in wound infection rates after replacing standard absorbable sutures with antibacterial sutures for repair of sternal and abdominal incisions.[7,8] A small RCT also demonstrated reduced infection rates when standard sutures were compared with triclosan based antibacterial sutures for wound closure after cerebrospinal fluid shunt surgery in children.[9] In many institutions these antibacterial sutures have replaced the comparable non-antibacterial sutures.

Wound Edema

Injured tissue will develop edema over the ensuing 24 to 48 hours after injury. Sutures that can stretch but return to their original length as the edema develops and resolves possess an advantage over sutures without this ability. Polybutester is one such suture.[10] Nylon, polypropylene, polyester, and silk will not stretch with swelling. As a result, they may lacerate or damage tissues that develop large amounts of edema, thereby increasing the likelihood of infection or suboptimal cosmetic result.

Ease of Suture Placement and Removal

One of the suture characteristics to consider is the coefficient of friction. Sutures with low coefficients of friction (such as polybutester) can be easily passed through the tissues and removed without requiring considerable force to separate the suture from the surrounding tissue.[11] Easy removal of sutures minimizes patient discomfort and the likelihood that sutures will break, leaving residual suture within the healing laceration. For the majority of lacerations and surgical incisions where sutures are in place for short periods, the ease of suture removal of the less costly nylon and polypropylene suture is quite adequate.

DETAILS OF SUTURE MATERIALS

The degradation properties of sutures separate them into two general categories. Sutures that undergo rapid degradation in tissues, losing their tensile strength within 60 days, are considered absorbable sutures. Sutures that generally maintain their tensile strength for longer than 60 days are classified as nonabsorbable sutures. It must be noted that even nonabsorbable sutures will lose some of their tensile strength during this 60-day interval.[12] A distinction must be made between the rate of absorption and the rate of tensile strength loss of the suture material. The rate of absorption is important with respect to complications such as sinus tracts and granulomas. The rate of tensile strength loss is of greater importance because the primary function of the suture is to maintain wound edge apposition during healing.

Nonabsorbable Sutures

Nonabsorbable sutures can be classified according to their origin as natural (e.g., silk) or synthetic (e.g., polyamides [nylon], polyesters [Dacron], polyolefins [polyethylene, polypropylene], polytetrafluoroethylene, or polybutester). Nonabsorbable sutures are also characterized by their physical configurations. Nylon, polypropylene, polybutester, polytetrafluoroethylene, and stainless steel are available as monofilament sutures (constructed from one filament). Silk and cotton sutures are available as multifilament (or braided) sutures. Only nylon and stainless steel sutures are available both as a monofilament and as a multifilament suture. Generally synthetic sutures are superior to sutures derived from natural sources. Table 13-1 summarizes the characteristics and common uses of nonabsorbable sutures.

Polypropylene

Polypropylene sutures have a low coefficient of friction that facilitates knot rundown (tying) and suture passage through the tissue.[10] They are inert in tissue and they retain in-vivo tensile strength for years. They exhibit a lower drag coefficient in tissue than do nylon sutures, making them ideal for use in continuous dermal and percutaneous suture closure. However, they stretch under high pressures with resultant widening of the suture loop, as edema resolves. This may allow wound edges to separate if sutures were placed during a period when a large amount of edema was present. Polypropylene is less stiff than nylon and may therefore be less irritating to the patient from the tail ends of the suture.

Nylon

Nylon is more pliable and easier to handle than polypropylene suture. There do not appear to be proven clinical differences between nylon and polypropylene sutures. Because the use of polypropylene sutures has a slightly lower propensity for erythema some physicians prefer them for patients at risk for inflammatory reactions or keloid formation. The largest clinical difference between polypropylene and nylon sutures might be the colors (nylon is black and polypropylene is blue).

Polybutester

Polybutester sutures have unique performance characteristics that are advantageous. They are as strong, exhibit similar degrees of elongation, and have the same knotting characteristics as the other monofilament sutures, but they are more elastic and flexible (stretch). The superior elasticity allows the suture to return to its original length once the load is removed. The increased stretch decreases tension on the wound, thereby reducing the tendency for hypertrophic scarring.[13]

Polyester

Polyester sutures are comprised of fibers of polyester, or poly (ethylene terephthalate), a synthetic linear polyester. Polyester sutures are synthetic braided sutures that last indefinitely in tissues. As a result, undyed sutures that are not likely to be visualized through the skin are primarily used for tendon lacerations in which the sutures remain within the tissue for long periods of time.

Absorbable Sutures

Absorbable sutures (Table 13-2) are made from either natural sources (collagen) or synthetic polymers.

Natural absorbable sutures

Collagen sutures are derived from the submucosal layer of sheep or the serosal layer of bovine small intestine (gut). **Chromic gut** is treated with a chromium salt to resist body enzymes making it more resistant to absorption. Gut is resorbed via lysosomal enzymes.[14]

Natural fiber absorbable sutures are seldom used for repair of traumatic lacerations and surgical incisions. They fray during knot construction and there is considerable variability in their tensile strength. These sutures are used for wounds involving mucosal surfaces subject to minimal tension. Nonabsorbable synthetic sutures are preferred for most epidermal nonmucosal skin closures.

Synthetic braided absorbable sutures

Synthesis of high-molecular-weight polyglycolic acid and polylactic acid produces **polyglycolic acid** and **Polyglactin 910** sutures. The copolymers of Polyglactin 910 are prepared by polymerizing nine parts of glycolide with one part of lactide, whereas the polyglycolic acid sutures are produced from the homopolymer. Because of the inherent rigidity of these copolymers, these high-molecular-weight polymers are extruded into thin filaments and braided.[15] The polyglycolic acid and Polyglactin 910 sutures degrade in an aqueous environment through hydrolysis of the ester linkage. **Lactomer glycolide/lactide** provides a high initial tensile strength with slow, uniform degradation in tissues. The smaller filaments in this braided suture enhance tensile strength, reduce coefficient of friction, and improve handling. The surfaces of these synthetic sutures have been coated to decrease their coefficient of friction.[12]

Synthetic monofilament absorbable sutures

Polydioxanone(PDS II) is a monofilament absorbable suture[16] that is processed into small granules and extruded into monofilaments. **Glycolide trimethylene carbonate** is a linear copolymer made by reacting trimethylene carbonate and glycolide with diethylene glycol as an initiator and stannous chloride dihydrate as the catalyst. **Polyglecaprone 25** is a synthetic absorbable suture that is one of the most pliable synthetic absorbable monofilament sutures commercially available. **Glycomer 631** is a monofilament synthetic absorbable suture that is significantly stronger than the braided synthetic absorbable suture over 4 weeks of implantation.[17] This monofilament suture also potentiates less bacterial infection than does the braided suture. The strength of the monofilament synthetic absorbable sutures is maintained in vivo much longer than that of the braided synthetic absorbable suture. These monofilament sutures retained approximately 70% of their breaking strength after implantation for 28 days, and still retained 13% of their original strength at 56 days. In contrast, braided absorbable sutures retained only 1% to 5% of their strength at 28 days.[16]

SURGICAL NEEDLES

Surgical needles are produced from stainless steel alloys. The surgical needle has three basic components: the swage, body, and needle point (Figure 13-1). The swage is the site of attachment of the suture. It provides a smooth juncture between the needle and suture minimizing the size of the hole made in the tissue. The body of the needle is the portion that is grasped by the needle holder. The shape of the cross-sectional area and the configuration of its length can categorize the needle body. There are circular, triangular, rectangular, and trapezoidal cross-sectional areas of the needle bodies (Figure 13-1). The curvature of the needle is described in degrees of the subtended arc. The radius is the distance from the center of the circle to the body of the needle. The curvature of the needle with one radius of curvature may vary from 90° to 225°. Needles with a curvature of 135° are generally used to approximate edges of traumatic lacerations. A 135° curvature will enable the needle to pass through the tissue with a limited rotation of the wrist. The 180° needle is ideally suited for use in deep body cavities where a more limited arc of wrist rotation will successfully pass the entire needle and provide sufficient exposure of the needle tip so that easy needle retrieval by the practitioner can occur.

The point of the needle is at its tip. There are several types of needle tips: cutting edges, taper points, or a combination of both, and blunt-tip needles. Cutting-edge needles have two or more opposing edges and are designed to penetrate tough tissue. The position of a third cutting edge categorizes the needle as either a conventional cutting-edge needle or a reverse cutting-edge needle (Figure 13-2). An inside cutting edge causes a linear cut that is perpendicular and close to the incision, against which the suture will exert a wound closure force that may ultimately cut through the tissue. In contrast, a reverse cutting edge cuts through

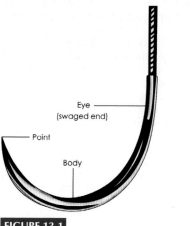

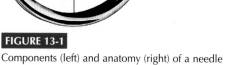

FIGURE 13-1
Components (left) and anatomy (right) of a needle

Conventional Cutting

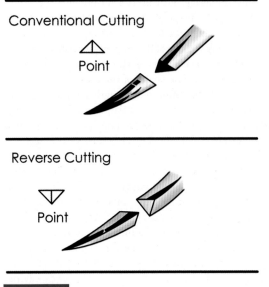

Point

Reverse Cutting

Point

FIGURE 13-2

A conventional cutting-edge surgical needle point has three cutting edges with its apical cutting edge on the inside concave surface of the needle. A reverse cutting-edge needle point has three cutting edges with its apical cutting edge on the outer convex surface of the needle.

skin leaving a wide wall of tissue, rather than an incision, against which the suture exerts its wound closure force. This wall of tissue resists suture cut-through.

The taper-point needle tapers to a sharp tip that spreads the tissue without cutting it. Taper-point needles are used in soft tissues that do not resist needle penetration, such as vessels, abdominal viscera, and fascia. They are not generally used for repair of traumatic lacerations in the emergency department or office setting. Blunt tip needles have traditionally been used in friable tissues such as liver but are being used more and more in muscle and fascia in an effort to reduce needle sticks.

REFERENCES

1. James GA, Swogger E, Wolcott R, et al. Biofilms in chronic wounds. *Wound Repair Regen.* 2008;16(1): 37–44.
2. Edlich RF, Tsung MS, Rogers W, Rogers P, Wangensteen OH. Studies in management of the contaminated wound. I. Technique of closure of such wounds together with a note on a reproducible experimental model. *J Surg Res.* 1968;8(12):585–592.
3. Edlich RF, Panek PH, Rodeheaver GT, Turnbull VG, Kurtz LD, Edgerton MT. Physical and chemical configuration of sutures in the development of surgical infection. *Ann Surg.* 1973;177(6):679–688.
4. Sharp WV, Belden TA, King PH, Teague PC. Suture resistance to infection. *Surgery.* 1982;91(1):61–63.
5. Ford HR, Jones P, Gaines B, Reblock K, Simpkins DL. Intraoperative handling and wound healing: controlled clinical trial comparing coated VICRYL plus antibacterial suture (coated polyglactin 910 suture with triclosan) with coated VICRYL suture (coated polyglactin 910 suture). *Surg Infect (Larchmt).* 2005; 6(3):313–321.
6. Ming X, Rothenburger S, Nichols MM. In vivo and in vitro antibacterial efficacy of PDS plus (polidioxanone with triclosan) suture. *Surg Infect (Larchmt).* 2008;9(4):451–457.
7. Fleck T, Moidl R, Blacky A, Fleck M, Wolner E, et al. Triclosan-coated sutures for the reduction of sterna wound infections: economic considerations. Ann Thorac Surg 2007;84:232–236.
8. Justinger C, Moussavian MR, Schlueter C, Kopp B, Kollmar O, Schilling MK. Antibiotic coating of abdominal closure sutures and wound infection. Surgery 2009;145:330–334.
9. Rozelle CJ, Leonardo J, Li V. Antimicrobial suture wound closure for cerebrospinal fluid shunt surgery: a prospective, double-blinded, randomized, controlled trial. J Neurosurg Pediatrics 2008;2:111–117.
10. Rodeheaver GT, Borzelleca DC, Thacker JG, Edlich RF. Unique performance characteristics of Novafil. *Surg Gynecol Obstet.* 1987;164(3):230–236.
11. Pham S, Rodeheaver GT, Dang MC, Foresman PA, Hwang JC, Edlich RF. Ease of continuous dermal suture removal. *J Emerg Med.* 1990;8(5):539–543.
12. Postlethwait RW. Long-term comparative study of nonabsorbable sutures. *Ann Surg.* 1970;171(6):892–898.
13. Trimbos JB, Smeets M, Verdel M, Hermans J. Cosmetic result of lower midline laparotomy wounds: polybutester and nylon in a randomized clinical trial. *Obstet Gynecol.* 1993;82(3):390–393.
14. Salthouse TN, Williams JA, Willigan DA. Relationship of cellular enzyme activity to catgut and collagen suture absorption. *Surg Gynecol Obstet.* 1969; 129(4):691–696.
15. Rodeheaver GT, Thacker JG, Edlich RF. Mechanical performance of polyglycolic acid and polyglactin 910 synthetic absorbable sutures. *Surg Gynecol Obstet.* 1981;153(6):835–841.
16. Ray JA, Doddi N, Regula D, Williams JA, Melveger A. Polydioxanone (PDS), a novel monofilament synthetic absorbable suture. *Surg Gynecol Obstet.* 1981; 153(4):497–507.
17. Rodeheaver GT, Beltran KA, Green CW, et al. Biomechanical and clinical performance of a new synthetic monofilament absorbable suture. *J Long Term Eff Med Implants.* 1996;6(3–4):181–198.

CHAPTER 14

Basic Suturing and Tissue Handling Techniques

Adam J. Singer, MD, and Lior Rosenberg, MD

The healing process of the cutaneous wound is a cascade of natural phenomena that evolved to restore the tissue defect that we call a "wound." The optimal course of these healing processes depends on several factors, but, first of all, on the integrity of the tissues involved. For generations, healers burned and purposely contaminated the wounds accepting severe complications as natural and even as the will of God. Ambroise Paré understood that boiling oil caused more harm than good and that leaving the wound lightly dressed would prevent, at least, good-intentioned iatrogenic disasters. He coined the slogan "I dressed the wound but God healed it," still very true to this very day: we may close the wound but the healing process is the one that will eventually close it permanently.

Before beginning our efforts to help the patient we first have to avoid additional harm. "Primum non nuocere" has been true since the first healer put his mind to helping the first patient. As long as we respect them, the healing tissues will be our partners in the healing process. However, once mistreated, they become the patient's worst enemies. The basis of the following chapter's technical details is this very simple truth: keep the tissue alive and happy!

GENERAL PRINCIPLES

The ultimate goal of wound closure is to achieve a good functional and cosmetically appealing result. This is best achieved by conscious and gentle handling of all tissues, avoiding additional trauma, matching each layer of the wound with its corresponding counterpart on the opposite side and providing the proper functional conditions that allow tissue survival and the healing processes. The tension should be released by subdermal and dermal sutures providing optimal conditions for a proper approximation of the more superficial dermal layers and the epidermis. The epidermis requires slight eversion of its wound edges and the dermis requires minimizing and optimizing of the amount of tension on the wound's edges.

As the wound heals and contracts and the swelling subsides, the wound will eventually flatten, becoming flush with the surrounding skin surface. Care should be taken to avoid an inverted or depressed scar, which, when shined upon, will cast a shadow that tends to accentuate the scar's width. Taking a larger bite at the depth of the wound than through the more superficial layers helps achieve wound eversion. Wound eversion is facilitated by use of mattress or deep sutures. For most wounds, simple interrupted percutaneous sutures, with or without interrupted dermal sutures, are all that are required.

Tissue Handling

Increasing the amount of trauma to the wound edges and its surrounding skin increases the likelihood of necrosis, infection, disruption, and suboptimal cosmetic scar appearance.[1] Therefore, it is very important to avoid any further damage by handling the traumatized tissues carefully during repair. This can be achieved by minimizing the amount of tissue handling and using the least destructive surgical instruments. Excessive twisting or bending of the base of tissue flaps should be avoided as this may reduce their blood flow.

The following are the commonest causes of tissue mishandling and the corrective or preventive actions that should be practiced:

1. Use of tooth forceps to grasp the wound's edges: When grasping the wound's edge with tooth forceps, very often the practitioner has to exert high pressure to hold and pull the wound's edges. This pressure is concentrated at the tips of the forceps' teeth. The pressure applied by the teeth crushes the tissue leaving typical necrotic points 1 mm to 3 mm from the edges. These necrotic points will slough and, under the best scenario, will heal with a separate scar from the main defect. These scars resemble and in many cases join and enhance the necrosis and scars ("cross marks") caused by tight stitches (see 3). In the worst scenario, these triangular necrotic areas (the base of the triangle is the wound's edge) will join causing wound infection and disruption.

    Nontraumatic grasping, approximation, elevation, and turning over of the wound edges may be achieved by the use of skin hooks (Figure 14-1) or temporary holding sutures. Fine-toothed forceps (such as the finest-toothed Adson forceps) may be used just to stabilize the tissues with one arm only, without closing the jaws in the same manner as

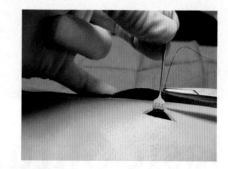

FIGURE 14-1

A skin hook is used to elevate the wound edge, facilitating suture placement.

using one's fingers (Figure 14-2). If holding tissues with toothed forceps cannot be avoided, only the deepest part of the dermis or subcutaneous tissue should be grasped and not the more superficial dermis–epidermis (Figure 14-2).

2. Monopolar electrocautery: The goal of hemostasis is to stop bleeding. There are very few (if any) large arteries in the skin that will not occlude by applying gentle pressure. The monopolar cautery leaves a sphere of charred tissue that may, or may not, include a bleeding vessel.[1] Charring enough tissue at the vicinity of the bleeder will eventually cauterize it but at a price: an area of necrotic burned tissue, several millimeters in size. Dead tissue will necrotize, become infected, and will not heal until disintegrated, sloughed, and phagocytized or débrided causing additional scarring and wound healing delay.

    Cutaneous hemostasis can be achieved very effectively by pressing on the wound, placing the subdermal or intradermal suture around the bleeder, or, if everything else fails, using bipolar cautery that will char only the tissue immediately between the two fine poles.

3. Tight sutures: The role of a suture is to approximate tissues (without harming them) to a distance that will allow healing processes to take place.

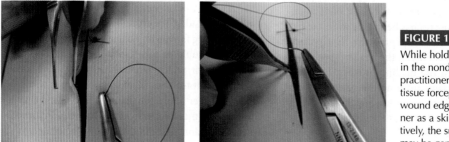

FIGURE 14-2

While holding the tissue forceps in the nondominant hand, the practitioner uses one arm of the tissue forceps to elevate the wound edge in the same manner as a skin hook (left). Alternatively, the subcutaneous tissue may be gently grasped (right).

Overtightening will strangulate and kill the tissues within the stitch in a typical triangular shape (see 1). An exception may be a subdermal or intradermal suture that was placed for hemostatic purposes (see 2). Such sutures will not harm the skin as they are below the papillary dermis with its rich capillary blood supply

Sutures should be tightened just enough to bring the healing surfaces into contact, bridging the healing distance. Blanching of the encircled tissues should be avoided. Continuous sutures can distribute the tension along the entire wound front preventing strangulation.

Use of Scalpels

The skin should always be cut with a sharp blade and smooth, continuous strokes. "Sawing" motions further traumatize the skin and should be avoided. The No. 15 blade is preferred for débridement of most small traumatic lacerations and for excision of dog ears. It allows the most accurate incisions, particularly those that are angular or irregular. The blade should enter the skin at a 90° angle using the blade's "belly" (its round part). The handle, preferably a round one, should be held like a pencil between the thumb and index finger supported by the middle finger of the dominant hand (Figure 14-3). The No. 10 blade is rarely used in the acute setting. Its rounded belly edge is mainly used to perform long, linear incisions in the more extensive operations. Traditionally, the No. 10 scalpel is held like a violin's bowstring (Figure 14-4), but it can also be held like a pencil especially for more accurate incisions.

BASIC SUTURING TECHNIQUES

Generally, the instrument tie with the needle holder is the preferred method for tying sutures when one is

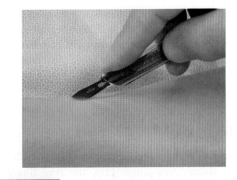
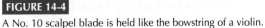

FIGURE 14-4

A No. 10 scalpel blade is held like the bowstring of a violin.

closing the skin. Instrument ties are more rapid and accurate, allowing better control of tension than most manual ties and can be used in recesses that do not allow manual tying. The major disadvantage to tying with instruments is the inability to apply continuous tension to the suture ends. As a result, the suture knots may slip and lose the required closure tension.

As previously mentioned, the wound should never be closed under tension. The closing tension should be distributed along the entire wound's length and three dimensionally, throughout the wound's structures. The strongest tissues should be used to approximate the edges starting with the subcutaneous fascia followed by the deep dermal layer. Using intradermal sutures at different layers will help distribute the tension over a greater number of sutures and tissue volume. To avoid slippage of the suture, the first knot may be a double loop, using a double throw. Hand tying should be considered when one is using large sutures (larger than 2-0), by those who have not mastered the instrument tie, and only rarely, in wounds subject to very large static tensions, being aware of the future, permanent cross-mark scars that result.

Choosing a Needle Holder

Straight surgical needles are almost never used in the acute setting. The curved surgical needles that are used require the use of a needle holder. Many needle holders have small teeth along their jaws to avoid slippage of the needle.[2] However, these teeth can damage or tear the suture material.[3] Needle holders with smooth jaws avoid these problems, but the needle may slip or rotate.[4] When available, specialized needle holders in which a hard tungsten–steel insert with a very fine texture of their jaws are a good option.[5] Such a fine-jaw needle holder should not be used for purposes other than holding fine needles. Closing and twisting the

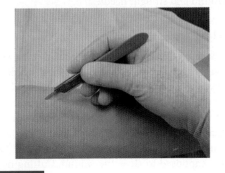

FIGURE 14-3

A No. 15 scalpel blade is held like a pencil.

fine jaws on a thick needle (>2–3/0) or even worse, using the fine-jaw needle holder as pliers to remove scalpel blades or to twist needles will destroy them. Additionally the needle may rotate in a mistreated needle holder with the suturing thread slipping through the maimed jaws.

Holding the Needle Holder

The needle holder may be held by one of two methods. In the thumb–ring finger grip, the ring finger is inserted in the lower ringlet of the needle holder (traditionally referred to as the "bow") and serves as the pivot point around which the instrument rotates. The tip of the thumb's distal ulnar–volar pad is positioned on the inner side of the upper bow, stabilizing it and facilitating the release of the ratchet mechanism (Figure 14-5). This grip allows controlled movement of the needle holder and an accurate and controlled disengagement of the ratchet mechanism when one is releasing the needle. This precise needle manipulation and avoidance of inadvertent motion during the release process is crucial for the accurate placement of sutures. This grip, in which the needle holder is held by the fingers and not palmed, may be a little difficult to master at first but it is worth learning because of its precision. The disadvantage is that the entire torque forces are transferred to the pivot fourth, ring finger limiting the use of the technique in sutures where a great amount of force is needed to penetrate thick layers or hard tissues (e.g., scars).

In the palm–thenar grip, the needle holder is grasped in the palm of the hand without inserting the tips of the thumb and ring fingers into the needle holder bow (Figure 14-6). In this position, the needle holder is palmed between the thenar eminence and the second to fifth fingers. The major advantage of this grip is its versatility and the possibility to apply

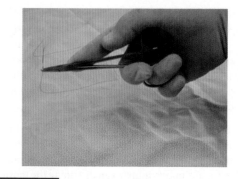

FIGURE 14-6

The thenar grip for a needle holder is shown.

controlled force by the palmed instrument, allowing even long needle holders to be accurately manipulated in difficult areas such as recessed cavities. Its major disadvantage is the skill needed to release the ratchet mechanism by the use of the thenar eminence and the potential loss of precision when one is disengaging the ratchet mechanism and uncontrolled movement of the needle when it is half through and still imbedded in the tissues. The thenar grip should only be used after one has mastered the thumb–ring finger grip and after thoroughly practicing the palm grip and especially the transition from one grip to the other.

Pushing the needle in a different vector than its curvature will result in "plowing" of the tissue, its uncontrolled cutting-through, and further trauma. This "plowing" motion may also bend or break the needle. The needle should be pushed and pulled through the tissues following the direction and radius of its curvature.

Choosing the Needle

Basically there are two kinds of needle tips and two kinds of needles. The "cutting" and "tapered" tips, and the round and straight needles.

Cutting tip

The needle is sharpened as a triangular lance with its cutting edge facing foreword ("cutting needle") or backward ("reverse cutting"). These needles will incise a minute slit through the skin to reduce resistance to their passage through the tissues. When "plowing" with such needles their cutting action and the slits they produce may entirely transect the thin tissue bridge that is supposed to close the wound. Cutting needles should be used properly in resistant tissues (skin and dermis).

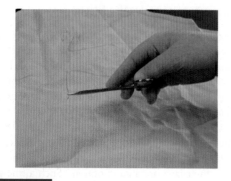

FIGURE 14-5

The thumb–ring finger grip for a needle holder is shown.

Tapered tips

The rounded tapering pinlike tip pushes its way through the tissue like a wedge through a pinpoint puncture. They are obviously less traumatic but can not be used in resisting tissues such as dermis as the applied force and torque will bend and even break the needle. They are mainly used in visceral–vascular surgery.

Round needles

These are the most common "surgical" needles (though their origin is the sail needle). Their shape is designed to follow a suturing course that will unite two edges on the same plane. There is an endless choice of needles having different radiuses and the practitioner should choose the radius that best fulfills the needle's course in the tissue. Usually smaller radiuses are chosen for intradermal sutures and flatter, larger radiuses will be the choice when a larger tissue bulk needs to be included in the stitch.

Straight needles

Originating in the classical tailor's sawing needle, these needles are rarely used in surgery, except for very specialized indications.

Simple Interrupted Percutaneous Sutures and Instrument Ties

The advantages and disadvantages of the various suturing methods are summarized in Table 14-1. The simple interrupted suture is the most commonly used method of closing cutaneous wounds.[6] In one series of more than 5000 traumatic lacerations (prior to

TABLE 14–1	Advantages and Disadvantages of Various Suturing Methods		
Suture Type	**Advantages**	**Disadvantages**	**Frequent Uses**
Interrupted percutaneous	Excellent approximation	Time-consuming May strangulate tissues Tedious suture removal	Low-tension wounds May be used with deep sutures for high-tension wounds
Continuous percutaneous	Rapid closure Accommodates edema Results in tension distribution Easy suture removal	Requires more skill and practice as it is less forgiving for inaccuracies If a single knot unravels, the wound may dehisce (if no deep sutures are placed)	Percutaneous closure in conjunction with deep-tension relieving sutures
Interrupted dermal	Reduces tension on wound surface Allows early removal of percutaneous sutures, avoiding hatch-marking May reduce scar width May be used for hemostasis	May increase infection in contaminated wounds	High-tension wounds Closure of dead space Dermal bleeding
Continuous dermal	Rapid Reduces tension on wound surface Allows early removal of percutaneous sutures, avoiding hatch-marking May reduce scar width	Technically difficult Less accurate approximation than interrupted sutures If a single knot unravels, the wound may dehisce	Closure of dead space

(Continued)

TABLE 14–1	Advantages and Disadvantages of Various Suturing Methods (Continued)		
Suture Type	**Advantages**	**Disadvantages**	**Frequent Uses**
Vertical mattress	Excellent wound edge eversion	May cause tissue strangulation	Thin or lax skin with little dermal or fascial tissue
	Combines advantages of deep and superficial sutures	May be difficult to remove	High-tension areas (e.g., extremities)
Horizontal mattress	More rapid than simple interrupted sutures	May cause tissue strangulation	Bleeding scalp wounds
	Excellent wound edge eversion	May be difficult to remove	Initial approximation of high-tension wounds
Half-buried, horizontal mattress	Less compromising to flap perfusion	Time-consuming Technically difficult	Corner stitches and flaps

introduction of tissue adhesives), 78% were repaired by simple interrupted sutures, 8% by using staples, 4% by using vertical mattress sutures, 3% by using adhesive tapes, 2% by using running sutures, and 1% by using horizontal mattress sutures.[7] The simple interrupted suture is most appropriate for closing the outer layers of the skin when the laceration or incision is under minimal tension. It is most forgiving to execute as each stitch can be done and undone until perfection is achieved resulting in meticulous apposition of the edges of the wound.

The needle is grasped with the tip of the needle holder approximately one half to one third of the distance from the attachment of the suture to the needle and the needle's tip, and the ratchet mechanism is engaged with one click (Figure 14-7). To insert simple interrupted sutures, the needle should be passed so that more tissue is included at the depth

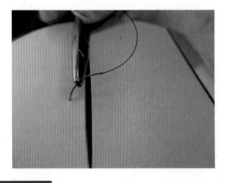

The needle is held by the jaws of the needle holder approximately one third to one half of the distance from the junction of the suture and needle. The needle enters the skin at a 90° angle.

of the wound than at the surface, resulting in a pear-shaped loop when the wound is viewed in cross-section (Figure 14-8). This procedure promotes eversion of the skin edges. It is best achieved by entering the skin at an angle of 90° (see Figure 14-7) and is facilitated by starting with the hand in full pronation and supinating the wrist during passage of the needle through the skin. Eversion of the skin edges is thought to avoid a depressed scar by opposing the tendency of the approximated wound edges to contract downward during healing.

For right-handed practitioners, the needle should usually enter the right or far side of the wound and exit through the middle of the wound. The needle is then grasped with the tip of the needle holder and rearmed by using a tissue forceps (Figure 14-9). When not in use, the tissue forceps may be held in the palm of the nondominant hand to maximize practitioner efficiency. The needle is then passed through the other side of the wound, starting at its depth and exiting through the skin's surface. The needle should enter and exit the skin at exactly the same levels and distances on either side of the wound to achieve accurate approximation and matching of the various levels of the skin.

When the wound edges are uneven, with one being less stable than the other (e.g., with a flap), the needle should first be passed through the less stable side. If this is on the left or near side of the wound, the practitioner should use a backhanded approach in which the wrist is fully supinated and the needle passed by pronating the wrist (Figure 14-10A). Note that with this approach, the needle should be loaded with its tip pointing to the right side of the needle holder (Figure 14-10B).

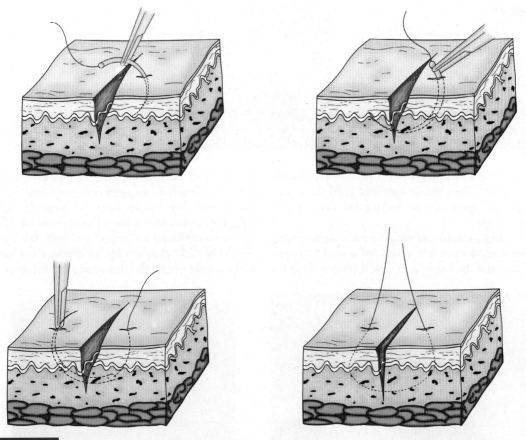

FIGURE 14-8

Cross section of wound demonstrating proper suture placement. The distance of the suture from the wound edge is greater at the depth of the wound than it is near its surface resulting in wound edge eversion after being tied.

After exiting the second side of the wound, the suture should be advanced through the tissue until only its distal 2 cm to 4 cm remains within the skin. This will ease loop formation. To avoid getting entangled when the thread is still very long, one may drop

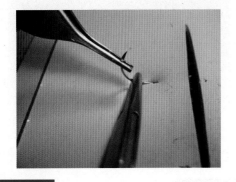

FIGURE 14-9

The needle is grasped by the forceps and rearmed within the jaws of the needle holder.

the needle with the loose thread on the surgical field and grasp the suture material approximately 10 cm to 20 cm away from the wound (Figure 14-11).

When one is tying the first knot, the fixed end of the suture should be wrapped twice around the tip of the needle holder in a clockwise direction with the nondominant hand (Figure 14-12). The free end of the suture is then grasped with the jaws of the needle holder. The tip of the suture is then pulled through the suture loop across the wound while the fixed end is also pulled across the wound in the opposite direction (Figure 14-13). The suture loop may be tightened by pulling on the suture ends. In this case, the knot will not slip. The knot may be further stabilized by pulling the end of the cut suture across the wound, thus locking it in this position (Figure 14-14). Alternatively, the first knot may be formed by creating a single loop around the needle holder and almost completely tightening it (Figure 14-15, left). A second loop is then created with the fixed end of the suture around the needle

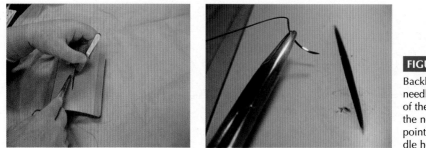

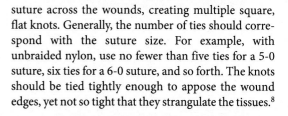

FIGURE 14-10
Backhand approach to inserting needle from the left or near side of the wound (left). Note that the needle is armed with its tip pointing to the right of the needle holder (right).

holder in the **same direction** (Figure 14-15, middle). The knot is then slowly tightened until the wound edges are apposed, thus locking the knot (Figure 14-15, right).

Additional ties are placed alternating the direction in which the suture is wrapped around the needle holder and the hands are crossed when pulling the suture across the wounds, creating multiple square, flat knots. Generally, the number of ties should correspond with the suture size. For example, with unbraided nylon, use no fewer than five ties for a 5-0 suture, six ties for a 6-0 suture, and so forth. The knots should be tied tightly enough to appose the wound edges, yet not so tight that they strangulate the tissues.[8]

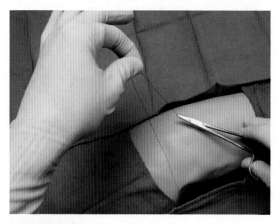

FIGURE 14-11
The suture material may be grasped at its center to avoid getting entangled when very long.

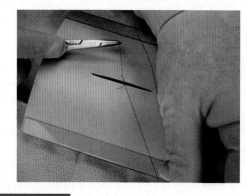

FIGURE 14-13
The tip of the suture is grasped with the needle holder and pulled across the wound. Note that the nondominant hand is pulling the fixed end of the suture in the opposite direction, creating a flat knot.

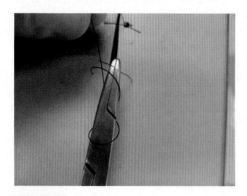

FIGURE 14-12
The first throw is formed by looping the fixed end of the suture twice around the tip of the needle holder in a clockwise direction.

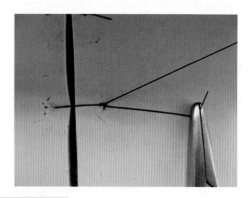

FIGURE 14-14
The knot is "locked" by pulling the end of the cut suture across the wound preventing its slippage.

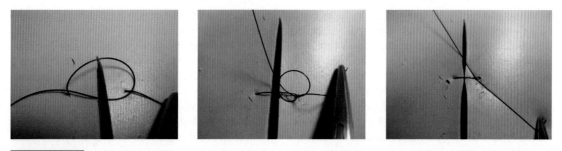

FIGURE 14-15

Alternative method of forming the first knot: The fixed end of the suture is wrapped once clockwise around the needle holder and partially tightened (left). A second loop is made in the same clockwise direction (middle). The knot is then completely tightened until the wound edges appose (right). In this manner, the knot does not slip.

The ends of the suture should be cut leaving ends that are shorter than the distance between sutures (usually 3 mm to 5 mm long) to facilitate removal and to avoid getting them entangled with neighboring stitches.

The first suture should be placed at the center of the wound. Additional sutures are then placed midway between the center of the wound and its corners. This process of bisecting the remaining limbs of the wound with sutures is continued until apposition of the wound edges is achieved (Figure 14-16). The first interrupted intradermal suture will bear much of the tension and its proper placement will ease the rest of the suturing process (see next paragraph). Because the presence of suture material increases the likelihood of infection,[9] the number of sutures should be kept at a minimum.

Simple Interrupted Dermal Sutures

Simple interrupted buried subdermal and dermal sutures are used to close the dermis. As these sutures should bear the wound's dehiscence force, the subcutaneous tissues should be closed as well to release the tension from the dermis. Subcutaneous fascia (e.g., Scarpa's fascia) should be closed first, bringing in the cutaneous mass connected to it followed by closing of the subcutaneous fat to fill depressions and cavities below the wound. These sutures are placed not only in wounds that are subject to large static tensions but also in deep wounds that are in line with the skin creases (minimal tension lines). The dermal sutures should bear the opening tension of the wound's edges reducing the tendency for these wounds to form wide scars or to dehisce. Using dermal sutures also allows early removal of the percutaneous sutures before the formation of unsightly suture marks (which generally occurs after the seventh day). Deep sutures should be used judiciously because they have been shown to increase infection rates in contaminated wounds.[10] For most deep sutures, an absorbable suture that remains in the wound for at least 4 to 6 weeks is required.

Deep sutures should be placed so that the knot is buried at the depth of the wound. This is accomplished

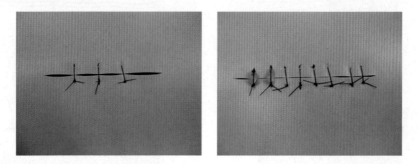

FIGURE 14-16

The first suture is placed at the center of the wound (left). The remaining limbs are sequentially bisected with additional sutures until wound apposition is complete (right).
By placing the first suture in the middle and then bisecting the rest of the wound accurate approximation is achieved. In the right picture, the first two left sutures are too tight and the gray areas represent the ischemic tissue caused by the constricting stitch. These sutures should be removed and replaced with less tight sutures.

by starting and ending suture placement at the depth of the wound. The deep suture is placed by entering the wound at the subdermal–reticular dermis and exiting beneath the dermal–epidermal junction on the left or near side of the wound (Figure 14-17). After exiting the first side of the wound and rearming the needle holder and pulling on the subdermal–dermal junction (using a hook if possible), the needle is then inserted on the other side of the wound immediately beneath the epidermal–dermal junction, exiting at the lower portion of the reticular dermis at exactly the same level on the contralateral side (see Figure 14-17).

After placement of the suture, a knot should be formed using four or five throws. When one is tying the knot, the hands should move in a direction parallel to the wound (Figure 14-18). The deep suture should then be cut close to the knot (approximately 1 mm) and the knot should be pushed down into the wound. To avoid premature unraveling of the suture because of very short tail ends, one additional throw

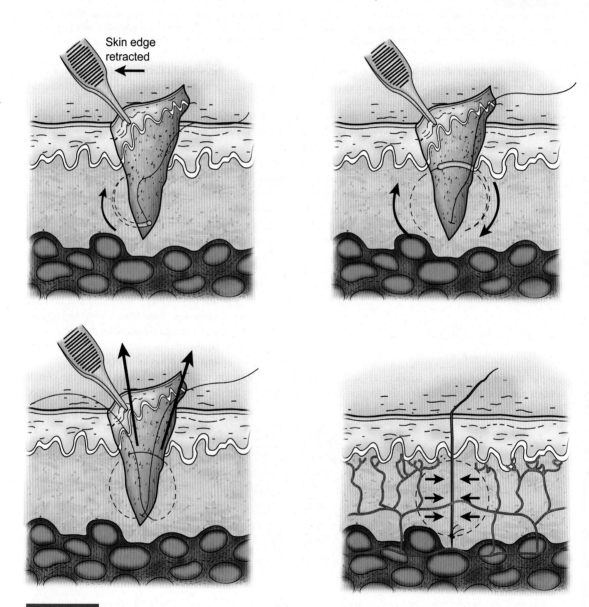

FIGURE 14-17

Placement of a deep suture: The needle is inserted at the depth of the dermis and directed upward, exiting immediately beneath the dermal–epidermal junction. The needle is then inserted through the opposite side of the wound, starting at the dermal–epidermal junction and exiting at the depth of the dermis.

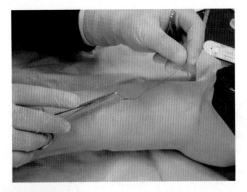

FIGURE 14-18

Tying the knot of a deep suture. The hands move in a direction parallel to the wound.

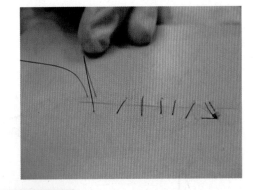

FIGURE 14-19

Continuous percutaneous sutures: The suture crosses the wound superficially at a 90° angle. The suture traverses the depth of the wound at a 65° angle.

should be added prior to cutting the suture.[11] With long wounds, several dermal sutures may be required. The first suture should be placed at the center of the wound, with sequential bisection of the remaining limbs of the wound as described earlier.

Continuous Percutaneous Sutures

With continuous sutures, the entire wound is closed before dividing the suture material. The major advantages of continuous sutures are their relative speed and the ability to adapt to progressive swelling of the wound. They are particularly useful for long linear wounds. It is less important to control the individual tension of each loop as eventually the tension will be distributed along the entire wound. This even tension distribution suffices also to stop any capillary bleeding from the edges. Some skill and expertise is needed to achieve perfect apposition of the wound edges. Continuous sutures should be used judiciously and not for irregular wounds or by the novice. This suture does not play a major role in the acute setting.

The first suture, similar to a simple interrupted percutaneous suture, is placed at one end of the wound. After completion of the first knot, the suture thread is not divided. The needle is then inserted next to the first suture at the opposite side of the wound, crossing the wound at a 90° angle (Figure 14-19). The needle then crosses the depth of the wound in a circular motion perpendicular to the wound, exiting on the opposite side approximately 3 mm to 5 mm from the wound edge. This process is repeated as needed until the entire wound is approximated. After the last suture is placed, a small loop is left, which serves as an anchor for tying the knot (Figure 14-20). The knot itself is constructed as described previously. To ensure knot security, at least five or six throws should be used.[12]

Continuous Dermal Sutures

Continuous dermal sutures are quite technically complex. When the technique is mastered, they allow excellent wound closure and excellent cosmesis with little or without any need for percutaneous sutures. This is particularly advantageous for frightened children, patients in whom suture removal is problematic, and patients with a tendency to form hypertrophic scars or keloids. Continuous dermal sutures are also very useful when the wound will be under a cast or splint precluding their early removal. Continuous dermal sutures are also appropriate for wounds subject to large dynamic or static tensions. If crushing of the skin with the forceps is avoided, there is no risk of suture marks with this method of closure. Dermal sutures have not been shown to reduce scar width in non-gaping wounds,[13,14] and their use may be associated

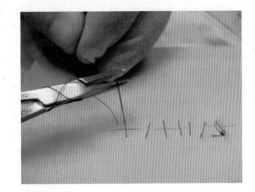

FIGURE 14-20

After the practitioner completes placement of the continuous percutaneous suture, the knot is formed by grasping a loop of suture. Note that the sutures are not placed equally; this is to compensate for variation in tension along the wound.

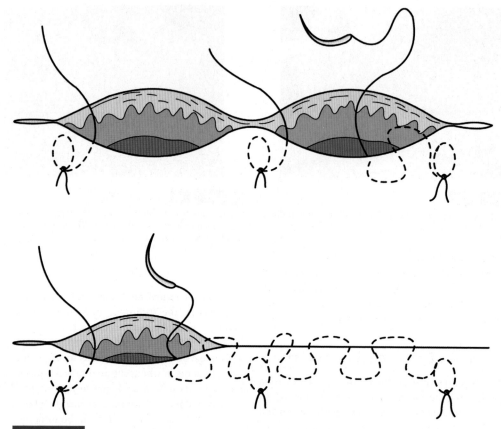

FIGURE 14-21

Placement of interrupted dermal sutures prior to a continuous dermal suture (upper figure): A long tail is left with each suture as an anchor for the more superficial continuous intradermal suture (lower figure).

with higher wound infection rates.[15] An alternative to continuous dermal sutures is a combination of interrupted dermal sutures and tissue adhesives.

Before placement of the continuous dermal suture, it is helpful to place several deep sutures every 2 cm to 5 cm along the wound to reduce tension and align the wound edges in an optimal position. One tail of these interrupted dermal sutures is left longer for anchoring of the continuous dermal suture (Figure 14-21). A deep suture is also placed at the corner of the wound to anchor the last continuous suture. When one is constructing a continuous dermal suture, the suture should first be anchored in the skin by entering the subcutaneous tissue at one end of the wound (usually on the right or farthest side in the case of a right-handed practitioner) and exiting in the lower dermis (Figure 14-22). A five-throw knot is tied and the end is cut.

The needle is then inserted below the epidermal–dermal junction on the far side of the wound and passed in a horizontal direction parallel to the wound

surface (Figure 14-23). After exiting the upper dermis, the needle in backtracked 1 mm or 2 mm and inserted on the near side of the wound through the upper dermis in a horizontal direction as before. This process is repeated using small bites, passing above the interrupted dermal sutures, intermittently tying the suture

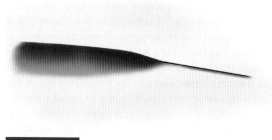

FIGURE 14-22

Placement of a continuous dermal suture. The suture is anchored at the apex of the wound.

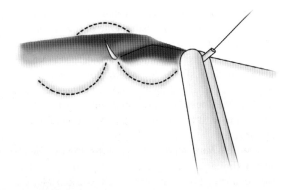

FIGURE 14-23

Placement of the continuous dermal suture. Small horizontal bites are taken beneath the dermal–epidermal junction. Slight backtracking of the needle path should be performed to ensure wound coaptation.

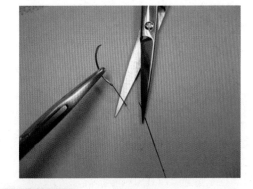

FIGURE 14-25

The knot is buried in the subcutaneous tissue by inserting the needle at the wound depth and exiting approximately 5 mm from the wound edge. The suture is pulled taut and then cut retracting beneath the skin surface.

to the long tail ends of the dermal suture that were placed for this purpose (see Figure 14-21) and cutting its remains above the knot until the wound is closed. Careful yet steady traction on the fixed end of the suture while progressing helps to approximate the wound edges.

When the last suture is passed, it is tied to the long tail of the last interrupted dermal suture (see Figure 14-21). With short or tension-free wounds, the practitioner may choose to place continuous dermal sutures without underlying interrupted dermal sutures. In this case, the last suture is tied by using a small loop of the suture to anchor the knot, similar to a continuous percutaneous suture (Figure 14-24). After the knot is tied, the suture is cut and buried beneath the skin by passing the needle and fixed end of the suture through the wound, exiting through the skin at a distance from the end of the wound (Figure 14-25). After tension is applied on the fixed end of the suture, the suture is cut flush with the skin and its end retracts beneath the surface.

SPECIAL SUTURES AND SITUATIONS

Mattress Sutures

Where approximation and eversion of the wound's edges is difficult, interrupted or continuous mattress sutures may also be used to close the skin. With *vertical mattress* sutures, the first bite is a large one, which includes equal amounts of tissue from either side of the wound, extending up to 1 cm outward from each side. The needle is then reversed and a smaller, more superficial, backhanded bite is taken 1 mm to 2 mm from the wound edges (Figure 14-26). Alternatively, vertical mattress sutures may be placed by starting with the small bite. After elevating the wound edges by traction on the first suture ends, the needle is reversed and a second, deep bite is taken.[16] This method is more rapid than the first, but the second bite is passed blindly, risking injury to underlying structures and creating asymmetry.

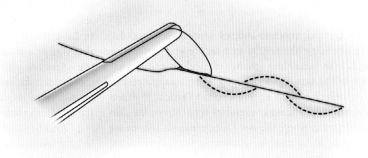

FIGURE 14-24

After the practitioner completes placement of the continuous dermal suture, the knot is tied by grasping a loop of suture material.

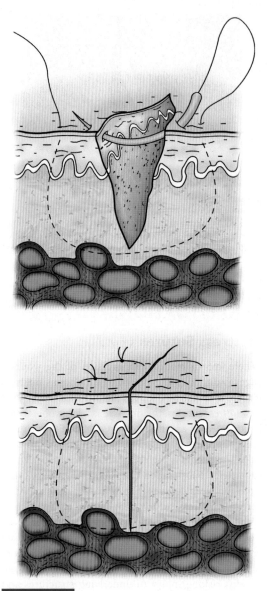

FIGURE 14-26

Formation of a vertical mattress suture: The first bite is taken far from the wound. The direction of the needle is reversed and a second bite is taken close to the wound edge.

Vertical mattress sutures serve two functions: (1) The large bite results in a secure grasp of tissue, and (2) the small bite achieves meticulous approximation of the skin–epidermal edges. This suture results in excellent wound edge eversion. Vertical mattress sutures are particularly useful in very thin or lax skin and in areas where the deep subcutaneous tissues are too poor to be used for anchoring tension-reducing sutures (for example, over the shin area). Vertical mat-

tress sutures also may be indicated when the wound edges tend to invert on closure. One of the major disadvantages of vertical mattress sutures, however, is that they may result in too much tension on the more superficial skin edges, which reduces blood supply to the skin. The ischemic skin may then undergo necrosis and become macerated, inviting infection, interfering with the healing process, and resulting in a poor scar.

With a *horizontal mattress* suture, the first bite is placed similar to a simple interrupted suture. Before one ties a knot, however, a second bite is taken adjacent to the first one by reversing the direction of the needle (Figure 14-27). This suture also results in wound edge eversion but the pressure on the skin that is caught within each horizontal bite may interfere with local circulation, resulting in necrosis. Initial placement of a horizontal mattress suture in the middle of the wound before closure with simple interrupted sutures makes it easier to obtain wound edge eversion. Horizontal mattress sutures can be used by the novice or in the case of difficult approximation as temporary sutures to facilitate wound edge eversion before initiating final repair with simple interrupted sutures. After placement of the simple sutures, the initial horizontal mattress suture can be removed and replaced with two simple interrupted sutures. This method facilitates excellent eversion that sometimes cannot be accomplished with simple sutures alone. The two horizontal and vertical mattress sutures may also be combined into an oblique mattress suture. As with all percutaneous sutures, special care should be taken to avoid tension to prevent cross-hatching marks.

Closing Wounds With Edges of Uneven Length

When the lengths of the two opposite sides of a wound are uneven, simple closure may result in distortion of adjacent skin, and sometimes formation of a dog ear at the wound's distal points. This may be avoided by placing the first suture in the exact midpoint of *each side* of the wound. Prior to tying the knot, it is helpful to hold the wound edges together with the suture that was placed in the middle of the wound to see if the edges are properly aligned. If the positioning is satisfactory, the knot is tied and the remaining sutures are placed by sequentially placing bisecting sutures in the remaining halves of the wound.

Another method to close wounds with uneven lengths without ending up with deformation or a dog ear is to place the sutures farther apart on the longer

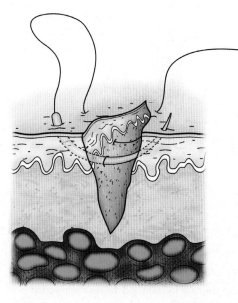

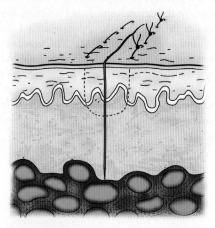

FIGURE 14-27

Formation of a horizontal mattress suture: The first bite is taken and the needle is reversed and a second bite is taken.

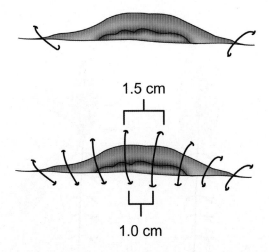

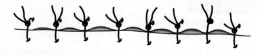

FIGURE 14-28

Alternative method for closing wounds whose edges are of uneven lengths: The distances between sutures on the longer side are greater than on the shorter side.

side of the wound (Figure 14-28). Once the central suture is placed and distal dog ears form, the rest of the sutures can be placed starting at the wound's ends and gradually advancing toward the center "stealing" longer segments from the longer wound edge and, thus, distributing the excess length equally along the entire length of the wound.

Sometimes, however, a dog ear is unavoidable. One method for managing a dog ear is presented in Figure 14-29. However, this method does elongate the scar.

Closing Wounds With Surfaces That Are Not Level

When one side of the wound is elevated and the other is depressed, deeper "bites" should be taken from the depressed side of the wound by inserting the needle at a deeper level on the depressed side (Figure 14-30). This will elevate that side.

Corner Stitches and Closure of Flaps

At times, the wound creates a flap or multiple flaps with narrow, poorly vascularized bases. This may occur, for example, with lacerations in the shape of a "V," "Y," or "X." Placement of percutaneous sutures through the end of such flaps may further compromise blood flow and cause necrosis of the skin at the tip. This outcome can be avoided by placing a half-buried, circular horizontal mattress suture in which the suture material is placed in the subcuticular region of the flap (Figure 14-31).

Placement of Buried Deep Sutures in Difficult Situations

Occasionally, placement of a buried deep dermal suture is difficult, especially when the dermis is partic-

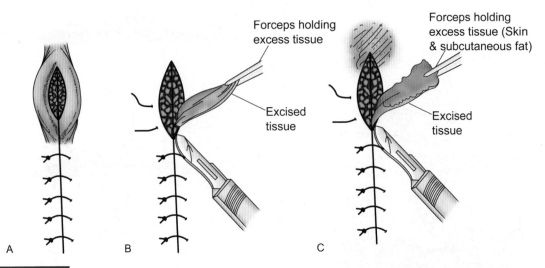

FIGURE 14-29

Method for managing a dog ear: The excessive tissue is removed with an elliptical incision and the resulting wound is closed. Undermining of the skin (as shown in red) facilitates a tension free closure.

ularly thin. In this situation a modified *buried* vertical mattress suture can be performed with a monofilament absorbable suture such as monocryl. The needle is inserted through the subcutaneous tissue on the left side of the wound and exits through the skin approximately 1 cm from the wound edge on the same side of the wound. The needle is then reversed and inserted through the same hole on the left side of the wound exiting just below the dermal–epidermal junction on the same side of the wound (Figure 14-32). The needle

is then inserted through the opposite, right side of the wound just below the dermal–epidermal junction and exits on that side through the skin approximately 1 cm from the wound edge (Figure 14-32). The needle is then reversed and inserted through the same hole and exits through the subcutaneous layer in the center of the wound. When the suture knot is formed and tightened, the suture material that pokes through the skin surface is pulled through the holes and, thus, is buried beneath the skin.

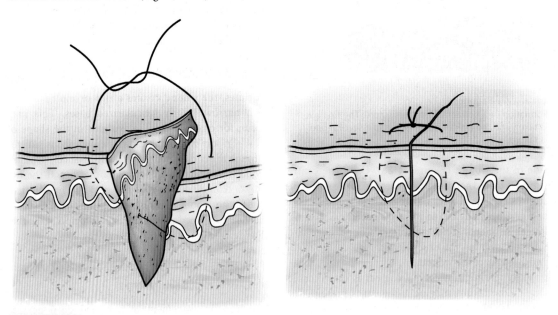

FIGURE 14-30

Closing wounds with surfaces on different levels: A "deeper" bite is taken from the depressed side, elevating it.

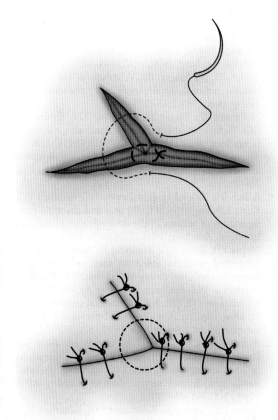

FIGURE 14-31

The half-buried horizontal mattress suture for closing corners and flaps: The needle is passed underneath the epidermis at the tip of the flap. The needle should enter and exit at the same level of the dermis on either side of the wound.

Tissue Undermining

Occasionally high tension on the wound makes it difficult to approximate wound edges. The amount of tension on the wound may be reduced by undermining the areas of the skin on either side of the wound. With undermining, tissue is recruited by cutting the attaching fibers and septi of the dermis and superficial fascia from deeper structures, which then allows a tension-free closure. The dissection should occur in the deep subdermal plane below the subdermal plexus (Figure 14-33). An upward scraping motion on the undersurface of the dermis is helpful when one is using a blade.

Undermining may be performed with scissors (either Iris or Metzenbaum scissors) or with a No. 15 scalpel. For accurate dissection, the skin to be undermined must be **pulled forward** following the direction

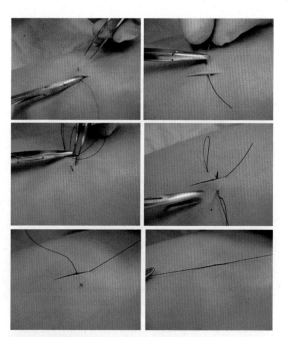

FIGURE 14-32

Placement of a buried vertical mattress suture. The needle is inserted through the subcutaneous tissue on the left side of the wound and exits through the skin approximately 1 cm from the wound edge on the same side of the wound (upper left). The needle is then reversed and inserted through the same hole on the left side of the wound exiting just below the dermal–epidermal junction on the same side of the wound (right upper). The needle is then inserted through the opposite, right side of the wound just below the dermal–epidermal junction and exits on that side through the skin approximately 1 cm from the wound edge (left middle). The needle is then reversed and inserted through the same hole and exits through the subcutaneous layer in the center of the wound (right middle). When the suture knot is formed and tightened, the suture material that pokes through the skin surface is pulled through the holes and (lower left), thus, is buried beneath the skin (lower right).

of the skin, not flipped backward as to expose the deeper tissues. The skin should be pulled forward with a skin hook, not forceps. If no skin hook is available, one can be fashioned by using forceps to bend back the point of a 21-gauge needle. As the skin is pulled a clear dissection plane is created and the scissors can be advanced along this plane (usually at the level of the deeper fascia) with preservation of the subcutaneous plexus and an even-thickness subcutaneous layer as a padding. Dissecting the subcutaneous layer and flipping the skin backward may bring the tip of the dissecting scissors into the very dangerous vicinity of the dermal plexus and sometimes may even penetrate the skin itself.

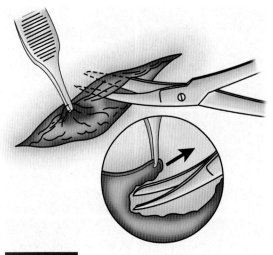

FIGURE 14-33

Method of tissue undermining: The superficial skin is pulled in the direction of the arrow and released from the deeper subcutaneous structure with scissors or by sweeping a No. 15 scalpel blade below the dermis.

REFERENCES

1. Singer AJ, Quinn JV, Thode HC Jr, Hollander JE; TraumaSeal Study Group. Determinants of poor outcome after laceration and incision repair. *Plast Reconstr Surg.* 2002;110(2):429–435.
2. Thacker JG, Borzelleca DC, Hunter JC, McGregor W, Rodeheaver GT, Edlich RF. Biomechanical analysis of needle holding security. *J Biomed Mater Res.* 1986; 20(7):903–917.
3. Stamp CV, McGregor W, Rodeheaver GT, Thacker JG, Towler MA, Edlich RF. Surgical needle holder damage to sutures. *Am Surg.* 1988;54(5):300–306.
4. Bond RF, McGregor W, Cutler PV, Becker DG, Thacker JG, Edlich RF. Influence of needle holder jaw configuration on the biomechanics of curved surgical needle bending. *J Appl Biomater.* 1990;1(1):39–47.
5. Abidin MR, Dunlapp JA, Towler MA, et al. Metallurgically bonded needle holder jaws. A technique to enhance needle holding security without sutural damage. *Am Surg.* 1990;56(10):643–647.
6. Hollander JE, Singer AJ, Valentine S, Henry MC. Wound registry: development and validation. *Ann Emerg Med.* 1995;25(5):675–685.
7. Hollander JE, Singer AJ, Valentine SM, Shofer FS. Risk factors for infection in patients with traumatic lacerations. *Acad Emerg Med.* 2001;8(7):716–720.
8. Myers BM, Cherry G. Functional and angiographic vasculature in healing wounds. *Am Surg.* 1970; 36(12):750–756.
9. Edlich RF, Panek PH, Rodeheaver GT, Turnbull VG, Kurtz LD, Edgerton MT. Physical and chemical configuration of sutures in the development of surgical infection. *Ann Surg.* 1973;177(6):679–688.
10. Mehta PH, Dunn KA, Bradfield JF, Austin PE. Contaminated wounds: infection rates with subcutaneous sutures. *Ann Emerg Med.* 1996;27(1):43–48.
11. Mazzarese PM, Faulkner BC, Gear AJ, Watkins FH, Rodeheaver GT, Edlich RF. Technical considerations in knot construction. Part II. Interrupted dermal suture closure. *J Emerg Med.* 1999;15(4):505–511.
12. Annunziata CC, Drake DB, Woods JA, Gear AJ, Rodeheaver GT, Edlich RF. Technical considerations in knot construction. Part I. Continuous percutaneous and dermal suture closure. *J Emerg Med.* 1999;15(3):351–356.
13. Winn HR, Jane RA, Rodeheaver G, Edgerton MT, Edlich RF. Influence of subcuticular sutures on scar formation. *Am J Surg.* 1977;133(2):257–259.
14. Singer AJ, Gulla J, Hein M, Marchini S, Chale S, Arora BP. Single-layer versus double-layer closure of facial lacerations: a randomized controlled trial. *Plast Reconstr Surg.* 2005;116(2):363–368.
15. Foster GE, Hardy EG, Hardcastle JD. Subcuticular suturing after appendectomy. *Lancet.* 1977;1(8022): 1128–1129.
16. Jones JS, Gartner M, Drew G, Pack S. The shorthand vertical mattress stitch: evaluation of a new suture technique. *Am J Emerg Med.* 1993;11(5):483–485.

Animal Bite Wounds

Esther H. Chen, MD

The true incidence of bite wounds from domestic and wild animals is difficult to estimate because many who sustain minor injuries do not seek medical evaluation unless an infection or other complication occurs. In the United States, an estimated 1 to 2 million animal bites are treated each year.[1] In 2001, an estimated 350,000 people were evaluated in emergency departments (EDs) for nonfatal dog bite injuries alone.[2] Not surprisingly, the majority of ED visits were for dog bites (60%), followed by cat bites (20%).[3] The goals of treatment are to restore function, ensure good cosmesis, facilitate healing, and prevent infection, the most common complication of bites. This chapter will focus primarily on the management of dog, cat, and human bite injuries and briefly discuss wild animal injuries.

Compared with adults, children have a higher risk of being bitten by dogs and less likely by cats.[2] Children often are bitten because they are small and ignorant about what is considered provocative behavior to a dog. Simple play or teasing may provoke a dog bite. For example, injured children were more likely to be petting, playing with, or feeding the animal, in contrast to adults who were more likely to be breaking up a fight between animals.[4] They are also three times more likely to be injured by other pets such as hamsters, gerbils, and rabbits.

By contrast, 80% of non-dog and non-cat bites (e.g., raccoon, rats, mice) occur in adults.[4] In particular, people in certain occupations (e.g., veterinarians, animal control workers, laboratory workers, zookeepers) and those that keep wild animals as pets have the highest risk of wild animal bites.[5]

Moreover, more pediatric injuries (75%) occur in the yard or home compared to 58% of adult bites.[4] For pediatric patients, more often than not the animal may be observed or its immunization history may be obtainable. In adult patients, however, one third of animal exposures occur in the park or public streets, where information about the animal would be difficult to obtain.

The injury pattern also differs between adults and children and by the type of animal. Injuries to the head, face, neck, and trunk are more commonly seen in children whereas upper-extremity injuries are more common in adults.[4] Almost all bat bites and 84% of rodent bites involve the hand or arm. Superficial wounds are seen in two thirds of the pediatric patients, compared with 50% of the adult wounds. In addition, dogs are more likely to cause lacerations because they have large teeth that can crush and tear tissue whereas the small sharp teeth of cats are more likely to cause puncture wounds.

BACTERIOLOGY

Dog and cat bite wounds are typically infected with mixed aerobic and anaerobic bacteria,[6] with a few pathogens that are unique to the biter's oral flora. The bacteriology of dog bites is more complex and polymicrobial than cat bites. The most common pathogen is *Pasteurella* species, isolated from 50% of dog and 75% of cat bites. In infected dog bites, the most common strain is *P canis* (26%) whereas *P multocida* (75%) is most commonly implicated in cat bites. Oral flora (e.g., *Streptococcus* species) dominate human skin flora (i.e., *Staphylococcus aureus*) in bite infection isolates, particularly for puncture wounds. Other anaerobic pathogens include *Fusobacterium nucleatum*, *Bacteroides tectum*, *Porphyromonas* species, and *Prevotella heparinolytica*. Aerobic isolates include *Moraxella*, *Corynebacterium*, and *Neisseria* species.[6]

An important pathogen associated with dog bites is *Capnocytophaga canimorsus*, a gram-negative bacillus found in the normal oral flora. It is a fastidious organism that can cause severe sepsis with disseminated intravascular coagulopathy, cutaneous gangrene, and multiorgan failure, especially in asplenic, immunocompromised, and chronic alcoholic patients, but also in healthy patients.[3] In a case series of septic patients for whom the mortality rate was 31%, more than 50% of infections were caused by dog bites, and 10% were attributable to licking.[7]

Pasteurella multocida, the major pathogen in cat bite infections, is a gram-negative coccobacillus that can incite an intense inflammatory response, typically within 24 hours of injury. It can cause serious infections such as necrotizing fasciitis, septic arthritis, and osteomyelitis.[3] Less commonly, it has been implicated in a variety of systemic illnesses including pneumonia in patients with underlying pulmonary disease, meningitis and brain abscesses in infants and elderly patients, spontaneous bacterial peritonitis in AIDS patients, and bacteremia in patients with liver dysfunction.[8]

Similar to animal bite infections, human bite wound infections are typically caused by mixed anaerobic and aerobic bacteria, most commonly *Streptococcus* species (84%), *Prevotella* species (36%), *Fusobacterium* species (34%), *S aureus* (30%), *Eikenella corrodens* (30%), and *Veillonella* species (24%).[9] Pure gram-negative infections are uncommon.[10]

Eikenella corrodens, a gram-negative rod, is the infecting organism in 7% to 29% of human bites and is very common in clenched-fist injuries (when the closed fist strikes the teeth of someone's mouth).[11] A local wound infection develops within 24 to 36 hours after the injury; systemic symptoms and signs are uncommon. *Eikenella* is an important cause of chronic infection, osteomyelitis, and loss of joint function in the hand[12] and has also been associated with abdominal abscesses, meningitis, endocarditis, and fatal gram-negative sepsis.[13]

CLINICAL PRESENTATION

Patients seek medical attention either immediately following the exposure for wound management or when infectious complications occur. Acute symptoms depend on the type of animal inflicting the injury.

Large animals such as dogs have teeth that can tear the skin and cause lacerations, whereas small animals such as cats or rodents have small, sharp teeth that can cause puncture wounds. Large animals can also inflict other blunt trauma either by direct impact with their body or by causing falls.[5]

Human bites are categorized as either occlusional bites (when the teeth sink into and crush the skin tissue) or clenched-fist injuries. Also known as "fight bites," clenched-fist injuries commonly involve the fourth metacarpophalangeal joint of the dominant hand. These wounds may appear minor on the surface of the skin, yet they may have underlying bone or metacarpal joint injury. Involvement of the deeper structures is easy to miss on initial assessment. Small lacerations over a dorsal metacarpophalangeal joint should be considered a human bite and evaluated accordingly.

Wound infections presenting with erythema, induration, lymphangitis, or purulent drainage can develop rapidly, within 24 to 72 hours after injury.[14] Infectious complications include local cellulitis, abcess, osteomyelitis, septic arthritis, and tenosynovitis.[14]

EVALUATION AND TREATMENT

The goals of wound management are to promote healing, prevent infection, restore function, and maintain aesthetics. Local wound care begins with a thorough evaluation of the injury and documentation of the location, number, type, and depth of the wounds, as well as any signs of wound infection.

Bite wounds are notoriously deceptive and wounds that appear minor may actually be more extensive and involve deeper structures. Wounds should be explored for foreign bodies and concurrent injury to tendons, joint spaces, and bone. Special attention should be paid to clenched-fist injuries. Because they are injured when the hand is clenched, the site of skin penetration will move proximal to the metacarpal head when the hand is extended during evaluation and the underlying joint capsule and tendon sheath may appear normal. To avoid missing a deeper tissue injury, the wound must be explored throughout the entire range of motion. In addition, if bony penetration or embedded foreign bodies (e.g., embedded teeth in cat bites) are suspected, a radiograph of the site of injury should be performed.

After examination, all wounds should be thoroughly cleaned and irrigated with normal saline. One prospective ED study showed that irrigation with a 1% povidone–iodine solution for 60 seconds decreased infection rates in sutured traumatic lacerations[15] whereas another ED study of traumatic wounds showed no difference in infection rate between normal saline, 1% povidone-iodine solution, and pluronic F-68 (Shur-Clens).[16] Nevertheless, because of the potential for disease transmission, irrigating with 1% povidone–iodine solution may be helpful in grossly contaminated bite wounds.

Some wounds require generous débridement with a scalpel of devitalized tissues, including tissue embedded with organisms, soil, and clots that may be difficult to remove by mechanical irrigation. After débridement, the wound should be irrigated again to remove any remaining contamination.

Superficial abrasions and puncture wounds should be covered with a topical antimicrobial agent, which reduces infection in traumatic lacerations.[17] Alternatively, abrasions may be covered with an absorbent, occlusive dressing, which creates a moist environment to promote healing[18] and reduce infection.[19] Patients should change the dressing daily and be followed closely for wound infection.

Most lacerations, even on the extremities, may undergo primary closure after good local wound care. Infection rates after wound closure have been reported in the literature to be 5.5% to 7.7%.[20,21] These rates are acceptable in wounds where cosmesis is important, such as facial wounds (Figure 15-1) or large extremity wounds[20] In a study of dog bites to the head and neck, the infection rate of wounds that were primarily

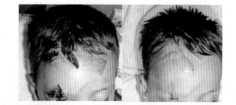

Laceration repair of facial dog bite wounds.

repaired and not treated with antibiotics was 1.4%.[22] Very small lacerations (<1.5 cm) may behave as puncture wounds and should be allowed to heal by secondary intent.[23] Large wounds requiring reconstructive surgery should be referred to the appropriate speciaist. Delayed primary closure may be used to treat lacerations that are heavily contaminated or that involve the hand, where bacteria are inoculated into the wound and trapped within the small compartments and numerous fascial planes. Injured extremities should be immobilized and elevated.

ANTIBIOTICS

Infected wounds should be treated with the appropriate antibiotics against the most likely offending organism (Table 15-1). Infections from dog and cat bites that develop within 24 hours are likely caused by

TABLE 15–1	**Antibiotic Recommendations for Outpatient Therapy and Prophylaxis**		
		Oral Antibiotic Regimen	
Bite	*Predominant Pathogens*	*Primary*	*Alternate*
Dog	*Pasteurella multocida* *Streptococcus* species *Staphylococcus aureus* *Capnocytophaga cani-morsus* Anaerobes	Amoxicillin–clavulanate 875/125 mg, twice daily	Clindamycin 300 mg orally three times daily + fluoroquinolone ciprofloxacin 500 mg twice daily (adults) or clindamycin 20-40 mg/kg/day divided three times daily + TMP/SMX 10 mg/kg/day TMP divided twice daily (children)
Cat	*P multocida* *S aureus*	Amoxicillin–clavulanate 875/125 mg, twice daily	Cefuroxime axetil 0.5 gm twice daily or doxycycline 100 mg orally, twice daily
Human	*S aureus* *Eikenella corrodens* Anaerobes	Amoxicillin–clavulanate 875/125 mg, twice daily	Clindamycin 300 mg three times daily + fluoroquinolone ciprofloxacin 500 mg twice daily (adults) or clindamycin 20-40 mg/kg/day divided three times daily + TMP/SMX 10 mg/kg/day TMP divided twice daily (children)

Note. TMP/SMX = trimethoprim–sulfamethoxazole.

P multocida whereas symptoms that develop after 24 hours are more likely caused by *Staphylococcus* or *Streptococcus* species.[6,23] Treatment of human bite infections should cover *S aureus, E corrodens*, and anaerobic bacteria.[9] Wound cultures should be obtained for all infections, if possible. Patients with local cellulitis, no deep structure involvement, or who lack systemic symptoms may be treated as outpatients. Amoxicillin–clavulanate is a good initial oral antibiotic of choice that provides broad coverage for all bite wounds. Patients with a penicillin and cephalosporin allergy may be given a fluoroquinolone, doxycycline, or macrolide antibiotic. Alternative regimens include clindamycin and either a fluoroquinolone (adults) or trimethoprim–sulfamethoxazole (children).[13] Outpatient oral treatment should continue for 7 to 10 days. Patients should be followed closely and re-evaluated every 2 days.

Patients with systemic symptoms and signs, complicated infections (e.g., tenosynovitis, osteomyelitis, lymphangitis), or failed outpatient therapy should be admitted for parenteral antibiotics and surgical consultation. Ampicillin–sulbactam, nafcillin, or imipenem–cilastatin with gentamicin (only if one suspects a gram-negative organism) are good antibiotic regimens.

Superficial bite wounds in adults and children do not benefit from antibiotic prophylaxis. Uninfected, high-risk wounds (Table 15-2) should be considered for antibiotic prophylaxis, even though prophylactic antibiotics have not been shown to significantly reduce infection rates of most bite wounds[24] (although the trials analyzed in this meta-analysis were small and very heterogeneous). Specifically, this study found no difference in infection rates when analyzed by animal type (dog versus human versus cat bites), injury type (puncture versus lacerations), or wound location (forearm

versus head and neck). The only subgroups for which antibiotic prophylaxis decreased the infection rate included patients with hand bites (2% [antibiotic] versus 28% [control]) and human bites (0% [antibiotic] versus 47% [control]).[24] For dog bite injuries, a meta-analysis of eight randomized trials of antibiotic prophylaxis showed that the relative risk for infection was extremely low (0.58)[25] and a subsequent study of the same data showed that it was not cost-effective to prescribe antibiotics for all uninfected dog bite wounds.[26]

Hand bites and human bites, especially clenched-fist injuries,[27] have such a high risk of infection that those patients should be given prophylaxis. Dog and cat bite wounds that are full-thickness and deep, contain devitalized tissue, or are heavily contaminated also should be given prophylactic antibiotics.

Once the decision is made to give antibiotics, some clinicians recommend that the first dose of antibiotics be administered parenterally to ensure rapid tissue penetration,[13] despite the lack of supporting data. This approach is reasonable but should not be considered the standard of care. The same antibiotics used to treat infections are also given for prophylaxis. Patients should be prescribed a 3- to 5-day course.

TETANUS AND RABIES IMMUNOPROPHYLAXIS

Do not forget to address the need for tetanus immunoprophylaxis. Bite wounds should be considered tetanus-prone injuries.

All patients with bite wounds should be assessed for the need for postexposure rabies immunoprophylaxis. Although animal bites are frequently encountered in the clinical setting, human rabies is a rare though fatal disease.[28] The virus is transmitted through a bite from a clinically ill animal, enters the central nervous system, and causes an acute, progressive encephalomyelitis. In the United States, most cases of human rabies occur from exposure to wild animals, primarily raccoons, skunks, foxes, and bats.[29] Rodents and lagomorphs (i.e., rabbits and hares) rarely harbor rabies. Over the past few years, the majority of cases have been from bat exposures. The Advisory Committee on Immunization Practices' recommendations for rabies prophylaxis should be followed (Table 15-3). Local and state public health officials may be consulted for individual cases.

Postexposure prophylaxis consists of human rabies immunoglobulin and the 4- or 5-dose series of rabies vaccine. In 2009, the Advisory Committee on Immunization Practices removed the fifth dose of vaccine for all immunocompetent persons; the fifth

TABLE 15–2	**Recommendations for Antibiotic Prophylaxis**

Wound location
  Hand or wrist; penetration into joint space
Wound type
  Deep puncture wounds; extensive crush injury; involvement of underlying tendon, muscle, or bone; retained foreign body
Patient characteristics
  Orthopedic prosthesis; immunocompromised state; prosthetic or diseased cardiac valve
Animal type
  Large wild cats, pigs

TABLE 15–3	Postexposure Rabies Immunoprophylaxis Guide: Advisory Committee on Immunization Practices Recommendations, 2008[29]	
Animal Type	**Animal Characteristics**	**Recommendations**
Domestic dogs, cats, and ferrets	Rabid	Immediate prophylaxis
	Healthy and can be confined and observed for 10 days	No prophylaxis unless the animal develops signs of rabies
	Unknown	Consult local health officials because rabies risk has regional variation
Raccoons, skunks, foxes, and most carnivores	All are considered to be rabid unless the animal is available for testing	Immediate prophylaxis unless the animal tested negative for rabies
Bats	Regarded as rabid unless the animal has tested negative; includes any bite or non-bite (e.g., sleeping with a bat in the room) exposure	Immediate prophylaxis
Small rodents (squirrels, mice, hamsters, gerbils), large rodents (chipmunks), and lagomorphs (rabbits, hares)	Rarely infected with rabies; risk only in areas where raccoon rabies is enzootic	Consult public health officials; rarely require prophylaxis

dose is still recommended for immunocompromised persons.[30] Immunization with rabies immunoglobulin provides passive immunity for a few weeks (half-life of 21 days) until the active antibody response to the vaccine develops (within 7 to 10 days).[29, 30] If anatomically feasible, as much of the immunoglobulin (20 IU/kg) should be administered into the wound and the remainder intramuscularly in the gluteal region. In adults, the vaccine should be administered in the deltoid region whereas in younger children, the outer aspect of the thigh should be used to ensure intramuscular administration. Patients should return for the remainder of the series on days 0, 3, 7, and 14, and, if immunocompromised, on day 28.

Reactions to the rabies vaccine are predominantly local and mild, including pain at the injection site, redness, swelling, and induration. Systemic symptoms include headache, dizziness, myalgias, nausea, and weakness. Serious systemic reactions such as anaphylaxis and neuroparalytic reactions are rare.

WILD ANIMALS

Wild animals can cause tearing, penetrating, and crushing injuries, combined with falls and other blunt trauma. All patients should have a thorough trauma evaluation for injuries that are less obvious than the bite wound.[5]

The management of wild animal bites is either extrapolated from studies of dog and cat bites or anecdotal. Because many exposures occur in remote or wilderness settings, the delay in seeking medical care increases the risk of infection. Moreover, certain animals (e.g., wild cats, pigs, large carnivores) inflict wounds that are prone to infection.[5] Similar to other animal bites, puncture wounds and wounds that are heavily contaminated or involve the hand should be treated with delayed primary closure or left to heal by secondary intent. All other lacerations may be repaired primarily. Prophylactic antibiotics are reasonable for extremity injuries, immunocompromised patients, large cat and pig exposures, puncture wounds, and severe crushing injuries.

COMPLICATIONS

As mentioned previously, the most frequent complication of bites is wound infection. Severe systemic diseases such as sepsis, osteomyelitis, meningitis, endocarditis, and peritonitis have been seen not only in patients with impaired immunity and chronic diseases, but also in healthy hosts. Animal bites can transmit other diseases including cat-scratch fever (*Bartonella henselae*), tularemia (*Franciscella tularensis*), leptospirosis, brucellosis, and rat-bite fever (*Spirillum minus*).[14] Human bites can transmit hepatitis B, hepatitis C, syphilis, herpes simplex, tuberculosis, actinomycosis, tetanus, and HIV.[14]

MANDATORY REPORTING

Finally, remember that many local governments mandate reporting of all domestic and wild animal bites to the health department. Public health departments can assist in coordinating follow-up with the animal, its owner, and the patient that was bitten.

REFERENCES

1. Weiss HB, Friedman DI, Coben JH. Incidence of dog bite injuries treated in emergency departments. *JAMA*. 1998;279(1):51–53.
2. Centers for Disease Control and Prevention. Nonfatal dog bite-related injuries treated in hospital emergency departments—United States, 2001. *MMWR Morb Mortal Wkly Rep*. 2003;52(26):605–610.
3. Oehler RL, Velez AP, Mizrachi M, Lamarche J, Gompf S. Bite-related and septic syndromes caused by cats and dogs. *Lancet Infect Dis*. 2009;9(7):439–447.
4. Steele MT, Ma OJ, Nakase J, et al. Epidemiology of animal exposures presenting to emergency departments. *Acad Emerg Med*. 2007;14(5):398–403.
5. Freer L. North American wild mammalian injuries. *Emerg Med Clin North Am*. 2004;22(2):445–473, ix.
6. Talan DA, Citron DM, Abrahamian FM, Moran GJ, Goldstein EJ. Bacteriologic analysis of infected dog and cat bites. Emergency Medicine Animal Bite Infection Study Group. *N Engl J Med*. 1999;340(2):85–92.
7. Pers C, Gahrn-Hansen B, Frederiksen W. Capnocytophaga canimorsus septicemia in Denmark, 1982-1995: review of 39 cases. *Clin Infect Dis*. 1996;23(1):71–75.
8. Weber DJ, Wolfson JS, Swartz MN, Hooper DC. Pasteurella multocida infections. Report of 34 cases and review of the literature. *Medicine (Baltimore)*. 1984;63(3):133–154.
9. Talan DA, Abrahamian FM, Moran GJ, Citron DM, Tan JO, Goldstein EJ; Emergency Medicine Human Bite Infection Study Group. Clinical presentation and bacteriologic analysis of infected human bites in patients presenting to emergency departments. *Clin Infect Dis*. 2003;37(11):1481–1489.
10. Zubowicz VN, Gravier M. Management of early human bites of the hand: a prospective randomized study. *Plast Reconstr Surg*. 1991;88(1):111–114.
11. Faciszewski T, Coleman DA. Human bite wounds. *Hand Clin*. 1989;5(4):561–569.
12. Schmidt DR, Heckman JD. Eikenella corrodens in human bite infections of the hand. *J Trauma*. 1983;23(6):478–482.
13. Nakamura Y, Daya M. Use of appropriate antimicrobials in wound management. *Emerg Med Clin North Am*. 2007;25(1):159–176.
14. Brook I. Management of human and animal bite wounds: an overview. *Adv Skin Wound Care*. 2005;18(4):197–203.
15. Gravett A, Sterner S, Clinton JE, Ruiz E. A trial of povidone-iodine in the prevention of infection in sutured lacerations. *Ann Emerg Med*. 1987;16(2):167–171.
16. Dire DJ, Welsh AP. A comparison of wound irrigation solutions used in the emergency department. *Ann Emerg Med*. 1990;19(6):704–708.
17. Dire DJ, Coppola M, Dwyer DA, Lorette JJ, Karr JL. Prospective evaluation of topical antibiotics for preventing infections in uncomplicated soft-tissue wounds repaired in the ED. *Acad Emerg Med*. 1995;2(1):4–10.
18. Field FK, Kerstein MD. Overview of wound healing in a moist environment. *Am J Surg*. 1994;167(1A):2S–6S.
19. Hutchinson JJ, Lawrence JC. Wound infection under occlusive dressings. *J Hosp Infect*. 1991;17(2):83–94.
20. Chen E, Hornig S, Shepherd SM, Hollander JE. Primary closure of mammalian bites. *Acad Emerg Med*. 2000;7(2):157–161.
21. Maimaris C, Quinton DN. Dog-bite lacerations: a controlled trial of primary wound closure. *Arch Emerg Med*. 1988;5(3):156–161.
22. Guy RJ, Zook EG. Successful treatment of acute head and neck dog bite wounds without antibiotics. *Ann Plast Surg*. 1986;17(1):45–48.
23. Dire DJ. Cat bite wounds: risk factors for infection. *Ann Emerg Med*. 1991;20(9):973–979.
24. Medeiros I, Saconato H. Antibiotic prophylaxis for mammalian bites. *Cochrane Database Syst Rev*. 2001(2):CD001738.
25. Cummings P. Antibiotics to prevent infection in patients with dog bite wounds: a meta-analysis of randomized trials. *Ann Emerg Med*. 1994;23(3):535–540.
26. Callaham M. Prophylactic antibiotics in dog bite wounds: nipping at the heels of progress. *Ann Emerg Med*. 1994;23(3):577–579.
27. Gilchrist J, Sacks JJ, White D, Kresnow MJ. Dog bites: still a problem? *Inj Prev*. 2008;14(5):296–301.
28. Moran GJ, Talan DA, Mower W, et al. Appropriateness of rabies postexposure prophylaxis treatment for animal exposures. Emergency ID Net Study Group. *JAMA*. 2000;284(8):1001–1007.
29. Manning SE, Rupprecht CE, Fishbein D, et al. Human rabies prevention—United States, 2008: recommendations of the Advisory Committee on Immunization Practices. *MMWR Recomm Rep*. 2008;57(RR-3):1–28.
30. Advisory Committee on Immunization Practices. Use of a reduced (4-dose) vaccine schedule for postexposure prophylaxis to prevent human rabies. *MMWR Recomm Rep*. 2010; 59(RR-2):1-12.

Foreign Bodies in Wounds

Anthony J. Dean, MD

Although most wounds heal without complications, those containing foreign bodies are at increased risk of delayed healing, prolonged inflammation, and infection.[1-5] Failure to identify foreign bodies is a leading cause of malpractice torts brought against emergency physicians.[6] One retrospective series determined that 38% of foreign bodies were overlooked on initial examination. Thus, the first step in the accurate identification of a foreign body is the consideration that it might exist: any wound should be approached as the potential site of an occult foreign body.[7,8]

There are a variety of difficulties associated with accurate identification and management of soft-tissue foreign bodies. In addition to patients' uncertainty or ignorance about the existence of the object, physical examination is unreliable, and may be limited in patients with altered sensorium. Although radiopaque foreign bodies (e.g., metal, glass, gravel) are usually identifiable on plain radiography, radiolucent objects such as wood and plastic are not, necessitating other imaging modalities that are more cumbersome and more time-consuming, and may also fail to identify many foreign bodies.[7,9,10] Conversely, unnecessary exploration for a foreign body is time-consuming, stressful to both physician and patient, and creates an iatrogenic wound, frequently in cosmetically and functionally important areas, leading to increased tissue damage, and the risk of complications.[3,5]

Although there is a continuum between microscopic debris and grossly identifiable foreign bodies, the discussion in this chapter will be limited to objects that are large enough to be visually identified and that are not removed by high-pressure irrigation and other routine techniques of wound cleansing discussed in detail in Chapter 4. With an appropriately high index of suspicion for foreign body when one is approaching any wound, management can be broken down into three phases: detection, clinical decisions about removal, and procedures for removal, if indicated.

FOREIGN BODY DETECTION

Clinical evaluation

As in most areas of clinical practice, decisions about testing and management are based on the history and physical examination. Although the goal is to identify all foreign bodies at the time of the patient's first presentation to the health care system (ideally immediately following the injury), some foreign bodies are either unidentifiable or overlooked, so that clinicians should be familiar with the delayed findings of retained foreign body. Clinical clues to both acute and chronic foreign bodies are listed in Table 16-1.

TABLE 16–1	Clinical Findings Suggestive of Acute and Chronic Foreign Body
History	**Physical Examination**
Acute/Immediate	**Acute/Immediate**
Laceration caused by glass	Palpable mass, raised deformity
Patient perception of object that broke in wound	Focal, discontinuous, or deep tenderness on superficial or indirect palpation of wound
Patient sensation of retained foreign body	Grating or resistance on blunt exploration of wound
Bullet, blast, or other high-velocity missile injuries	Discontinuous or deep tenderness on palpation of anesthetized wound
Proximity to high-pressure hydraulic or injection devices	
Blunt oral trauma with tooth fractures	
Injuries to knuckles (suspected clenched-fist injury)	
Delayed	**Delayed**
Occurrence of infection in low-risk wounds	Chronic tenderness, swelling, erythema, mass
Recurrent infections	Abscess formation
Delayed nerve, vessel, or tendon injuries	Chronic draining sinus
Nonhealing wounds	Distal neurovascular effects including ischemia, edema, neuropathy
Persistent pain, especially with activity	Musculoskeletal effects including decreased range of motion

A common-sense approach combined with an understanding of high-risk injuries is necessary. Injuries caused by unbroken sharp metal objects (such as tools and knives) are unlikely to harbor a foreign body. Conversely, wounds caused by friable or frangible objects, especially glass, are at high risk.[11] Thin needles, thorns, and spines often penetrate soft tissue deeply before breaking off. Any but the most superficial wood splinter injuries are highly prone to retained foreign body, and those in the sole of the foot or hand should be viewed with particular suspicion for two reasons. First, the puncturing forces involved are often considerable, resulting in deeply buried foreign bodies. Second, foreign bodies in these locations that become infected may result in the most disabling sequellae. Injuries in which the patient states that he or she thinks that the injuring object broke in the wound or that he or she can feel a foreign body are at significantly increased risk.[11,12]

A useful question to ask patients after any laceration is "was the object that caused this wound broken before, during, or after your injury?" Although many patients will respond that they are "not sure," an affirmative answer may be the only clue to the presence of an occult foreign body, whereas a definitely negative answer can be reassuring. Bites, clenched-fist injuries, and intraoral lacerations may contain tooth fragments.

Finally, the history will be the basis for recognition of high-pressure injected liquid foreign body, which should be suspected in patients presenting with unexplained painless swelling of the hand and an occupation in proximity to high-pressure hydraulic or injection equipment. These initially innocuous-appearing injuries can be devastating and require emergent operative débridement with massive saline lavage (Figure 16-1).[13]

On examination, linear lacerations, especially if the base of the wound can be inspected and is no deeper than the subcutaneous fat, are less likely to contain a foreign body, whereas puncture wounds are more so.[11,12,14] Wounds that extend beyond the dermis are at significantly greater risk of harboring a foreign body, even with careful inspection.[15] Raised irregularities in the vicinity of a wound suggest a foreign body, especially if palpation causes deep tenderness. Because any wound is locally tender, a technique of indirect palpation is often useful. The examiner tries to get a sense of deeper injuries or foreign body by palpation at a point removed from the immediate area of pain and swelling. This may not be possible over bony structures, but is usually possible in areas where the soft tissues are loose and palpation can be performed perpendicular to the path of a penetrating object. It is also important to consider this technique when one is eval-

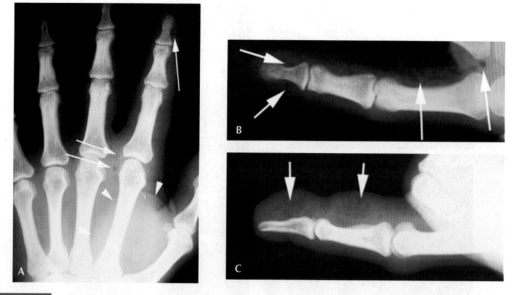

FIGURE 16-1

This patient presented with painless swelling of his index finger and thumb. The patient's occupation working with high-pressure hydraulic equipment was confirmed. Plain radiographs revealed extensive soft tissue gas (arrows), a collection of fluid in the thenar region (arrowheads, A), and a metallic foreign body (thumb web-space, A). The fluid was drained operatively, and the patient was able to return to work despite permanent impairment of the range of motion of his index finger and thumb.

uating wounds caused by high-velocity objects, which may result in foreign bodies that are unexpectedly distant from the site of a puncture wound that they caused. This is attributable to the fact that an object that has the kinetic energy to penetrate the skin, which is highly resilient, can travel remarkable distances when it reaches the looser areolar subdermal tissues (see Figure 16-2).

Most wounds cannot be effectively explored without local anesthesia. To avoid anesthetization twice, many clinicians will obtain imaging studies after completion of the clinical examination, and prior to exploration if the wound is at risk for a foreign body. If the nature and location of a foreign body is known with certainty it may be more expeditious to proceed directly to exploration.

Any wound with unexplained delayed or impaired healing is suspicious for retained foreign body (Table 16-1). Findings may include abscess formation, recurrent infections, fistulae, or abnormal and increasing fibrosis manifested by an enlarging indurated or granulomatous mass at the site of a wound. The historical factors discussed previously should be reviewed. Puncture wounds to the feet, especially through the rubber sole of a shoe, are notoriously prone to pseudomonal infections, including osteomyelitis, frequently with a delayed onset of months.[16,17] In evaluating chronic wounds at risk for retained foreign bodies, the clinician should bear in mind that, by their nature, puncture wounds are both less effectively lavaged and less thoroughly explored at the time of original injury, which, in addition to the mechanism itself, renders them more susceptible to a retained foreign body.

Detection of Foreign Body by Diagnostic Imaging Studies

Diagnostic imaging should be considered in the management of wounds with any of the following indications:

1. History of possible or definite foreign body
2. History of injury or puncture wound by an object at risk for fragmentation
3. History of injury at risk for multiple foreign bodies
4. After removal of multiple or friable or fragmented foreign body

The choice of imaging modality will depend on the nature of the presumed foreign body, and its location. The advantages and disadvantages of each are discussed in detail subsequently and are summarized in Table 16–2. As a general rule, foreign bodies become harder to identify by any modality as they become

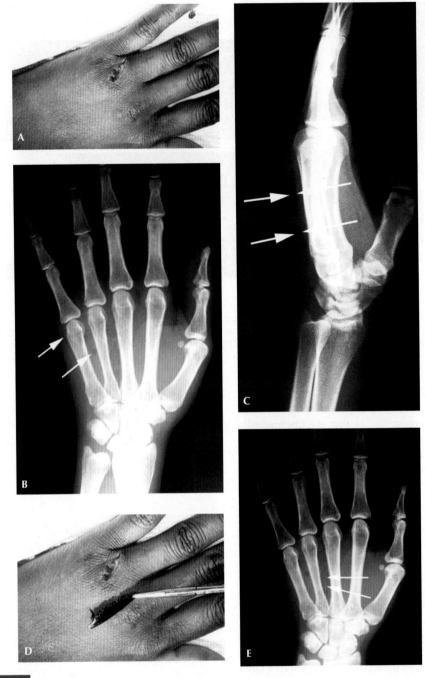

FIGURE 16-2

This patient presented with an injury after putting his hand into the moving plastic blades of an electric fan. The patient did not have the sensation of a foreign body but stated that "the blade went everywhere." His presenting wound appeared as a simple laceration of the knuckle (A). Radiographs showed soft tissue gas (arrows B and C) but no definite foreign body. In view of the potential for foreign bodies, meticulous efforts with optimal lighting were made to examine the entire depth of the wound, which tracked along the tendon sheaths of the dorsum of the hand. The search revealed the presence of a foreign body almost 4 cm proximal to the skin defect. This was removed (D). Retrospective review of the anteroposterior radiograph showed a questionable foreign body shadow (arrowheads, E).

TABLE 16–2	Comparison of Imaging Modalities for the Detection of Foreign Bodies	
Imaging Modality	**Advantages**	**Disadvantages**
Plain radiography	Readily available Easy to interpret Shows most foreign bodies	Two-dimensional Organic material not identified Ionizing radiation
Ultrasound	No radiation Bedside availability for many clinicians Can assist in localization and removal	Operator dependency Many causes of false-positive or false-negative examinations
Fluoroscopy	Real-time exploration Can assist in localization and removal	More ionizing radiation than plain film (patient and clinician) Organic material not identified Limited availability
Computed tomography	Improved sensitivity for radiolucent foreign bodies Shows relationship of foreign bodies to surrounding anatomic structures	More costly More ionizing radiation than fluoroscopy Need to specify fine (1 mm to 2 mm) cuts for small foreign body: more ionizing radiation More organic materials identified than fluoroscopy, but many missed
Magnetic resonance imaging	May be more sensitive than computed tomography May identify wider range of materials Shows relationship of foreign body to surrounding anatomic structures No radiation	Limited scientific data More costly Must exclude the possibility of metallic foreign bodies Limited availability

smaller and their density approaches that of surrounding soft tissues. For this reason, absolute rules about the reliability of the various imaging modalities cannot be made because of idiosyncratic features of wounds and foreign bodies. Such features include size, thickness, composition, orientation, the type of surrounding soft tissues, time elapsed since injury (causing changes in both surrounding tissues and the foreign body itself, if organic), proximity of bones, and presence of gas in the wound. Thus, negative findings in any imaging test should be used with caution, and further steps taken if warranted by the clinical suspicion.

Plain radiography

Of all the imaging studies used, plain radiography is the most readily available, easiest to interpret, and least expensive. Metal, bone, teeth, pencil graphite, certain plastics, glass, and gravel are visible on most plain radiographs (Figures 16-3, 16-4, 16-5, and 16-6).[9,10,18,19] Sometimes radiolucent foreign bodies such as sand, fish bones, wood, and aluminum are

sufficiently large or dense, or surrounded by gas, to allow them to be distinguished from surrounding soft tissues, so plain radiography may be the initial imaging modality of choice even with such foreign objects, as long as the limitations of a negative study are not overlooked.

Almost all glass fragments of 2 mm or larger, and more than half of glass fragments between 0.5 mm and 2.0 mm, are visible on radiographs.[9] Glass does not have to contain lead to be visible on plain films.[19] Long, thin foreign bodies appear smaller but are more easily detected if they lie parallel to the x-ray beam, because they cause greater attenuation of the x-ray beam. The contrast between foreign bodies and surrounding tissue is enhanced by using "soft tissue technique" (underpenetrated compared to typical skeletal x-ray intensity), although this makes it harder to identify foreign bodies that are overlying bone.[20] A wound known to have been caused by metal or glass with no foreign body on wound exploration or plain film is unlikely to harbor a foreign body. Radiopaque foreign bodies are difficult to identify adjacent to, or embedded within, bone.

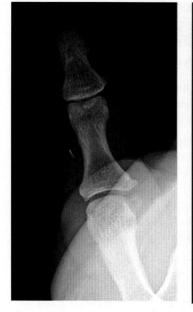

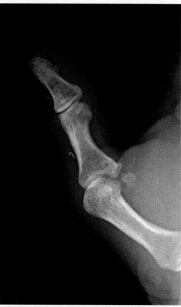

FIGURE 16-3

This plain film shows a wire foreign body adjacent to the proximal phalanx of the thumb.

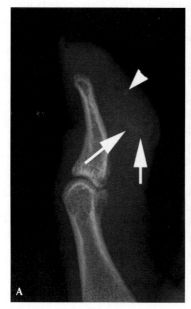

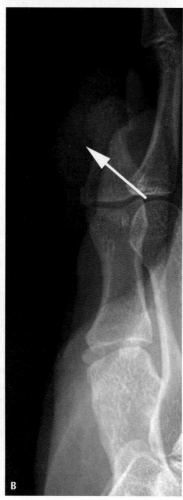

FIGURE 16-4

This plain film of a thumb laceration caused by breaking glass shows how much the appearance of a thin glass foreign body differs in appearance when viewed *en face* (A arrowhead) or on edge (B arrow). This film also demonstrates the appearance of soft tissue densities in wounds (in this case caused by clotted blood: A, arrows), which may be mistaken for foreign bodies. Foreign bodies can usually be distinguished by the presence of a complete perimeter and the presence of "on edge" density as in B.

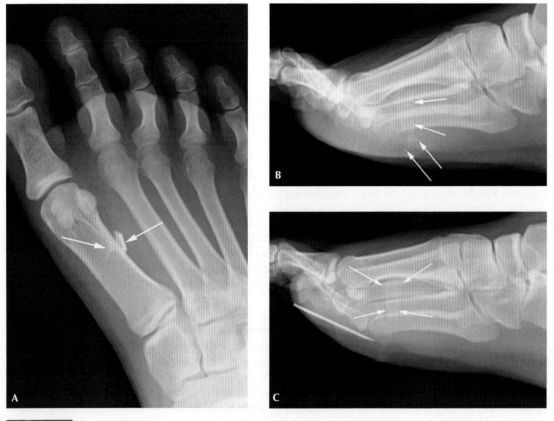

FIGURE 16-5

This patient presented with a foot laceration caused by a piece of glass. The initial anterior-posterior plain film shows two obvious foreign bodies (A). The lateral film (B) shows a third foreign body, and also indicates that the largest of the fragments is approximately 2 cm long, and deep within the space between the first and second metatarsal. After the first attempt at removal a subsequent film (C; note the presence of a locator needle) shows that the largest fragment has not been removed. After another attempt, the final film showed no evidence of retained glass.

The depth and position of radiopaque foreign bodies can be estimated by using radiopaque skin markers such as lead circles, paper clips, or hypodermic needles and obtaining images in two or more projections (see Figure 16-5C). Prior to placing the skin markers, their location should be marked using an indelible pen so that if a foreign body is found, the marker location is identifiable after the

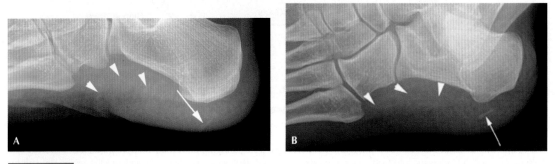

FIGURE 16-6

This patient presented stating that he had trodden on glass 2 weeks previously, "but I thought I got it all out." The foreign body on the lateral (A) and oblique (B) plain films was easily removed. The sharp margins of this foreign body make it easy to distinguish from the dense fibrous bands of the foot, which can be seen on these films (arrowheads).

marker has been removed for exploration of the wound. Alternatively, needle markers can be placed directly into the tissues as described in the wound exploration section of this chapter.

Fluoroscopy

Fluoroscopy can be used to identify a foreign body, although it is more commonly used as an adjunct in the operating room in the removal of deep or difficult-to-access foreign bodies. Surface and deeper tissue needle markers can be used as for plain film and ultrasonography (see Figures 16-7 and 16-5C).[21] Radiation exposure can be minimized by brief, intermittent imaging and appropriate shielding.[22] Fluoroscopy is not available in most emergency departments (EDs), although portable C-arm systems, using low doses of radiation, may lead to its increasing utilization.[23]

Computed tomography

Computed tomography (CT) is capable of resolving objects in tissues with more subtle variations of radiodensity than is plain film radiography, and is therefore of greater value in the diagnosis of suspected radiolucent foreign body than is traditional radiographs.[20,24,25] Computed tomography also has the advantage of demonstrating the location of the foreign body with respect to surrounding landmarks and neurovascular structures. Computed tomography findings of foreign body include soft tissue air and linear densities that are close to but dissimilar from the surrounding tissue. (They may be either more or less radiopaque, depending on both the nature and the duration of the foreign body.) However, these findings can be confused with soft tissue changes arising from acute trauma, or chronic healing, and studies suggest that the sensitivity and specificity of CT for radiopaque foreign body detection do not exceed 90%, and that sensitivity is much lower for smaller wooden foreign bodies.[26]

Typical conditions in the ED may reduce the performance characteristics of CT even further. First, many studies have investigated the use of CT in limited and well-defined anatomic regions such as the orbit and esophagus. Second, CT studies are done in ideal conditions with well-rested expert imaging specialists focusing on foreign body identification using high-resolution monitors with the capacity for fine adjustments of the imaging windows (only possible if the CT images are being reviewed in digital format).[27]

Third, the majority of ED patients and foreign bodies present during the 128 hours (of the 168-hour week) that radiologists are not available in most hospitals. During these hours, in many EDs, CT studies are not reviewed by imaging specialists at all until the following day. If they are reviewed in real time, this happens remotely (by the imaging specialist at home or a "night hawk" service on another continent) without the capability of digital adjustment, often on inferior-quality monitors.

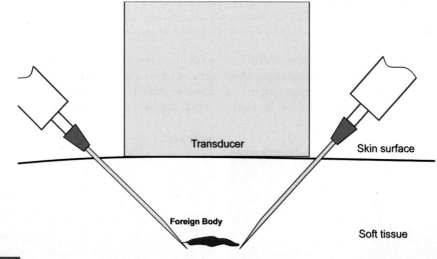

FIGURE 16-7

Use of anesthetic needles to localize a foreign body under real-time sonographic or fluoroscopic guidance is shown. Although the technique seems intuitively easy, the fine 27-gauge needles preferred for anesthetization may be difficult to detect on ultrasound, and if more than one needle is used, they can rarely be placed in the same plane. Prior to placement of the needles and provision of deeper anesthesia, the entire area should be pre-anesthetized by injections via the wound (*not* through intact skin). This may allow for localization by using slightly larger (21-gauge) needles. With ultrasound, orienting the bevel toward the probe may render the needle tip more echogenic, and, thus, easier to localize.

Finally, the high reported accuracy of CT in foreign body detection depends on stipulation of fine cuts on the CT order, and a technician performing the scan who is meticulous about keeping the patient absolutely still. These conditions are rarely met after hours in a high-volume CT scanning suite of the ED with typical ED patients, many of whom may be agitated, uncooperative, and afflicted with other more significant injuries, some of which may cause foreign bodies to be overlooked by those reading the films in a remote location. An additional concern of CT is the incremental doses of ionizing radiation needed for the fine cuts of high-resolution scanning, frequently over extensive regions of the body if multiple lacerations are involved (See Figure 16-8).

Ultrasonography

Ultrasonography can detect both radiopaque and radiolucent foreign bodies, although its use is particularly attractive in the evaluation of wounds caused by

organic objects (including plastic and all biological materials) that are almost uniformly radiolucent.[28,30] Studies investigating the accuracy of ultrasound in the detection of foreign bodies have reported sensitivities ranging from 50% to 100%, and specificities from 47% to 97%.[4-7,28,30-35] This wide range reflects the fact that in vivo studies lack an absolute criterion standard (foreign body can never be excluded with complete certainty) and in vitro study models lack the variety of foreign bodies, tissues, and the injuries that are encountered in clinical practice. The fibrous bands found especially in the body parts most prone to a foreign body (the hands and feet), are highly echogenic and may cause shadowing, making them easily mistaken for foreign body. False-positive ultrasound exams can also be caused by the pockets of air in many wounds, gas-containing abscesses, sesamoid and other small bones of the extremities, and soft-tissue calcifications.[34,36]

Although one should bear these limitations in mind, ultrasonography does have a role in the

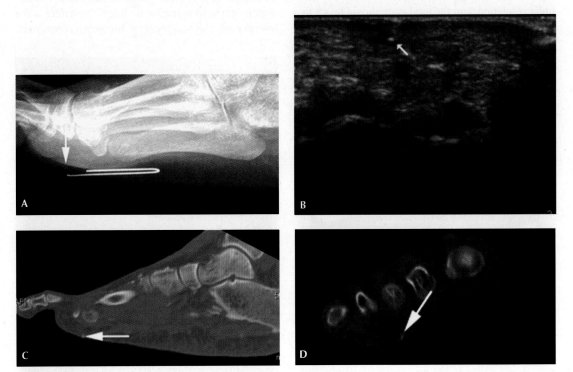

FIGURE 16-8

This patient presented with complaints of pain in her sole with a "lump" for a week since stepping on an unknown sharp object at night. Plain film (A) was read as negative by both the emergency physician and radiologist, although with the benefit of subsequent studies the foreign body can probably be made out at the tip of the paper-clip marker (arrow). A bedside ultrasound was done that showed a hypoechoic track leading to a punctate hyperechoic focus (B). Uncharacteristically, the foreign body displayed neither shadowing nor reverberation artifact, although its location and discontinuous nature argued for its identity as the foreign object. To confirm its identity and obtain more information about the size and nature of the foreign body a CT scan was performed that showed the object apparently at the skin surface (arrows, C and D). It was easily removed with ultrasound guidance.

management of foreign bodies for several reasons. Compared with other techniques, especially when used by the practicing clinician at the bedside, ultrasonography can be rapidly deployed and is available around the clock without the use of ionizing radiation. In the event that a probable foreign body is identified clinically, ultrasonography can be used in real time with blunt instruments or with a needle to confirm or exclude the diagnosis. Ultrasound permits guided anesthetization and localization of the foreign body and provides additional information about its size and orientation, and can be used for real-time guidance during removal.

With the increase in utilization of bedside sonography in emergency practice, a brief review of soft-tissue ultrasound technique is in order. A high-frequency linear array probe should be used if available; if not, other high-frequency transducers can be used, with or without the additional use of a "stand-off" or spacer.[37] For all but the deepest wounds, the highest available frequency should be selected to maximize resolution, and the focal zone should be set to a depth within 2 cm of the skin. To avoid contamination of the ultrasound equipment (and of the wound), the probe should be covered with a sterile impermeable cover (or a sterile nonpowdered examination glove if no such cover is available). When the full extent of possible locations for a retained foreign body has been identified, the region should be evaluated with slow, methodical systematic sweeps first in one, then in an orthogonal plane. The findings of a soft-tissue foreign body are one or more of the following (see Figures 16-8, 16-9, and 16-10):

1. A discontinuous echogenic object that is not consistent with normal anatomic structures
2. A shadowing object in the soft tissues
3. An object in the soft tissues causing reverberation ("ring-down") artifact

Although the three commonest forms of foreign body tend to have characteristic sonographic signatures (wood predominantly shadow, metal predominantly reverberation, and glass either or both), the most important task is to recognize the presence of one or more of the sonographic findings. The nature of the foreign body will become apparent once it is removed.

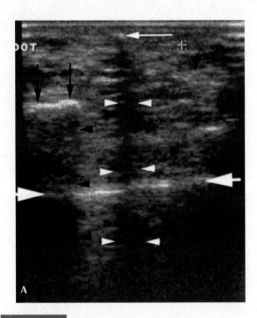

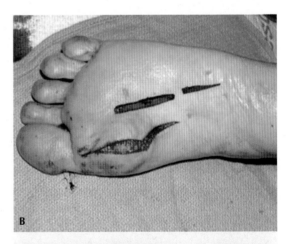

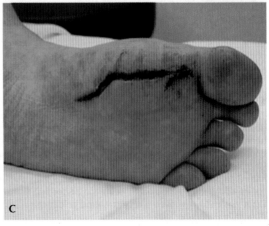

FIGURE 16-9

This patient presented to the ED after impaling his foot on a splinter from a rough wood floor. The ultrasound (A) showed 2 separate echogenic foci (in plane: black arrows, and perpendicular to scanning plane: small white arrow) each with shadowing (arrowheads). The deeper echogenic band (between large white arrows) is a fascial band, and can be distinguished from foreign bodies by the absence of shadowing. The two pieces of splinter and the necessary incision are shown in B. The patient's laceration was not closed until 4 days later when it was seen to be granulating without sign of infection (C).

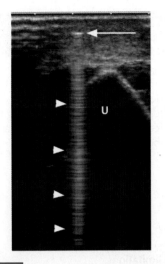

A metallic foreign body (arrow) in the forearm shows strong posterior reverberation artifact (arrowheads) that persist through the shadowing caused by the ulna (U).

It might be anticipated that these findings would be unequivocal and easily identified; however, this is frequently not the case. Any person who is familiar with the challenges of ultrasound-guided peripheral intravenous access, which requires the recognition of a foreign body that is being manipulated by the clinician) will know how easily a small foreign body can be overlooked. It is essential to perform the examination in a darkened room with optimal depth, focus, and gain settings adjusted so that normal muscle fascia and striations appear white, normal interlobular fat septations appear gray, and normal fat lobules and muscle tissue appear almost black. Image optimization will enable detection of smaller objects and facilitate the distinction between the echoes and shadowing caused by a foreign body compared with those of normal fibrous bands (especially in the palm and sole). The scan should be repeated in at least two orthogonal planes and, if the index of suspicion is high, followed by rescanning using different angles of insonation, which may be necessary to reveal the presence of an anisotropic foreign body (one that reflects ultrasound selectively based on the angle of the incident beam). In this context, it is important to bear in mind that, as the orientation of linear foreign bodies gets closer to perpendicular to the skin surface, it is increasingly difficult to identify them (Figure 16-11). Sonographic

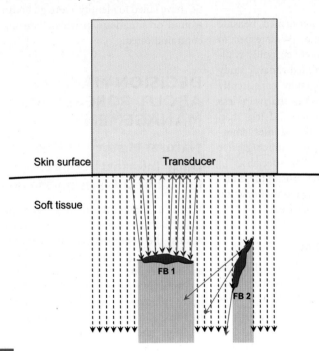

The effect of angle of insonation on sonographic detection of foreign bodies: Two identical foreign bodies (FB) at the same depth but at different angles with respect to the ultrasound beam will not be equally identifiable. FB1 is oriented perpendicular to the incident ultrasound beam (broken black lines), causing reflected echoes (red) directed toward the transducer, resulting in a strong signal and more likely detection. FB2 is almost parallel with the incident beam resulting in few or no echoes being reflected toward the probe. Note that both FBs cause shadowing (gray), but that the shadow of FB2 will be much smaller than that of FB1, adding to the difficulty of its detection. In some cases the operator can overcome this problem by scanning the foreign body from a different direction.

TABLE 16–3	**Common Causes of Inaccurate Ultrasound Examination for Foreign Body**	
Causes of False-Negative Exams		**Causes of False-Positive Exams**
Operator-dependent errors		**Operator-dependent errors**
Failure to scan slowly and methodically through all tissue planes in two orthogonal directions		Misidentification of small bones as foreign bodies
Failure to consider reverberation or shadowing alone as evidence of foreign body		Misidentification of fibrous tissue bands as foreign bodies
Failure to optimize resolution (maximize frequency)		
Failure to optimize depth and focus settings		
Failure to optimize gain settings		
Misidentification of foreign body as small bone		
Technical limitations		**Technical limitations**
Limit of resolution of ultrasound equipment		Presence of pockets of gas in wound

signal distortion from the foreign body itself, gas, blood, or pus may create additional impediments.[34-36] Commonly encountered reasons for diagnostic error with ultrasonography for foreign body localization are listed in Table 16–3.

The accuracy of clinician-performed bedside sonography is still under investigation. With respect to foreign body size and the resolution of currently available equipment, a recent unembalmed cadaver study demonstrated bedside ultrasonography consistently *unreliable* in detecting foreign bodies that were less than 2.5 mm^3 in maximum volume and less than 5 mm in maximum length.[33] In other studies, emergency physicians have performed with much greater accuracy and comparably to imaging specialists in detection of foreign bodies.[31,38] The basis of these discordant results, as with other investigations of imaging tests in foreign body detection, is not clear.

Magnetic Resonance Imaging

There are limited data on the test characteristics of magnetic resonance imaging (MRI) in foreign body detection. It may identify some organic foreign bodies that are missed by ultrasound and CT, and, with its ability to define soft tissue structures, may have a special role to play in the evaluation of chronic foreign bodies. Magnetic resonance imaging is contraindicated with metallic foreign bodies in the orbit or other regions with complex neurovascular structures.[39] Because gravel frequently contains ferrometallic material, the use of MRI to detect these types of foreign

bodies in neurovascularly vulnerable regions is contraindicated. Because of its limited availability in most EDs at this time and its marginal advantages over CT, MRI is reserved for situations in which other modalities have failed to identify a foreign body in a high-risk wound or situations in which ionizing radiation is contraindicated.

DECISION-MAKING ABOUT FOREIGN BODY MANAGEMENT

Natural History of Foreign Body Injuries: Implications for Clinical Decision-Making

When a foreign body has been identified, the physician must weigh the risk of leaving it in place against the potential harm of attempting to remove it. Not all foreign bodies need to be removed, and not all that require removal must be extracted during the initial evaluation. Decision-making about foreign body removal is based on considerations relating to the nature of the foreign body, its anatomical location, and patient factors such as comorbidities and the ability to comply with discharge and follow-up plans.

Immediate damage caused by a foreign body is usually limited to local soft tissues. Injuries caused by missiles or broken glass are exceptions and may cause vascular, tendon, nerve, or bone damage. Delayed

TABLE 16–4	Described Complications of Retained Foreign Bodies

Damage to vessels, resulting in:

- Erosion or perforation with hemorrhage
- Occlusion with distal ischemia
- Pseudoaneurysm formation

Damage to nerves, tendons, ligaments, or joints
Intravascular migration or embolization
Chronic pain, impaired function, or secondary
   disuse syndromes
Inflammatory mass
Chronic or recurrent infections

---

consequences of foreign bodies can be divided into direct effects and inflammatory sequellae. The most common direct effects are caused by compression or laceration of local structures, which can occur months or years after the injury.[40–42] This is the rationale for the removal of most sharp foreign bodies, especially glass, particularly in regions that are subject to extensive or repetitive motion (all major joints) or are susceptible to repetitive pressure (hands, feet, knees, or elbows). Conversely, foreign bodies that are deep within tissues (such as a bullet lodged within a muscle belly) that do not have significant surrounding neurovascular structures can often be left in place. Many other chronic direct effects have been described including vascular occlusion, erosion, thrombosis, and migration to distant sites (Table 16-4).[43]

Any foreign body causes some degree of inflammation. The nature, location, and extent of the inflammatory response are major considerations in the clinical management of foreign bodies. With respect to the nature of the response, a "chemical" inflammation can be provoked by even completely sterile foreign bodies.[2] In general, inorganic or synthetic materials with smooth, nonporous surfaces cause less inflammation, whereas organic matter, especially animal or vegetable materials, cause more. For this reason, bullets and shrapnel are frequently left in wounds, and permanent steel and polypropylene sutures used in surgical procedures are usually tolerated indefinitely. Glass has a low inflammatory potential but, as noted above, is usually removed because of its proclivity for causing direct damage if left in place. In addition to the chemical response, many foreign bodies cause inflammation as a result of infection.

The same organic materials that are most likely to provoke a sterile inflammatory response are also most likely to harbor bacteria, and, thus, cause infection. It should be noted that even sterile foreign bodies increase the susceptibility of a wound to infection.[44] Because the chemical and infectious properties of organic foreign bodies such as wood splinters, thorns, and spines from marine animals predispose them to both acute and chronic inflammation, attempts to remove them are usually undertaken as soon as possible after an injury. There are three possible outcomes for a chronically retained inflammatory foreign body:

1. At any time it may cause a recurrent acute inflammatory response, resulting in abscess formation (usually sterile, but possibly infectious). This may result in any of the complications associated with an abscess, but also may lead to extrusion of the foreign body at the time of drainage.

2. It may cause a smoldering chronic inflammatory response, with or without granuloma formation, leading to chronic discomfort, swelling, and erythema. Retained foreign bodies with infectious potential can also cause secondary infections of local soft-tissue structures or bones.[2,8,16,17]

3. It may result in the formation of a stable fibrotic capsule ("cyst") that is sequestered from the immune system and, thus, becomes asymptomatic except for swelling.[2] Such lesions, however, are susceptible to "reactivation" for idiopathic reasons, by local trauma, or as a result of hematogenous infection.

In addition to its intrinsic pathogenic effects, chronic inflammation can cause secondary damage to, or compression of, local structures, resulting in tendonitis, synovitis, bursitis, contractures, ischemia, edema, thrombosis, or neuropathy. Consideration of the foreign body location determines its potential for causing secondary damage. Thus, foreign bodies that directly involve, or are in close proximity to bones, tendons, ligaments, nerves, or vascular bundles are more likely to need early removal. Because these structures are highly represented in the head, neck, hands, and feet, foreign bodies in these locations are usually removed. The functional and cosmetic importance of nearby structures is also a consideration when one is deciding whether to remove the foreign body in the ED or refer the patient to a specialist. With a reliable patient, inert objects such as glass may be left in place for follow-up care by a specialist with the extremity immobilized and protected

TABLE 16–5	Foreign Body Features Mitigating *for* Removal

Foreign body characteristics

- High inflammatory potential
- High infectious potential
- Organic or chemically reactive material
- Potential for tattooing

Location

- Proximity to nerves, vessels, joints, or tendons
- Hands, feet, head, or neck
- Proximity to bone fracture

Other clinical features

- Heavily contaminated wound
- Patient at risk for impaired healing or infection: diabetes, vascular insufficiency, steroid use, immunocompromise, etc.
- Signs or symptoms of retained foreign body (see Table 16–2)
- Cause of pain or psychological distress
- Evidence of allergic reaction
- Migration toward important structures

Toxicity

- Spines with venom
- Heavy metals

from use by splints and/or crutches. Indications mitigating *for* attempted foreign body removal are summarized in Table 16-5.

MANAGEMENT OF FOREIGN BODIES

Wound Exploration

If the decision has been made to attempt removal of a known or probable foreign body, a frank discussion with the patient about the risks and benefits of the procedure is essential. The components of such a discussion differ slightly depending on whether the foreign body is known for certain or only suspected (see Table 16-6). In all cases, however, the key element to be addressed is *the possibility of failure to remove the*

foreign body. Vocalizing this potential outcome creates a win-win situation in which the patient is additionally appreciative if the foreign body is retrieved, and, if it is not (or if complications occur), is prepared for this eventuality.

When a practitioner is approaching a wound that contains a foreign body either identified by imaging studies or strongly suspected by history, optimal lighting and a bloodless field are prerequisites. As with most ED procedures, time spent in preparation is time saved, and reassures the patient about the professionalism of the effort in the event of a failed attempt. For foreign bodies of the sole, placing the patient prone provides optimal visualization, allows for effective venous drainage prior to application of the tourniquet, and spares the patient the anxiety of witnessing the procedure. Blood pressure cuff tourniquets can be

TABLE 16–6	Risks and Benefits of Foreign Body Removal to be Addressed Prior to the Procedure	
Risks		**Benefits**
If the presence of foreign body is known with certainty: All risks of invasive surgical procedure and local anesthesia AND - Potential damage to local structures - Failure to find foreign bodies - Incomplete removal of foreign bodies If the presence of foreign body is *not* known with certainty: All risks of invasive surgical procedure and local anesthesia AND - Potential damage to local structures - Potential risk without benefit if no foreign body is present - Possibility of being unable to find foreign body that is actually there - Possibility of incomplete removal of foreign body		Removal may avoid all the complications of retained foreign bodies listed in Table 16-4.

applied to the arm, forearm, thigh, or calf, with more distal sites chosen for hand or foot, respectively. Prior to inflating the cuff (to 20 mm Hg above systolic pressure), the venous compartment should be drained of blood by elevating the extremity for 30 seconds. Although minimal tourniquet time is the goal, ischemic effects in a previously well-perfused extremity do not occur for several hours. As the duration of local anesthesia is about 30 minutes, and the time available to most emergency physicians for such procedures is even less, extremity ischemia should not be an issue.

The most frequent locations of foreign bodies are the hands and feet, where the skin is frequently heavily soiled. The region of the wound should be cleansed, and, if necessary, scrubbed, with bactericidal soap. The discomfort caused by effective irrigation of a wound usually mandates the prior administration of local anesthetic. This should be done *without digital exploration of the wound if there is a possibility of a sharp foreign body*. After preparation of the wound, a sterile field should be created around the planned surgical site. Because the exact location of most foreign bodies is not known, it is advisable to have additional local anesthetic drawn up on the sterile field.

If bedside ultrasound is available, the machine should be placed in a convenient location, and the transducer and wire placed in a sterile cover, with sterile coupling gel, on the operative field. Even for foreign bodies identified by other imaging modalities, ultrasound provides additional real-time information about the orientation and depth of the object. For deeper foreign bodies, ultrasound can also be used in conjunction with a needle placed on a syringe containing local anesthetic simultaneously to locate the object, anesthetize the tissues between it and the skin surface, and anesthetize the tissues surrounding the foreign body under direct visualization. The latter procedure has the additional benefit of enhancing the sonographic visualization of the foreign body as it becomes surrounded by anesthetic fluid and edematous tissue. A needle that is directly touching or slightly deep to the foreign body can be removed from the syringe and left in place as a direct guide for exploration. The needle guide should be placed in the plane of the long axis of the foreign body (unless the incision for its recovery cannot be made in this plane), and a second needle can be placed in a similar fashion from the opposite end of the long axis of the foreign body (see Figure 16-7).

When as much information as possible has been obtained about a foreign body's location, a linear incision is made parallel with its long axis, and adjacent to its most superficial location. The foreign body should be located by using gentle probing with needles or a closed hemostat. Those not experienced in the removal of foreign bodies from regions with dense connective tissue (such as the palm or sole) should be forewarned that the "scratching" quality of a blunt instrument exploration caused by a metallic or glass foreign body is almost indistinguishable from that caused by fibrous tissue. Conversely, the absence of foreign body sensation with blunt instrument probing does not exclude the presence of foreign body.[11]

Although probing to locate a foreign body can be done through a relatively small incision, once the object has been located *a common error is in making too small an incision for its extraction*, which both decreases the likelihood of success (by impeding visualization of the tissues) and increases the likelihood of iatrogenic harm (by prolonging the procedure and increasing the tendency to blind probing). With fairly superficial wood splinters or thorns, there is a temptation to make a short incision at the site of entry in order to grasp and remove the object. Although minimal iatrogenic harm is always the goal, such an approach can result in occult residual fragments in the deepest, most problematic part of the wound. A careful history about the type and condition of the wood that gave rise to the splinter may be reassuring, but in most cases it is more prudent to create an incision that goes down to the foreign body for its entire length, allowing visual confirmation of complete removal as well as thorough lavage of the wound tract. A removed wood splinter should be visually inspected: if the penetrating end is not sharp a residual broken fragment should be suspected.

In locations with nearby neurovascular or musculotendonous structures, it may be necessary to make the incision (and any subsequent sharp dissection) parallel with the course of these structures to minimize the likelihood of damage. In most circumstances, instrument dissection is limited to blunt spreading; however, after location of a friable or fragile foreign body, it is often necessary to cut some of the surrounding tissues to remove it intact. *Blind grasping for a foreign body in a wound should be avoided*: it is ineffective and increases the risk of iatrogenic injury.

After the successful removal of a foreign body, the wound should be thoroughly lavaged. If the clinician believes there is a significant risk of retained radiopaque foreign body, repeat ultrasonography can be performed in the field or repeat plain film can be ordered (see Figure 16-5C). For acute injuries at low risk for infection, the wound can be closed primarily. Other wounds should be left open for delayed primary or secondary closure. Sterile dressings should be applied, and the patient should be instructed to have the wound reassessed in 2 days by a physician (in the

ED if a primary care provider is not available). Neurovascular function should be rechecked at the completion of the procedure.

Special Situations and Techniques

Many special procedures and techniques have been described to manage specific foreign body injuries including fish-hooks, Taser darts, rings, body-piercing jewelry, zipper entrapment, toxic thorns, cactus injuries, marine stings, and envenomations. Detailed description of these techniques is beyond the scope of this chapter. Management of plantar wounds is discussed in Chapter 17.

Wounds that are grossly contaminated or that contain a friable foreign body, such as a sea urchin spine, should be considered for tissue excision. In most cases this can be performed in one of two ways. The preferred technique is to excise an approximately 5 mm by 15 mm ellipse of tissue (size will depend on the area and likely depth of foreign material), which can be excised to the depth of contamination under direct visualization. Caveats regarding skin incisions are as discussed previously in "Wound Management." A "coring" technique has also been described in which a No. 11 scalpel blade is buried to the hub and drawn in a 3 mm to 4 mm diameter circle to remove a cone of tissue usually a little more than a centimeter deep. The disadvantage of this technique is that the 11-blade is used blindly, so that deeper structures are at greater risk of injury.

Antibiotic Use

The benefit of prophylactic antibiotics in cases of occult retained foreign body has not been studied. After removal of an acute foreign body the same considerations regarding the use of antibiotics apply to the wound as to other soft tissue injuries. For a retained foreign body presenting as an abscess, definitive treatment is likely to be complete with drainage and removal of the foreign body, although extensive surrounding cellulitis may sometimes benefit from treatment with antibiotics.

DOCUMENTATION

Documentation of care should reflect the actions and thought processes of the treating physician in each of the key areas discussed in this chapter: the clinical setting, diagnostic imaging, decision-making regarding exploration, and interventions. The charting should reflect the conversations described previously about

exploration, and discharge instructions should emphasize the possibility of retained foreign body. Any patients at more than negligible risk for retained foreign body should have their wound rechecked in 2 days.

REFERENCES

1. Hollander JE, Singer AJ, Valentine SM, Shofer FS. Risk factors for infection in patients with traumatic lacerations. *Acad Emerg Med.* 2001;8(7):716–720.
2. Hirsh BC, Johnson WC. Pathology of granulomatous diseases. Foreign body granulomas. *Int J Dermatol.* 1984;23(8):531–538.
3. Lammers RL. Soft tissue foreign bodies. *Ann Emerg Med.* 1988;17(12):1336–1347.
4. Hill R, Conron R, Greissinger P, Heller M. Ultrasound for the detection of foreign bodies in human tissue. *Ann Emerg Med.* 1997;29(3):353–356.
5. Gooding GA, Hardiman T, Sumers M, Stess R, Graf P, Grunfeld C. Sonography of the hand and foot in foreign body detection. *J Ultrasound Med.* 1987;6(8):441–447.
6. Schlager D. Ultrasound detection of foreign bodies and procedure guidance. *Emerg Med Clin North Am.* 1997;15(4):895–912.
7. Anderson MA, Newmeyer WL 3rd, Kilgore ES Jr. Diagnosis and treatment of retained foreign bodies in the hand. *Am J Surg.* 1982;144(1):63–67.
8. Strömqvist B, Edlund E, Lidgren L. A case of black-thorn synovitis. *Acta Orthop Scand.* 1985;56(4):342–343.
9. Courter BJ. Radiographic screening for glass foreign bodies: what does a "negative" foreign body series really mean? *Ann Emerg Med.* 1990;19(9):997–1000.
10. Chisholm CD, Wood CO, Chua G, Cordell WH, Nelson DR. Radiographic detection of gravel in soft tissue. *Ann Emerg Med.* 1997;29(6):725–730.
11. Steele MT, Tran LV, Watson WA, Muelleman RL. Retained glass foreign bodies in wounds: predictive value of wound characteristics, patient perception, and wound exploration. *Am J Emerg Med.* 1998;16(7):627–630.
12. Montano JB, Steele MT, Watson WA. Foreign body retention in glass-caused wounds. *Ann Emerg Med.* 1992;21(11):1360–1363.
13. Bekler H, Gokce A, Beyzadeoglu T, Parmaksizoglu F. The surgical treatment and outcomes of high-pressure injection injuries of the hand. *J Hand Surg Eur Vol.* 2007;32(4):394–399.
14. Avner JR, Baker MD. Lacerations involving glass. The role of routine roentgenograms. *Am J Dis Child.* 1992;146(5):600–602.
15. Orlinsky M, Bright AA. The utility of routine x-rays in all glass-caused wounds. *Am J Emerg Med.* 2006;24(2):233–236.
16. Brand RA, Black H. Pseudomonas osteomyelitis following puncture wounds in children. *J Bone Joint Surg.* 1974;56(8):1637–1642.

17. Riegler HF, Routson GW. Complications of deep puncture wounds of the foot. *J Trauma*. 1979;19(1):18–22.

18. Ellis GL. Are aluminum foreign bodies detectable radiographically? *Am J Emerg Med*. 1993;11(1):12–13.

19. Felman AH, Fisher MS. The radiographic detection of glass in soft tissue. *Radiology*. 1969;92(7):1529–1531.

20. Roobottom CA, Weston MJ. The detection of foreign bodies in soft tissue—comparison of conventional and digital radiography. *Clin Radiol*. 1994;49(5):330–332.

21. Ariyan S. A simple stereotactic method to isolate and remove foreign bodies. *Arch Surg*. 1977;112(7):857–859.

22. Cohen DM, Garcia CT, Dietrich AM, Hickey RW Jr. Miniature C-arm imaging: an in vitro study of detecting foreign bodies in the emergency department. *Pediatr Emerg Care*. 1997;13(4):247–249.

23. Levine MR, Yarnold PR, Michelson EA. A training program in portable fluoroscopy for the detection of glass in soft tissues. *Acad Emerg Med*. 2002;9(8):858–862.

24. Kjhns LR, Borlaza GS, Seigel RS, Paramagul C, Berger PE. An in vitro comparison of computed tomography, xerography, and radiography in the detection of soft-tissue foreign bodies. *Radiology*. 1979;132(1):218–219.

25. Bauer AR Jr, Yutani D. Computed tomographic localization of wooden foreign bodies in children's extremities. *Arch Surg*. 1983;118(9):1084–1086.

26. Mizel MS, Steinmetz ND, Trepman E. Detection of wooden foreign bodies in muscle tissue: experimental comparison of computed tomography, magnetic resonance imaging, and ultrasonography. *Foot Ankle Int*. 1994;15(8):437–443.

27. Reiner B, Siegel E, McLaurin T, et al. Evaluation of soft-tissue foreign bodies: comparing conventional plain film radiography, computed radiography printed on film, and computed radiography displayed on a computer workstation. *AJR Am J Roentgenol*. 1996;167(1):141–144.

28. Friedman DI, Forti RJ, Wall SP, Crain EF. The utility of bedside ultrasound and patient perception in detecting soft tissue foreign bodies in children. *Pediatr Emerg Care*. 2005;21(8):487–492.

29. Blankstein A, Cohen I, Heiman Z, et al. Ultrasonography as a diagnostic modality and therapeutic adjuvant in the management of soft tissue foreign bodies in the lower extremities. *Isr Med Assoc J*. 2001;3(6):411–413.

30. Graham DD Jr. Ultrasound in the emergency department: detection of wooden foreign bodies in the soft tissues. *J Emerg Med*. 2002;22(1):75–79.

31. Orlinsky M, Knittel P, Feit T, Chan L, Mandavia D. The comparative accuracy of radiolucent foreign body detection using ultrasonography. *Am J Emerg Med*. 2000;18(4):401–403.

32. Crawford R, Matheson AB. Clinical value of ultrasonography in the detection and removal of radiolucent foreign bodies. *Injury*. 1989;20(6):341–343.

33. Crystal CS, Masneri DA, Hellums JS, et al. Bedside ultrasound for the detection of soft tissue foreign bodies: a cadaveric study. *J Emerg Med*. 2009;36(4):377–380.

34. Manthey DE, Storrow AB, Milbourn JM, Wagner BJ. Ultrasound versus radiography in the detection of soft-tissue foreign bodies. *Ann Emerg Med*. 1996;28(1):7–9.

35. Gilbert FJ, Campbell RSD, Bayliss AP. The role of ultrasound in the detection of non-radiopaque foreign bodies. *Clin Radiol*. 1990;41:109–112.

36. Banerjee B, Das RK. Sonographic detection of foreign bodies of the extremities. *Br J Radiol*. 1991;64(758):107–112.

37. Dean AJ, Gronczewski CA, Costantino TG. Technique for emergency medicine bedside ultrasound identification of a radiolucent foreign body. *J Emerg Med*. 2003;24(3):303–308.

38. Lyon M, Brannam L, Johnson D, Blaivas M, Duggal S. Detection of soft tissue foreign bodies in the presence of soft tissue gas. *J Ultrasound Med*. 2004;23(5):677–681.

39. Bodne D, Quinn SF, Cochran CF. Imaging foreign glass and wooden bodies of the extremities with CT and MR. *J Comput Assist Tomogr*. 1988;12(4):608–611.

40. Browett JP, Fiddian NJ. Delayed median nerve injury due to retained glass fragments. A report of two cases. *J Bone Joint Surg Br*. 1985;67(3):382–384.

41. Jablon M, Rabin SI. Late flexor pollicis longus tendon rupture due to retained glass fragments. *J Hand Surg Am*. 1988;13(5):713–716.

42. Meurer WJ. Radial artery pseudoaneurysm caused by occult retained glass from a hand laceration. *Pediatr Emerg Care*. 2009;25(4):255–257.

43. Dadsetan MR, Jinkins JR. Peripheral vascular gunshot bullet embolus migration to the cerebral circulation. Report and literature review. *Neuroradiology*. 1990;36(6):516–519.

44. Zimmerli W, Zak O, Vosbeck K. Experimental hematogenous infection of subcutaneously implanted foreign bodies. *Scand J Infect Dis*. 1985;17(3):303–310.

CHAPTER 17

Plantar Puncture Wounds

David F. Gaieski, MD, and Martin Camacho, MSN, ACNP-BC

The plantar puncture wound is one of the most common lower-extremity injuries seen in the emergency department (ED). Plantar puncture wounds are penetrating injuries to the plantar, or weight-bearing, surface of the foot, which can often appear as trivial, innocuous injuries.[1] They are characterized by a depth of penetration that exceeds the diameter of the visible surface injury. Patients with plantar puncture wounds seek medical attention in the ED for a variety of reasons including concern for retained foreign bodies, tetanus immunization, pain control, development of infection, or possible accompanying musculoskeletal injuries including fractures. Health care providers have widely divergent views on the management of plantar puncture wounds. Some prefer expectant therapy, reacting to complications as they develop. Others pursue potential foreign bodies with relatively invasive exploration, hoping to prevent unusual but devastating infections. This chapter highlights the evaluation, treatment, and controversies surrounding the management of plantar puncture wounds.

EPIDEMIOLOGY

Plantar puncture wounds can be sustained in diverse environments including the home, recreational settings, and the workplace. They are most commonly caused by a penetrating nail but can also be caused by broken glass, sharp metal objects, projectiles including bullets (Figure 17-1), pieces of wood, and other organic material.[2] Occasionally, plantar puncture wounds are caused by arthropod or mammalian bites, spiny processes on aquatic animals, and high-pressure injections from industrial tools.

PATHOPHYSIOLOGY

When a sharp, penetrating object punctures the plantar surface of the foot, it transmits a shearing force through the epidermis and dermis into the subcutaneous tissue layers, which causes disruption and devitalization of tissue and has the potential to introduce bacteria and debris into a sealed-off, anaerobic environment.[3] This mechanism produces the ideal setting for the proliferation of bacteria and development of infection.[4] The depth of the penetrating injury can also cause damage to periosteum and bone, ligamentous and tendonous structures, articular cartilage, and joint capsules. Injury to these structures can lead to osteochondritis, osteomyelitis, septic arthritis, and loss of function.[3] These risks are theoretically increased with forefoot puncture wounds, where joint structures and tissue are impacted by the transmission of body weight to the plantar surface.[3,5–7] The incidence of infection is increased by factors that hamper appropriate

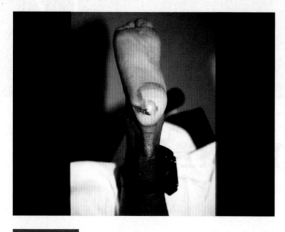

FIGURE 17-1

Plantar puncture wound resulting from gunshot.

wound healing including diabetes mellitus, peripheral vascular disease, immunosuppression, previous trauma or devitalization of tissue, preexisting dermatologic infections, and peripheral neuropathy.[7]

COMPLICATIONS OF PLANTAR PUNCTURE WOUNDS

The complication rate from plantar puncture wounds is higher than the rate for puncture wounds in the remainder of the lower extremities. One reason is the short distance from the plantar skin surface to the bones and joints of the feet. The most common complication of plantar puncture wounds is superficial soft tissue infection. Other complications include retained foreign bodies; tendon, ligament, and cartilage damage; deep space infections; osteochondritis; septic arthritis; and osteomyelitis.[8]

MICROBIOLOGY OF INFECTED PLANTAR PUNCTURE WOUNDS

Gram-positive organisms, particularly *Staphylococcus aureus* and beta-hemolytic streptococci, are the most common isolates from plantar puncture wound infections.[9,4] *Pseudomonas aeruginosa* is the next most common isolate. It is associated with wounds sustained through the rubber soles of footwear such as work boots, tennis shoes, and beach sandals, where a hot, moist environment is conducive to its growth and sustainability.[8,10–14] *Pseudomonas* is believed to have a

predilection for cartilage, leading to osteochondritis and osteomyelitis. Although uncommon, clostridial infections also can develop in deep, closed wounds such as those caused by nail punctures.

EVALUATION

In general, the depth of penetration will dictate management, as superficial punctures pose nearly trivial risk, whereas deeper puncture injuries have a higher potential to lead to deep space infections.[15] An appreciation of the mechanism of injury and circumstances surrounding the injury can help identify risk factors for and the probability of accompanying bony injuries and subsequent infection.

As part of the initial evaluation it is important to ascertain the following:

1. Environment where the injury occurred
2. Description of the penetrating object, if known
3. Location of the injury on the plantar surface
4. Presumptive depth of the penetration (jump vs walk-step vs high-pressure injection injury)
5. Type of footwear worn at the time of injury, if any
6. Postinjury care
7. Presence of suspected foreign body
8. Timeframe between injury and clinical presentation
9. Past medical and surgical history
10. Medications, including status of tetanus immunization

The physical evaluation of the wound includes an inspection of the site of penetration and surrounding tissue.[1] The presence of visible foreign bodies and material should be noted. Adequate, direct lighting along with careful manipulation of the plantar surface and wound edges can allow for a better appreciation of the depth of the penetration; however, the exact extent of the injury is difficult to ascertain without more invasive and, therefore, not generally recommended, exploration.[16] Careful palpation sometimes reveals evidence of a retained foreign body not seen on visual inspection.[10] Range of motion at nearby joints as well as distal neurovascular status should be assessed. If the patient presents several hours to days after sustaining the injury a careful evaluation for evidence of infection should be performed.[1,10] Signs and symptoms of infection include fever, tachycardia, tachypnea, surrounding erythema, color, fluctuance, edema or induration, pain out of proportion to physical exam findings, decreased range of motion, drainage, and limited ability or complete inability to bear weight.[17]

The decision to obtain radiographs is dictated primarily by the history and physical examination. Radiographs are warranted for plantar puncture injuries caused by broken glass; metal objects including nails, needles, and metallic industrial debris; and fragile materials that may have shattered during penetration.[15] Organic material such as wood, thorns, and cactus spines present more difficult challenges for detection because they have radiodensities similar to soft tissue and do not appear as radiopaque foreign bodies on radiographs. Computed tomography and ultrasonography may provide immediate information about the presence or absence of retained foreign bodies[18]; magnetic resonance imaging (MRI) is less often available emergently but MRI is considered the most sensitive imaging modality for evaluation of retained foreign bodies.[19,20] In addition, MRI allows for an extensive evaluation of soft tissue infections and the presence of osteomyelitis.[20]

OUTCOMES

In a retrospective analysis of 2325 patients presenting to an ED with punctures, Houston and coworkers[21] reported a 2% infection rate with early treatment of these wounds, and a 10% rate if patients presented late. The rate of osteomyelitis was 0.04%.

However, Fitzgerald and Cowan[22] reported a study of 887 plantar puncture wounds, primarily in children, 98% of which were caused by nails. Foreign bodies were found in 3%; half of the foreign bodies were pieces of shoe or sock, and the other half were rust, gravel, grass, straw, or dirt. Of the 774 patients who were treated in the ED within 24 hours, 8.4% either already had or subsequently developed cellulitis. In the group of patients who presented for treatment 1 to 7 days after injury, 57% had cellulitis or another soft tissue infection. Almost 7% of the infections failed to respond to antimicrobial therapy and eventually required incision and drainage of an abscess. Of all the patients in this series, 4% developed serious infections; osteomyelitis occurred in almost 2%. In some cases, osteomyelitis developed despite the use of antibiotics. *Pseudomonas* was isolated in 81% of these infections.

The true risk of infection in all victims of puncture wounds of the feet is unknown, because many people never seek medical care for these injuries. Weber[23] surveyed 200 ED patients about prior episodes of plantar puncture wounds; 44% reported having punctured their foot at some time during their life; 50% of those had sought medical care. Ten subjects reported having had infections, 9 of whom had sought medical care. The infection rate in patients who had presented for treatment was 20.5% whereas the overall infection rate in patients reporting a history of plantar puncture wound was 11.4%. She concluded that because many wounds never come to medical attention, the actual infection rate from plantar puncture wounds is lower than that reported. Nevertheless, the self-reported infection rate was higher than in previous retrospective studies.

MANAGEMENT OF THE UNINFECTED PLANTAR PUNCTURE WOUND

A review of relevant literature yields little concrete, evidence-based guidance for the management of plantar puncture wounds.[4] Nevertheless, basic premises about the mechanism of injury dictate several general recommendations:

- *Tetanus immunization*
  Review immunization status and administer tetanus toxoid (as per Chapter 23) when immunization status is not up to date.
- *Removal of visible foreign bodies*
  Superficial debris and visible foreign material should be carefully, mechanically removed. The skin in this region is thick, relatively rigid, and quite sensitive. Most visible foreign bodies in plantar puncture wounds can be removed with tweezers; soaking the injured foot in warm water and epsom salts can facilitate foreign body removal.
- *Antibiotics*
  Whether to administer prophylactic antibiotics is based upon the degree of wound contamination, timing of presentation, functional impairment, and comorbidities potentially contributing to inadequate wound healing. When provided, antibiotic prophylaxis for plantar puncture wounds sustained through rubber-soled shoes should include coverage for *P aeruginosa*. There is a lack of data from well-performed studies to support prophylactic antibiotic use, despite it being commonly done.[24,25]
- *Wound management*
  Local anesthetics should be considered to provide comfort and facilitate the examination and probing of the wound.[15] However, the anatomy of the plantar surface of the foot often makes injection of adequate local anesthesia difficult. One of the unresolved controversies about plantar puncture wounds is whether to explore all of these wounds for foreign bodies; another is whether probing constitutes a sufficient exploration. Schwab and Powers[10] reported a 3% rate of retained foreign bodies after

initial surface cleansing without wound exploration. Some authors recommend enlarging the puncture wound to allow deeper exploration and irrigation,[12] particularly if bone or joint contact is suspected.[26] Others believe that excising a block or cone of tissue down to the subcutaneous layer, or "coring out" the wound with a punch biopsy, allows adequate visualization of accessible foreign bodies and removal of most of the contaminated tissue.[27] Others simply trim jagged epidermal skin edges with tissue scissors or scalpel.[28] Simple probing and blind grasping have unknown false-negative rates[5] and may force foreign objects and bacteria deeper into the wound.[4] It is not clear what percentage of unexpected foreign bodies will be discovered and removed during the initial visit if this more invasive approach is utilized. Healing of the puncture wound may be delayed somewhat by excising or incising the wound, but infection will delay healing even more.

Antiseptic solution and wound irrigation should be the standard for plantar punctures. However, most plantar puncture wounds, by definition, cannot be completely irrigated. Although there is no evidence with regard to the use of low- versus high-pressure irrigation, theoretically, low-pressure irrigation prevents small debris and bacterial organisms from tracking further into the wound. In summary, at present, the use of wound probing and coring has not been shown to provide better outcomes, is a more invasive and complicated process, and cannot be recommended as a routine management strategy.[5]

MANAGEMENT OF THE INFECTED PLANTAR PUNCTURE WOUND

The management of the infected puncture wound involves careful assessment for complicated infections including deep space infections, septic arthritis, and osteomyelitis. Signs and symptoms of sepsis and severe sepsis should be assessed and the patient resuscitated in a timely fashion. Initial antibiotic coverage for *S aureus* and beta-hemolytic streptococci is usually sufficient.[19] However, in appropriate circumstances, coverage should be broadened to include gram-negative and anaerobic organisms.[19] Superficial fluctuant areas should be drained through conventional incision and drainage. Wound cultures and tissue and fluid specimens should be obtained in cases of unusual puncture injuries or with infections refractory to initial therapy.

Several clinical trials have established that a 7- to 14-day course of antibiotic therapy provides sufficient antimicrobial therapy for the majority of infected plantar puncture wounds.[25,29] Ciprofloxacin (400 mg intravenously [IV] twice daily for the first 24 hours, followed by 750 mg orally twice daily) was found to be effective at treating cellulitis after 7 days and early osteomyelitis after 14 days.[29] Outcomes were superior when ciprofloxacin was combined with aggressive wound management, including irrigation, surgical exploration, and débridement. In a clinical trial evaluating infected plantar puncture wounds in children caused by *P aeruginosa*, early surgical intervention coupled with the intravenous ciprofloxacin therapy showed significant improvement in infection after 7.5 days.[30]

Historically, ciprofloxacin has demonstrated excellent *P aeruginosa* coverage; however, recent emergence of fluoroquinolone-resistant *Pseudomonas* has decreased its effectiveness. Empiric use of ciprofloxacin for plantar puncture wounds should be supported by, and modified as needed in response to, culture results. In most regions, fluoroquinolones continue to have acceptable activity against *P aeruginosa*, staphylococci, streptococci, and some clostridial species.[29,31] Local resistance patterns should be taken into account in treatment decisions.

DECISION-MAKING AND FOLLOW-UP

When the optimal management of a problem in medicine is unknown, it is best to actively involve the patient in the decision-making process. Because plantar puncture wounds are so difficult to explore and clean, physicians should clearly explain to the patient the limitations of current management strategies and clearly outline the potential complications of these injuries. Schedule patients for re-evaluation for infection within 2 to 3 days and aggressively search for a retained foreign body if infection develops at any time. Development of infection in a plantar puncture wound is highly suggestive of a retained foreign body.

REFERENCES

1. Haverstock BD, Grossman JP. Puncture wounds of the foot. Evaluation and treatment. *Clin Podiatr Med Surg.* 1999;16(4):583–596.
2. Baldwin G, Colbourne M. Puncture wounds. *Pediatr Rev.* 1999;20(1):21–23.
3. Chudnofsky CR, Sebastian S. Special wounds. Nail bed, plantar puncture, and cartilage. *Emerg Med Clin North Am.* 1992;10(4):801–822.

4. Reinherz R, Hong DT, Tisa LM, et al. Management of puncture wounds in the foot. *J Foot Surg.* 1985;24(4): 288–292.

5. Chisholm CD, Schlesser JF. Plantar puncture wounds: controversies and treatment recommendations. *Ann Emerg Med.* 1989;18(12):1352–1357.

6. Patzakis M, Wilkins J, Brien WW, Carter VS. Wound site as a predictor of complications following deep nail punctures to the foot. *West J Med.* 1989;150(5): 545–547.

7. Armstrong DG, Lavery LA, Quebedeaux TL, Walker SC. Surgical morbidity and the risk of amputation due to infected puncture wounds in diabetic versus nondiabetic adults. *J Am Podiatr Med Assoc.* 1997; 87(7):321–326.

8. Fisher MC, Goldsmith JF, Gilligan PH. Sneakers as a source of Pseudomonas aeruginosa in children with osteomyelitis following puncture wounds. *J Pediatr.* 1985;106(4):607–609.

9. Joseph WS, LeFrock JL. Infections complicating puncture wounds of the foot. *J Foot Surg.* 1987;26(1 suppl):S30–S33.

10. Schwab RA, Powers RD. Conservative therapy of plantar puncture wounds. *J Emerg Med.* 1995;13(3): 291–295.

11. Saha P, Parrish CA, McMillan JA. Pseudomonas osteomyelitis after a plantar puncture wound through a rubber sandal. *Pediatr Infect Dis J.* 1996; 15(8):710–711.

12. Inaba AS, Zukin DD, Perro M. An update on the evaluation and management of plantar puncture wounds and Pseudomonas osteomyelitis. *Pediatr Emerg Care.* 1992;8(1):38–44.

13. Rahn KA, Jacobson FS. Pseudomonas osteomyelitis of the metatarsal sesamoid bones. *Am J Orthop (Belle Mead NJ).* 1997;26(5):365–367.

14. Graham BS, Gregory DW. Pseudomonas aeruginosa causing osteomyelitis after puncture wounds of the foot. *South Med J.* 1984;77(10):1228–1230.

15. Lammers RL, Magill T. Detection and management of foreign bodies in soft tissue. *Emerg Med Clin North Am.* 1992;10(4):767–781.

16. Steele M, Tran LV, Watson WA, Muelleman RL. Retained glass foreign bodies in wounds: predictive value of wound characteristics, patient perception, and wound exploration. *Am J Emerg Med.* 1998; 16(7):627–630.

17. Krych SM, Lavery LA. Puncture wounds and foreign body reactions. *Clin Podiatr Med Surg.* 1990;7(4): 725–731.

18. Nyska M, Pomeranz S, Porat S. The advantage of computerized tomography in locating a foreign body in the foot. *J Trauma.* 1986;26(1):93–95.

19. Lavery LA, Walker SC, Harkless LB, Felder-Johnson K. Infected puncture wounds in diabetic and nondiabetic adults. *Diabetes Care.* 1995;18(12): 1588–1591.

20. Lau LS, Bin G, Jaovisidua S, Dankner W, Sartoris DJ. Cost-effectiveness of magnetic resonance imaging in diagnosing Pseudomonas aeruginosa infection after puncture wound. *J Foot Ankle Surg.* 1997;36(1): 36–43.

21. Houston AN, Roy WA, Faust RA, Ewin DM. Tetanus prophylaxis in the treatment of puncture wounds of patients in the deep South. *J Trauma.* 1962;2: 439–450.

22. Fitzgerald RH Jr, Cowan JD. Puncture wounds of the foot. *Orthop Clin North Am.* 1975;6(4):965–972.

23. Weber EJ. Plantar puncture wounds: a survey to determine the incidence of infection. *J Accid Emerg Med.* 1996;13(4):274–277.

24. Pennycook A, Makower R, O'Donnell AM. Puncture wounds of the foot: can infective complications be avoided? *J R Soc Med.* 1994;87(10):581–583.

25. Harrison M, Thomas M. Towards evidence based emergency medicine: best BETs from the Manchester Royal Informary. Antibiotics after puncture wounds to the foot. *Emerg Med J.* 2002;19(1):49.

26. Riegler HF, Routson GW. Complications of deep puncture wounds of the foot. *J Trauma.* 1979;19(1): 18–22.

27. Edlich RF, Rodeheaver GT, Horowitz JH, Morgan RF. Emergency department management of puncture wounds and needlestick exposure. *Emerg Med Clin North Am.* 1986;4(3):581–593.

28. Mahan KT, Kalish SR. Complications following puncture wounds of the foot. *J Am Podiatry Assoc.* 1982;72(10):497–504.

29. Raz R, Miron D. Oral ciprofloxacin for treatment of infection following nail puncture wounds of the foot. *Clin Infect Dis.* 1995;21(1):194–195.

30. Jacobs R, McCarthy R, Elser J. Pseudomonas osteochondritis complicating puncture wounds of the foot of children: a 10-year evaluation. *J Infect Dis.* 1989;160:657–661.

31. Ramirez-Ronda CH, Saavedra S, Rivera-Vazquez CR. Comparative, double-blind study of oral ciprofloxacin and intravenous cefotaxime in skin and skin structure infections. *Am J Med.* 1987;82(4A): 220–223.

CHAPTER 18

Cutaneous and Subcutaneous Abscesses

Subhasish Bose, MD, MRCP, and
Charles V. Pollack, Jr, MD, MA, FACEP, FAAEM, FAHA

Cutaneous and subcutaneous abscesses are surgical lesions within the dermis and deeper subcutaneous tissues. They are localized collections of inflammatory and infectious products completely or nearly completely encapsulated by firm granulation tissue. The typical cutaneous manifestations of abscesses are erythema, tenderness, and induration, with or without fluctuance.

EPIDEMIOLOGY

According to a 2007 report from the National Center for Health Statistics, infections of the skin are the seventh most common reason for emergency department (ED) visits, with cellulitis and abscesses accounting for nearly 2.7 million visits to the ED in 2005. Emergency department visits for abscesses have become much more common since 1996, owing at least in part to lay concern over resistant bacteria such as "flesh-eating Strep" and methicillin-resistant *Staphylococcus aureus* (MRSA).[1]

RISK FACTORS

Skin abscesses can develop in healthy individuals with no predisposing conditions other than skin or nasal carriage of *S aureus*; spontaneous infection caused by community-acquired MRSA (CA-MRSA) may occur with greater frequency than abscesses caused by other pathogens.[2] Individuals in close contact with others who have active infection with skin abscesses, furuncles, and carbuncles are at increased risk, as well, even if otherwise healthy. Moreover, any process leading to a breach in the skin barrier can predispose to the development of an abscess. Cutaneous abscesses are more common in patients with inflammatory bowel disease and various immune deficiencies such as chronic granulomatous disease and HIV infection. Skin and soft tissue infections are the most common cause of hospital admission of injection drug users (IDUs) who resort to injection directly into skin ("skin popping") or muscle when they are no longer able to inject intravenously.[3]

ANATOMICAL DISTRIBUTION

Anatomical location is an efficient determinant for the classification of abscesses, unlike other infectious processes, which are typically classified by microbiologic etiology. Abscesses occur throughout the body, on cutaneous and mucosal surfaces; approximately 20% occur on the head and neck, 25% in the buttock and perineal area, 25% in the axillae, 15% in the inguinal area, and 18% elsewhere on the extremities.[4] In immunocompetent patients, cutaneous and subcutaneous abscesses are typically local phenomena, caused by staphylococcal and streptococcal skin flora, and are not associated with systemic toxicity. Signs of infection beyond local erythema and associated lymphangitis should prompt suspicion of deeper tissue involvement or bacteremia.[5,6] Abscesses in immunocompromised patients should be approached with great respect. Early recognition is essential to effective management, and the nature of the immune deficiency may mask typical cutaneous signs of severity.[6]

PATHOGENESIS

Cutaneous abscesses are particularly prone to occur around hair follicles, after abrasions or lacerations, after self-treatment for abrasions (which frequently results in maceration of the skin), and around foreign bodies such as sutures, which allow bacteria to gain ready access to subcutaneous tissues usually protected by intact epidermis.[4,5] Whether this microbial penetration results in cellulitis or abscess formation depends upon the size of the inoculum, the virulence of the organism, and a variety of host factors. The body's attempt to sequester the infection and resulting inflammation may result in abscess formation.

MICROBIOLOGY

Skin abscesses can be caused by one or more than one pathogen and may include skin flora as well as organisms from adjacent mucous membranes. They originate from a breakdown in the usual epidermal defenses. Most cutaneous abscesses, therefore, are caused by skin flora: staphylococci in most areas, and anaerobic bacteria in the perioral (usually gram-positive) and perianal (usually gram-negative) regions.[7] Important exceptions to this rule include abscesses resulting from trauma, such as a bite wound, when foreign bacteria are injected under the epidermis. Less commonly, a deep tissue abscess may extend into the skin. Much rarer are hematogenously seeded skin infections such as that classically ascribed to bacterial endocarditis in IDUs.

For the past few years, there has been a gradual change in the microbiology of cutaneous abscesses.

TABLE 18–1	Risk Factors for MRSA Skin Infections
Recent hospitalization	Hemodialysis
Residence in a long-term care facility	Incarceration
	Military service
Recent antibiotic therapy	Sharing needles, razors, or other sharp objects
HIV infection	
Men who have sex with men	Sharing sports equipment
Injection drug use	Previous history of MRSA

Methicillin-resistant *S aureus* is now the most common cause of cutaneous abscesses in the United States.[8] Health care–associated MRSA (HA-MRSA) and CA-MRSA differ with respect to their clinical and molecular epidemiology. The former is associated with severe, invasive disease in hospitalized patients. Recently, several reports also describe a rise in CA-MRSA. It has been described as "an emerging epidemic."[9] A list of risk factors for MRSA skin infections is presented in Table 18-1.

DIAGNOSIS

Skin abscesses manifest as painful, tender, and erythematous nodules. They are frequently surmounted by a pustule and surrounded by a rim of erythematous swelling, and may be associated with regional reactive lymphadenopathy. They are often fluctuant, and spontaneous drainage of purulent material may occur. Fever, chills, and systemic toxicity are uncommon in immunocompetent hosts. A thorough history and physical examination should always precede treatment of all but the most minor and obvious cutaneous abscesses. Issues of interest include any evidence of immune compromise, any systemic symptoms that may give clues to the diagnosis of an underlying disease more complex than the abscess, and characteristics of the abscess (such as the presence of vesicles) that may suggest an alternative diagnosis.

If one is not sure whether an area of induration and erythema represents an abscess (when fluctuance is lacking, for example), diagnostic needle aspiration can be considered. If pus is identified, formal incision and drainage should then be performed. Ultrasound may also prove to be useful in identifying

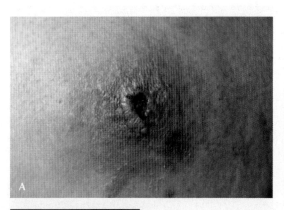

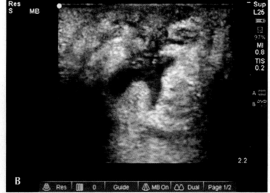

FIGURES 18-1A and 18-1B

Cellulitis with underlying abscess: The superficial appearance of this spontaneously draining cellulitic process leaves unclear the potential depth of tissue involvement below. Ultrasound, however, clearly demonstrates the purulent abscess underneath. Images courtesy of Jason Nomura, MD, Christiana Medical Center.

local collections of pus (Figure 18-1). Ultrasound is an efficient, noninvasive diagnostic tool that can augment the physician's clinical examination. Ultrasound has been shown to be superior to clinical judgment alone in determining the presence or the absence of occult abscess formation, differentiating between cellulitis and abscess, and helping to ensure appropriate management and limit unnecessary invasive procedures.[10,11] Ultrasonographic diagnosis of soft-tissue abscesses at different sites of the body can also help with an urgent choice of surgical procedure.[12] In case of suspected breast abscess, ultrasound can not only efficiently characterize the collection, but also can augment needle aspiration as an alternative to surgical incision and drainage.[13,14]

Soft tissue imaging with ultrasonography is best achieved with 7.5 to 10+ MHz linear transducers (3.5 to 5 MHz curved transducers may be helpful with deeper abscesses), using a probe cover to prevent cross-contamination. Fluid collections should be scanned in two planes to define their shape; gentle pressure over the abscess with the probe may yield a positive "squish sign." Subcutaneous tissue usually appears hypoechoic with hyperechoic strands of connective tissue distributed throughout. Cellulitis is characterized by diffuse thickening of the subcutaneous layer caused by edema; the edema and the hypoechoic septae between fat and connective tissue produce a characteristic "cobblestone" appearance. The appearance of abscesses is more variable, ranging from anechoic to irregularly hyperechoic; they may be round or irregular and are sometimes lobulated; more consistently, though, posterior acoustic enhancement is seen (Figures 18-2 and 18-3).

TREATMENT

Treatment of cutaneous and subcutaneous abscesses is attended by several significant questions:

1. Can the infection be treated with antimicrobials alone, or should a drainage procedure be performed?
2. If a drainage procedure is chosen, should antibiotics be given before the procedure, in case the procedure itself causes a seeding bacteremia?
3. If a drainage procedure is chosen, is needle aspiration sufficient, or should formal incision and drainage be performed?
4. If incision and drainage is chosen, how should the procedure be performed?
5. If incision and drainage completely empties the abscess cavity, is subsequent antibiotic therapy indicated?
6. Should immunocompromised patients be managed differently from immunocompetent patients?
7. Are there abscesses or similar-appearing cutaneous and subcutaneous lesions that should be managed differently in the ED?

The Role of Antibiotics

Antibiotics alone are inadequate treatment for a localized collection of pus.[15] The body encapsulates cutaneous and subcutaneous abscesses with dense fibrous tissue in an effort to prevent them from spreading, and, in so doing, also effectively reduces the blood supply to the infectious focus. Antibiotics do not concentrate sufficiently in these highly inflamed areas to ensure bactericidal effect.[15]

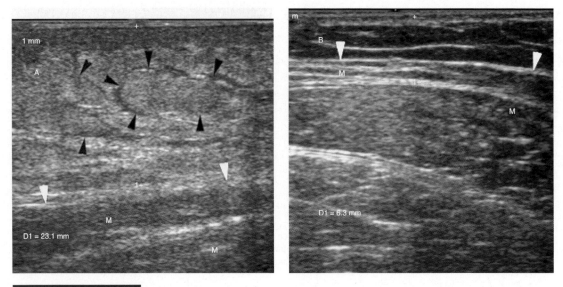

FIGURES 18-2A and 18-2B

Cellulitis with contralateral normal comparison: Image A shows the characteristic sonographic findings of cellulitis with thickening and echogenicity of the soft tissues (measured between the skin surface and the superficial muscle fascia, 23.1 mm), blurring of the muscle fascia (white arrowheads), and "cobblestoning" (black arrowheads) resulting from accumulation of edema in the interlobular septa of the adipose tissue. In comparison, contralateral normal subcutaneous tissue (B) is thinner (6.3 mm), and less echogenic, with septal architecture appearing echogenic (delicate white lines) and with crisp muscle fascia (white arrowheads). Note. M = muscle. Images courtesy of A.J. Dean, MD, University of Pennsylvania.

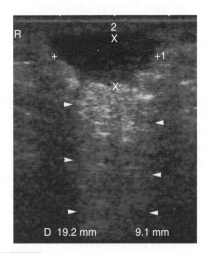

FIGURE 18-3

Abscess: Typical sonographic appearance of an abscess with heterogeneous echogenicity and irregular internal margins is shown. The internal echoes are caused by debris and occasionally gas. The artifact of posterior acoustic enhancement (arrowheads) is an important aid in recognizing abscesses that are isoechoic with surrounding soft tissues because of the presence of extensive internal debris. Image courtesy of A.J. Dean, MD, University of Pennsylvania.

On initial presentation, however, abscesses may not be amenable to drainage. Premature incision into an abscess before it is well localized may in fact allow the harmful spread of infection into adjacent and deeper tissues. In these situations, it may be appropriate to treat with antibiotics for 24 to 48 hours while the abscess "ripens," perhaps with the help of warm compresses. Resolution of the lesion during this time implies retrospectively that the pathologic process was cellulitis and not abscess, and should not be construed as supporting nonsurgical management of true cutaneous and subcutaneous abscesses.

In individuals at risk for endocarditis (immunocompromised patients or patients with artificial heart valves or joints, for instance), it is reasonable to administer empiric antimicrobial prophylaxis (with activity against MRSA) before incision and drainage.[16,17] Older studies have suggested that sharp instrumentation of an abscess has the potential to seed the bloodstream with bacteria from the abscess, even in immunocompetent patients.[18] Later studies, however, have refuted this theory.[19] In at-risk patients, intravenous vancomycin (1 g) 60 minutes prior to instrumentation is preferred. Other regimens may be appropriate as well.

Patients with multiple lesions, extensive surrounding cellulitis, immunosuppression, risk for MRSA,

TABLE 18–2	**Antimicrobial Therapy for Skin and Soft Tissue Infections Caused by Methicillin-Resistant *Staphylococcus aureus* in Adults**	
	Preferred	**Alternative**
Parental therapy	Vancomycin (30 mg/kg IV every 24 hours in 2 equally divided doses, not to exceed 2 g in 24 hours unless concentrations in serum are inappropriately low)	Daptomycin (4 mg/kg IV once daily) Linezolid (600 mg IV twice daily) Tigecycline (100 mg IV once, thereafter 50 mg IV every 12 hours)
Oral therapy	TMP-SMX* (2 double-strength tablets orally twice daily) Doxycycline or minocycline (100 mg orally twice daily) Clindamycin (300 mg to 450 mg orally every 6 to 8 hours)	Linezolid (600 mg orally twice daily)

* TMP–SMX = trimethoprim–sulfamethoxazole.

or systemic signs of infection should be managed with incision and drainage as well as antimicrobial therapy.[20] A list of suggested initial antibiotic choices for patients with abscesses is presented in Table 18-2.

Surgical Management

Needle aspiration

Thorough drainage of an abscess is achieved only by incision and drainage (I&D), not by aspiration. The only reasonable indication for needle aspiration of a suspected abscess is for diagnostic confirmation of the presence of pus when fluctuance is lacking, or when sterile hematoma or seroma are differential diagnostic considerations. If pus is found, then a formal I&D should follow. As noted previously, ultrasound can be used to guide needle placement and delineate the extent of the abscess cavity, and is both more sensitive and more specific than the clinical exam alone.[11,21] Incomplete drainage is painful and inefficient and needlessly prolongs the patient's course of treatment. Abscesses in cosmetically important areas can often be drained from the mucosal side (for example, a facial abscess may be drained through the buccal mucosa), but even when this is not possible, the inadequacy of needle aspiration still argues against its use as sole surgical therapy.

Incision and drainage

Incision and drainage is an exquisitely painful procedure performed in an area already rife with inflammation

and pain. After consideration of prophylactic antibiotic coverage, the clinician's next efforts should be directed at adequate anesthesia and analgesia. This is not only a humane approach, but also facilitates thorough exploration of the abscess cavity and destruction of any septations inside.

Typical infiltrated local anesthetics such as lidocaine are notoriously ineffective in areas of inflammation, increased tissue pressure, and thin skin.[22] Gentle subcutaneous infiltration across the dome of the abscess will anesthetize the patient to the incision, but not to the deeper exploration and dissection. Systemic analgesia or procedural sedation is generally effective for abscess drainage in the ED (see Chapter 6). Ethyl chloride spray is a poor choice of anesthetic agent in all but the most superficial of lesions.

It is generally true that the larger the abscess, the more analgesia is needed, but only up to a practical limit. Larger, more complex abscesses, those in particularly frail, ill, or immunocompromised patients, or those in exquisitely well-innervated areas such as the perineum should be considered for formal surgical I&D in the operating room under the influence of more powerful anesthetics. Occasionally, performance of a field block around the abscess will allow a relatively painless I&D procedure.

After anesthesia or analgesia and identification of anatomic structures that may obstruct the course of action (such as superficial blood vessels, nerves, or muscles and tendons), a single stab wound extended into a linear (not cruciate) incision is made across the length of the fluctuant area with a No. 11 scalpel blade.

The abscess cavity should be entered with the stab; avoid "sawing" or "probing" to find pus. Whenever possible, the direction of the incision should be parallel to the lines of minimal tension to optimize scarring after drainage. Beware of incision of a pulsatile abscess or one over large blood vessels. If there is concern for aneurysm or pseudoaneursym, ultrasound of the lesion can help confirm the presence of a true abscess; vascular structures should, of course, never be incised. Once the cavity is opened, it is essential that it be thoroughly and systematically explored. This should be done bluntly, with a hemostat or (size allowing) a gloved finger, and is the most painful portion of the procedure for the patient. Often, additional local anesthesia will be required. Through the years, various authors have recommended irrigating the cavity with saline, dilute hydrogen peroxide, or dilute povidine-iodine solution, but none of these have been associated with a change in outcome.

Liberated pus can be irrigated or suctioned away. Although Gram staining and cultures of pus from cutaneous and subcutaneous collections were not obtained routinely prior to the increased prevalence of MRSA,[23] it is now reasonable to send material obtained from I&D for culture and susceptibility testing.[24] In acutely toxic and immunocompromised patients, specimens for microbiologic study (including anaerobic cultures) to detect atypical or resistant pathogens are best obtained by sterile needle aspiration before I&D. The microbiology data are important for both clinicians and epidemiologists to guide both antimicrobial therapy for the patient, and prevention and control measures for the public health.

The incision should not be closed, even in cosmetically important areas. To prevent the opposing edges of the incision from touching, ribbon gauze should be placed into the wound, protruding out like a wick; it is not necessary to pack the cavity tightly; this practice traps purulence in the cavity and may enlarge the eventual scar. The goal is to apply the packing gauze to all surfaces of the cavity, so that its surface is gently débrided when the gauze is removed. Packing also generally promotes hemostasis, although abscess I&D is not typically a bloody procedure.

The gauze should be removed in 48 hours. This should be done in a prearranged wound-check examination scheduled at the time of incision and drainage. If purulent drainage persists, the cavity should be re-explored, irrigated, and re-wicked. Once the gauze removed is dry and clean, further packing is of no benefit. A recent study suggests that routine packing of drained abscesses in the ED is not only unnecessary but also more painful than no packing.[25]

Postprocedure Antibiotic Treatment

Thorough drainage of an abscess often obviates the need for antibiotic therapy. Patients with evidence of extensive skin involvement or systemic toxicity should receive parenteral antimicrobial therapy that includes empiric coverage for gram-positive pathogens including MRSA as well as gram-negative and anaerobic organisms, pending culture and susceptibility results. The duration of antimicrobial therapy should be tailored to clinical improvement; about 5 to 7 days is usually sufficient. Longer duration of therapy may be warranted for patients with severe disease; in such cases, duration should be tailored to clinical resolution of symptoms. Patients treated initially with parenteral therapy with resolving signs of infection may complete antimicrobial therapy with an oral agent.

Extra caution should be taken for the following patients with high-risk conditions and broad-spectrum antibiotic coverage should be instituted as early as possible to avoid bacteremia and worsening of the local tissue damage:

- systemic toxicity (fever, chills, rigors)
- recurrent abscesses
- significant surrounding cellulitis or proximal lymphangitis
- abscesses in high-risk areas, such as the central face
- any condition for which preprocedure antibiotics are deemed appropriate, even if the drainage is apparently successful.

SPECIAL CONSIDERATIONS, DIFFERENTIAL DIAGNOSIS, AND DIFFERENTIAL MANAGEMENT

1. Much anecdotal experience and worrisomely scant good data support the use of empiric antibiotic therapy as an adjunct to I&D for treatment of abscesses in immunocompromised patients. A broad definition of "immunocompromise" is appropriate in this regard, and includes patients with HIV/AIDS, patients with diabetes, those with chronic use of corticosteroids, organ transplant patients taking immunosuppressants, patients receiving chemotherapy for malignancy, alcoholics, malnourished patients, and even patients with significant liver, heart, or lung disease, whose overall humoral immunity might be questionable.

    As stated previously, for immunocompromised patients, it is reasonable to perform Gram stain and culture of the abscess contents, both to direct empiric therapy and to provide good alternative choices should initial treatment fail. Antibiotics should be given until the infection resolves.

2. Apart from the usual suspicion of MRSA, special considerations in the ED care of cutaneous and subcutaneous abscesses include specific predilections for nonstaphylococcal, nonstreptococcal etiologies. Isolation of multiple organisms (including gram-negatives and anaerobes) is more common in patients with skin abscesses involving the perioral, perirectal, or vulvovaginal areas. Organisms of oral origin, including anaerobes, are seen most frequently among IDUs.[7] Additional pathogens include *Pseudomonas, Candida* species, and others. Individuals exposed to whirlpool footbaths at nail salons are at risk for mycobacterial furunculosis.

3. Some skin lesions may appear to be simple cutaneous abscesses but in fact are not. Apparent abscesses that must be approached with great caution include those overlying the frontal bone and sinus, the chest wall, and the peritoneal cavity. Patients with some systemic diseases, such as malignancies or sarcoidosis, also should be carefully evaluated before drainage of an apparent cutaneous abscess is attempted.

   ■ ***Folliculitis, furuncles, and carbuncles:*** Folliculitis is a superficial bacterial infection of the hair follicles with purulent material in the epidermis, mostly caused by *S aureus*. Simple folliculitis typically responds to local cleansing and wound care. A furuncle (or "boil") is an infection of the hair follicle in which purulent material extends through the dermis into the subcutaneous tissue, where a small abscess forms. A carbuncle is a coalescence of several furuncles into a single inflammatory mass with purulent drainage from multiple hair follicles.[20] Furuncles are treated with I&D in a conventional fashion; carbuncles frequently require formal surgical drainage in the operating room.

   ■ ***Hidradenitis suppurativa*** is a chronic follicular occlusive disease involving the apocrine glands of the intertriginous skin of the axillary, groin, perianal, and inframammary regions. Secondary infection typically results in extensive abscess formation and fistulization. Recurrent I&Ds cause significant scarring, and wider drainage procedures eventually are indicated. Although anaerobic bacteria are frequently isolated from hidradenitis suppurativa, staphylococci remain the most common cause of infection. There is no simple cure for hidradenitis suppurativa, but medical and surgical strategies can help to eliminate existing lesions and prevent development of new lesions. No large randomized trials have addressed treatment and no single treatment is effective in all patients. The choice of medical and surgical therapy is based upon patient preferences, the outcome of previous treatments, and severity of current lesions graded according to Hurley's staging.[26] Patients should be counseled to avoid tight or synthetic clothing over affected area, prolonged exposure to hot humid environments, and use of deodorant or depilation in affected areas. Weight reduction and smoking cessation can also help.

   ■ ***Pilonidal cyst abscesses***: Pilonidal sinuses, cysts, and abscesses are relatively common findings in the sacrococcygeal region. Pilonidal sinuses are congenital lesions, but usually are not evident until adolescence, when body hair starts to increase. Drainage of a pilonidal abscess should always include a search for and removal of hair and follicular tissue at the base of the cavity. Because of the possibility of fecal soiling, these lesions may occasionally require broad-spectrum antibiotic coverage. Simple I&D will relieve symptoms temporarily, but formal excision of the cyst cavity is usually required to prevent recurrence.

   ■ ***Breast abscesses***: Although mastitis and breast abscess during breast feeding are common, non-puerperal mastitis is actually more frequently encountered. All these are typically managed with routine I&D, although periareolar abscesses are more problematic because they tend to be polymicrobial and because fluctuance may be deep and difficult to appreciate. Deeper breast abscesses typically require formal surgical drainage.[27] If the infection does not resolve within several days, inflammatory breast cancer should be considered.

   ■ Management of ***Bartholin's gland abscesses*** differs in two ways from the management of other cutaneous and subcutaneous processes: firstly, cultures of the Bartholin's abscess typically show polymicrobial infection[28] but usually with gram-negative organisms, particularly coliforms and gonococci. Cervical cultures should be taken for gonorrhea when the abscess is treated. Secondly, a specific device, the Word catheter, is used in the drainage of the abscesses; it fosters complete drainage and subsequent fistulization of the abscess. The incision, through the mucosal surface of the labia, should be made only large enough to admit the uninflated catheter tip, and the balloon should be filled with a sufficient volume of water to prevent extrusion without causing persistent pain. Prior to insertion of the catheter, all purulent material should be drained. The Word catheter is intended to be left in place for 6 to 8 weeks to allow proper epithelialization and fistulization to occur and therefore to prevent recurrence.[29] Persistent infection, especially in older patients, should raise the possibility of an inflammatory cancer.

- *Lymphogranuloma venereum* is a sexually transmitted disease caused by L1, L2, and L3 serotypes of *Chlamydia trachomatis*. It typically manifests as unilateral, painful, swollen, suppurative inguinal or femoral lymph nodes. Although these lesions may look like abscesses, they should not be drained, as fistulization is a likely undesirable sequela. Serology or immunology is more accurate in making the diagnosis than is aspiration and culture, which is notoriously unreliable. Ultrasound is useful to demonstrate the absence of abscess. The preferred treatment is oral doxycycline 100 mg twice daily for 21 days.[30]

- *Paronychia* are infections of the potential space between the nail cuticle and the nail root. They typically occur around the fingernails but may also affect toenails. A paronychium is usually a staphylococcal infection, but anaerobes may be found, particularly in patients who suck their fingers or bite their fingernails. The usual progression of illness is hangnail, to cellulitis, to abscess. Adequate I&D of paronychia typically does not require removal of the nail. Local anesthesia may be necessary and is best effected by a digital approach. These lesions are most readily drained by inserting a No. 11 blade scalpel just under the eponychium, parallel to the nail. A small ribbon gauze wick may be used to keep the wound open for 1 to 2 days. Persistence of symptoms for weeks should prompt investigation for osteomyelitis of the distal phalanx.[31]

- *Felons* are infections of the pulp space of the fingertip. They often result from trauma with or without a retained foreign body, although sometimes the patient cannot identify a specific traumatic cause. Felons are notoriously difficult to drain because of limiting fibrous septations and because of the potential for adverse functional and cosmetic sequelae with improper surgical approach. Drainage through a lateral incision is preferred. The incision should be performed just lateral to the nail fold and the fibrous septa should be broken down, keeping the exploration dorsal to the neurovascular bundle. Antibiotic coverage is usually recommended.[22]

- *Herpetic whitlow* is a viral infection of the distal phalanx that is caused by herpes simplex virus. At some point in their natural history these infections will manifest typical herpetic vesicles, but on ED presentation these are not always evident, and the fingertip may appear to be abscessed. Obtaining a detailed history for the presence of vesicles is important because whitlow does not respond to I&D. In fact, it may worsen after I&D owing to bacterial superinfection.[32] The natural history of herpetic whitlow is to improve on its own in 2 to 3 weeks.[33] Many recommend treatment with oral acyclovir (400 mg three times a day) for 10 days, although the efficacy of this approach is unproven in controlled trials.[34]

- *Pott's puffy tumor* is a subperiosteal abscess of the frontal bone that occurs as a complication of frontal sinusitis. Classically this lesion is manifest as an indolent, puffy, circumscribed swelling of the forehead. Fully developed, Pott's puffy tumor has the appearance of an abscess of the forehead. It is increasingly rare in this era of broad-spectrum antibiotics. Surgical drainage is the treatment of choice but should not be performed without a preceding CT scan of the head to determine the extent of frontal bone involvement. These infections tend to be polymicrobial and antibiotic therapy is guided by culture results.[35]

- *Granulomata*: A number of granulomatous syndromes may manifest skin lesions that appear to be cutaneous or subcutaneous abscesses. Wegener's granulomatosis may present with perirectal or perianal lesions; sarcoidosis may cause erythema nodosum and other skin lesions that may be mistaken for routine abscesses.[36] Careful attention should be paid to obtaining a thorough history in patients with abscess and any other skin lesions, otherwise unexplained pulmonary or gastrointestinal symptoms, or systemic symptoms consistent with chronic disease.

- *Skin lesions of Crohn's disease*: Likewise, Crohn's disease is sometimes accompanied by skin lesions, which may variably appear as nodules, abscesses, or ulcers. These are not known to precede the gastrointestinal symptoms. These lesions may become secondarily infected, but otherwise routinely respond to antiinflammatory medications.[37]

■ **Neoplastic extension**: There are occasional case reports of internal malignancies presenting as cutaneous abscesses.[38] Biopsy of the abscess wall may reveal the underlying diagnosis, but is not likely to be performed in the ED or the primary care setting. Again, this unusual relationship reinforces the value of a thorough history and physical examination in patients with cutaneous and subcutaneous abscesses; concern should be raised from recurring or resistant lesions.

■ **Deep abscess extension**: Likewise, untreated deep abscesses may manifest cutaneously. This should be suspected particularly in patients with diabetes or other immunocompromising conditions. When abscesses occur on the abdominal wall or chest wall, CT scanning should be considered before I&D is attempted and the deep tissues are inadvertently exposed.[39]

■ **Vibrio infection**: Although classically presenting as skin necrosis with bullous lesions, skin infections with *Vibrio vulnificus* may present early as abscesses. These patients tend to be rather ill and their prognosis without aggressive surgical treatment is poor. A history of any exposure of a wound to salt water or any recent ingestion of raw shellfish should be sought. Patients with liver disease and *Vibrio* infection may have particularly rapid downhill courses.[40]

■ **Necrotizing soft tissue infections** (panniculitis, necrotizing fasciitis, myositis, osteomyelitis) may present early with simple cutaneous abscess. This may be more likely in IDUs.[5] These illnesses can be detected early only with a thorough history and physical examination and close follow-up.

■ **Furuncular myiasis** is caused by invasion of viable skin by the larval maggots of various species of flies, such as the human botfly and the tumbu fly. These lesions will most often be seen in natives of, or recent visitors to, Africa or Central or South America. Unlike abscesses, myiasis lesions have a central opening through which the maggot breathes. In addition, the patient experiences lancinating pain when the maggot moves. The most atraumatic treatment for such lesions is to suffocate the maggot by covering the breathing opening for several hours. When the maggot tries to come out for air, it can be extruded by firm lateral pressure on the lesion.[41] Larvae are sometimes discovered unexpectedly upon routine abscess I&D.[42] A positive travel history is necessary to make the diagnosis before intervening.

REFERENCES

1. Taira BR, Singer AJ, Thode HC Jr, Lee CC. National epidemiology of cutaneous abscesses: 1996 to 2005. *Am J Emerg Med.* 2009;27(3):289–292.

2. Lee, MC, Rios, AM, Aten, MF, et al. Management and outcome of children with skin and soft tissue abscesses caused by community-acquired methicillin-resistant Staphylococcus aureus. *Pediatr Infect Dis J.* 2004;23(2):123–127.

3. Ebright JR, Pieper B. Skin and soft tissue infections in injection drug users. *Infect Dis Clin North Am.* 2002;16(3):697–712.

4. Peter G, Smith AL. Group A streptococcal infections of the skin and pharynx (first of two parts). *N Engl J Med.* 1977;297(6):311–317.

5. Callahan TE, Schecter WP, Horn JK. Necrotizing soft tissue infection masquerading as cutaneous abscess following illicit drug injection. *Arch Surg.* 1998; 133(8):812–817.

6. Bisno AL, Stevens DL. Streptococcal infections of skin and soft tissues. *N Engl J Med.* 1996;334(4): 240–245.

7. Summanen, PH, Talan, DA, Strong, C, et al. Bacteriology of skin and soft-tissue infections: comparison of infections in intravenous drug users and individuals with no history of intravenous drug use. *Clin Infect Dis.* 1995;20(suppl 2):S279–S282.

8. Moran GJ, Krishnadasan A, Gorwitz RJ, et al. Methicillin-resistant S. aureus infections among patients in the emergency department. *N Engl J Med.* 2006;355(7):666–674.

9. Cohen PR, Grossman ME. Management of cutaneous lesions associated with an emerging epidemic: community-acquired methicillin-resistant *Staphylococcus aureus* skin infections. *J Am Acad Dermatol.* 2004;51(1):132–135.

10. Ramirez-Schrempp D, Dorfman DH, Baker WE, Liteplo AS. Ultrasound soft-tissue applications in the pediatric emergency department: to drain or not to drain? *Pediatr Emerg Care.* 2009;25(1):44–48.

11. Squire BT, Fox JC, Anderson C. ABSCESS: applied bedside sonography for convenient evaluation of superficial soft tissue infections. *Acad Emerg Med.* 2005;12(7):601–606.

12. Buianov VM, Ishutinov VD, Rodoman GV, Za'vianov BG, Ionova EA. The role of ultrasonic diagnosis in selecting the surgical tactics in suppurative-inflammatory diseases of soft tissues [in Russian]. *Sov Med.* 1989;(9):35–39.

13. Elagili F, Abdullah N, Fong L, Pei T. Aspiration of breast abscess under ultrasound guidance: outcome obtained and factors affecting success. *Asian J Surg.* 2007;30(1):40–44.

14. Tiu CM, Chiou HJ, Chou YH, et al. Sonographic features of breast abscesses with emphasis on "hypoechoic rim" sign. *Zhonghua Yi Xue Za Zhi (Taipei).* 2001;64(3):153–160.

15. Llera JL, Levy RC, Staneck JL. Cutaneous abscesses: natural history and management in an outpatient facility. *J Emerg Med.* 1984;1(6):489–493.

16. Dijani AS, Taubert KA, Wilson W, et al. Prevention of bacterial endocarditis. Recommendations by the American Heart Association. *JAMA.* 1997;277(22): 1794–1801.

17. Wilson, W, Taubert, KA, Gewitz, M, et al. Prevention of infective endocarditis: guidelines from the American Heart Association: a guideline from the American Heart Association Rheumatic Fever, Endocarditis, and Kawasaki Disease Committee, Council on Cardiovascular Disease in the Young, and the Council on Clinical Cardiology, Council on Cardiovascular Surgery and Anesthesia, and the Quality of Care and Outcomes Research Interdisciplinary Working Group. *Circulation.* 2007;116(15): 1736–1754.

18. Le Frock JL, Molavi A. Transient bacteremia associated with diagnostic and therapeutic procedures. *Compr Ther.* 1982;8:65–71.

19. Bobrow BJ, Pollack CV Jr, Gamble S, Seligson RA. Incision and drainage of cutaneous abscesses is not associated with bacteremia in afebrile adults. *Ann Emerg Med.* 1997;29(3):404–408.

20. Stevens DL, Bisno AL, Chambers HF, et al. Practice guidelines for the diagnosis and management of skin and soft-tissue infections. *Clin Infect Dis.* 2005; 41(10):1373–1406.

21. Baurmash HD. Ultrasonography in the diagnosis and treatment of facial abscess. *J Oral Maxillofac Surg.* 1999;57(5):635–636.

22. Stapczynski JS. Skin and soft-tissue infections. In: Brillman JC, Quenzer RW, eds. *Infectious Disease in Emergency Medicine*, 2nd ed. Philadelphia, PA: Lippincott-Raven; 1998:755–790.

23. Meislin HW, McGehee MD, Rosen P. Management and microbiology of cutaneous abscesses. *JACEP.* 1978;7(5):186–191.

24. Miller LG, Quan C, Shay A, et al. A prospective investigation of outcomes after hospital discharge for endemic, community-acquired methicillin-resistant and -susceptible Staphylococcus aureus skin infection. *Clin Infect Dis.* 2007;44(4):483–492.

25. O'Malley GF, Dominici P, Giraldo P, Aguilera E, Verma M, Lares C, Burger P, Williams E. Routine packing of simple cutaneous abscesses is painful and probably unnecessary. *Acad Emerg Med.* 2009 May;16(5):470–3.

26. Hurley HJ. Axillary hyperhidrosis, apocrine bromhidrosis, hidradenitis suppurativa, and familial benign pemphigus: surgical approach. In: Roenigk RK, Roenigk HH, eds. *Dermatologic Surgery.* New York, NY: Marcel Dekker Inc.;1989:729.

27. Watt-Boolsen S, Rasmussen NR, Blichert-Toft M. Primary periareolar abscess in the nonlactating breast: risk of recurrence. *Am J Surg.* 1987;153(6): 571–573.

28. Tanaka K, Mikamo H, Ninomiya M, et al. Microbiology of Bartholin's gland abscess in Japan. *J Clin Microbiol.* 2005;43(8):4258–4261.

29. Word B. Office treatment of cyst and abscess of Bartholin's gland duct. *South Med J.* 1968;61(5): 514–518.

30. Ward H, Martin I, MacDonald N, et al. Lymphogranuloma venereum in the United Kingdom. *Clin Infect Dis.* 2007;44(1):26–32.

31. Zook EG, Brown RE. The perinychium. In: Green DP, Hotchkiss RN, Pederson WC, eds. *Operative Hand Surgery.* 4th ed. New York, NY: Churchill Livingstone; 1999:1353–1380.

32. Feder HM, Long SS. Herpetic whitlow. Epidemiology, clinical characteristics, diagnosis, and treatment. *Am J Dis Child.* 1983;137(9):861–863.

33. Walker LG, Simmons BP, Lovallo JL. Pediatric herpetic hand infections. *J Hand Surg (Am).* 1990;15; 176–180.

34. Kesson AM. Use of acyclovir in herpes simplex virus infections. *J Paediatr Child Health.* 1998;3 4(1):9–13.

35. Babu RP, Todor R, Kasoff SS. Pott's puffy tumor: the forgotten entity. Case report. *J Neurosurg.* 1996;84(1): 110–112.

36. Mañá J, Marcoval J, Graells J, Salazar A, Peyrí J, Pujol R. Cutaneous involvement in sarcoidosis. Relationship to systemic disease *Arch Dermatol.* 1997;133(7):882–888.

37. Hackzell-Bradley M, Hedblad MA, Stephansson EA. Metastatic Crohn's disease. Report of 3 cases with special reference to histopathologic findings. *Arch Dermatol.* 1996;132(8):928–932.

38. Mann GN, Scoggins CR, Adkins B. Perforated cecal adenocarcinoma presenting as a thigh abscess. *South Med J.* 1997;90(9):949–951.

39. Bobrow BJ, Mohr J, Pollack CV Jr. An unusual complication of missed appendicitis. *J Emerg Med.* 1996;14(6):719–722.

40. Pollack CV Jr, Fuller J. Update on emerging infections from the Centers for Disease Control and Prevention. Outbreak of *Vibrio parahaemolyticus* infection associated with eating raw oysters and clams harvested from Long Island Sound—Connecticut, New Jersey, and New York, 1998. *Ann Emerg Med.* 1999;34(5):679–680.

41. Kain KC. Skin lesions in returned travelers. *Med Clin N Am.* 1999;83(4):1077–1102.

42. Johnston M, Dickinson G. An unexpected surprise in a common boil. *J Emerg Med.* 1996;14(6): 779–781.

CHAPTER 19

Soft Tissue Injuries of the Hand

Breena R. Taira, MD, MPH, Mark Gelfand, MD, and
Alexander B. Dagum, MD, FRCS(C), FACS

The hand is very complex both in structure and function. Hand injuries account for 15% of emergency room visits. It is, therefore, critical for the emergency medicine practitioners and other acute care practitioners to have a good understanding of hand injuries.[1] When one approaches a patient with soft tissue injury of the hand, a careful history is essential. The history must include hand dominance, occupation, circumstances of the trauma with position of hand at the time of injury, time elapsed since injury, and symptomatology (location of pain, numbness, weakness, and loss of mobility in the hand).[2] Identification of injury mechanism can help to evaluate risk of foreign body within the wound. Foreign body sensation, however, as reported by the patient is unreliable in determining the presence of retained foreign body.[3] In addition, as in all patients with wounds, past medical history, medications, allergies, and tetanus status should also be discussed.[4]

On physical examination, if direct pressure and elevation are inadequate to control bleeding, a blood pressure cuff can be temporarily inflated to 10 mm Hg to 20 mm Hg above systolic blood pressure to help achieve hemostasis. Blind attempts at clamping vessels should be avoided.[5] If bleeding is controlled, the first aspect of physical examination is observation. One hint on physical examination of a tendon injury is disruption of the natural cascade of the fingers (Figure 19-1).[2] Next, overlying tissue should be inspected as débridement of devitalized tissue is necessary to aid healing and reduce risk of infection.[2] Nerve and vascular examinations should always be documented.

Nerve examination should include two-point discrimination and should be compared with the contralateral (uninjured) side as subjective examination is often unreliable. Vascular examination should include CTTC (capillary refill, temperature, turgor, and color). If there is any doubt about the vascular status of the digit, it should be pricked with a 22-gauge needle at the fingertip. Slow, bright-red bleeding should be observed (no bleeding is indicative of arterial insufficiency; fast, dark-blue bleeding is indicative of venous insufficiency). In general, radiographs should always be obtained in any hand injury to rule out a fracture, injury to a joint, or presence of a foreign body.[4] Any rings should be removed from an injured hand as the inevitable postinjury swelling may prevent their future removal and can cause ischemia to the digit.

There are very few evidence-based studies on the management of soft tissue injuries of the hand.[1] The majority of this chapter, therefore, is a synopsis of current practice, which is based on tradition and expert opinion. The remainder of this chapter will focus on the identification and treatment of common soft tissue injuries of the hand.

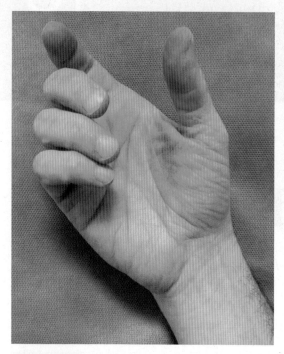

FIGURE 19-1
Disruption of the natural cascade of the digits.

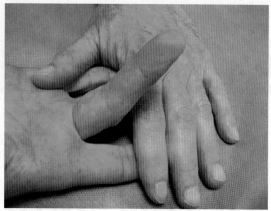

FIGURE 19-2
Evaluation of the flexor digitorum superficialis.

FLEXOR TENDON INJURIES

On physical examination, careful inspection of the wound with débridement of devitalized tissue is necessary. If the tendon sheath has been lacerated, one must have a high index of suspicion of a flexor tendon injury. On initial inspection, flexor tendon injury may be suspected if the affected finger does not assume a flexed position when one is inspecting the natural cascade of the fingers, which shows increased finger flexion from index to small finger.[6] Loss of the tenodesis effect (i.e., increased flexion of the digits with wrist extension) is also characteristic of a flexor tendon injury. Palpation of the extremity may identify a tender area that corresponds to a retracted tendon.[5] It is important to assess both the flexor digitorum superficialis (FDS) and the flexor digitorum profundus (FDP) functions separately. The FDS can be evaluated by holding the adjacent fingers in extension and thus blocking the FDP and asking the patient to flex the affected finger (Figure 19-2). The FDP is tested by holding the midportion of the finger in extension and asking the patient to flex the distal interphalangeal (DIP) joint (Figure 19-3). Flexor tendon injuries are particularly common in rock climbers.[7] The zones of flexor tendon injury were originally described by Verdan[8] and the classification still maintains clinical relevance (Table 19-1).

Partial tendon lacerations are generally repaired if more than 60% of the tendon is lacerated. They are diagnosed by visualization of the injury. Clues that a partial tendon injury might be present include the subjective complaint of weakness, pain with flexion against resistance, or a sensation of triggering of the digit with flexion.[6]

If definitive care of the flexor tendon injury by a hand surgeon will not be immediate, the wound should be irrigated and closed loosely with 5-0 nylon suture.[6] A posterior splint should be applied so that the wrist is maintained in 30° of flexion, the metacarpophalangeal (MCP) joints are in 70°, and the interphalangeal joints are at 15° (Figure 19-4). This will prevent further damage and proximal retraction of the flexor tendon.[6] Patients with grossly contaminated wounds requiring operating room débridement, patients with associated open fractures or joints, and those with high-pressure injection injuries should be admitted to the hospital. Problems requiring the patient to see a hand surgeon immediately in the emergency department (ED) rather than the clinic include

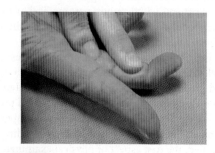

FIGURE 19-3
Evaluation of the flexor digitorum profundus.

TABLE 19–1	Flexor Tendon Injury Zones	
Zone	**Anatomy**	**Considerations**
I	Distal to the FDS insertion	FDP is susceptible to laceration or avulsion
II ("No man's land")	Within the limits of the flexor tendon sheath between the A1 pulley and the insertion of FDS	FDS and FDP injuries are common because of their proximity within the sheath
III	Within the palm between the distal edge of the transverse carpal ligament and A1 pulley	Adjacent tendons, nerves, and vessels are frequently involved
IV	Portion within the carpal tunnel	Lacerations are uncommon in this area
V	Forearm proximal to the carpal tunnel	

Note. FDS = flexor digitorum superficialis; FDP = flexor digitorum profundus.

all of the aforementioned in addition to patients with wounds that cannot be closed and those with arterial laceration. All other acute injuries of the tendons should be referred to be seen by a hand surgeon within 24 to 48 hours. Flexor tendon injuries can be repaired acutely up to 2 weeks after injury. After this point, contraction of the tendon makes primary repair difficult if not impossible. Chronic injuries presenting to the ED (i.e., greater than 2 weeks old) can be referred to a hand surgeon for routine follow-up.[5]

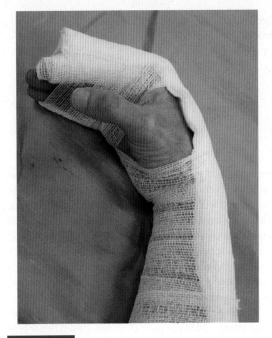

FIGURE 19-4

Splinting of a flexor tendon injury.

EXTENSOR TENDON INJURIES

Because the extensor tendons are superficial, they are susceptible to injury even with minor lacerations. A thorough history is essential as the clenched fist injury with a tooth (the so-called "fight bite" or human bite) is a common mechanism of extensor tendon injuries and can lead to a severe joint infection.[4] The physical examination should again begin with the natural lie of the hand. If this seems abnormal, a high likelihood of tendon injury exists. In an unconscious patient or child where active extension cannot be tested, loss of the tenodesis effect in the involved digit (flexion of the finger with wrist extension and extension of the finger with wrist flexion) should alert the practitioner to an extensor tendon injury. All open wounds on the dorsum of the hand are suspect for extensor tendon injury.[4] Placing the patient's hand palm down on the examination table allows easy examination of extensor tendon function. The tendons should be palpated and then each extensor should be checked by asking the patient to extend the fingertips against resistance. Examination of the tendons directly through the wound requires a local anesthetic, optimal lighting, and sterile technique.[4] This is important as motor function can appear to be intact with partial tendon injuries and, thus, might not be appreciated without direct visualization.

Most clinicians apply the data for partial flexor tendon lacerations to partial extensor tendon lacerations as well and thus advise repair of any injury greater than 50%.[1] Extensor tendon injuries are classified by the location in which the injury occurs. Certain extensor tendon injuries may be repaired by a trained

TABLE 19–2	Extensor Tendon Injury Zones		
Zone	**Anatomy**	**Considerations**	**Treatment**
I	Distal phalanx	Presents as mallet deformity Untreated can lead to a flexion deformity of the distal interphalangeal (DIP) joint and a swan neck deformity	If closed injury, splint DIP joint in extension for 6 weeks
II	Middle phalanx	Presents as mallet deformity Untreated can lead to a flexion deformity of the DIP joint and a swan neck deformity	If closed injury, splint DIP in extension for 6 weeks
III	Proximal interphalangeal (PIP) joint	Untreated leads to boutonnière deformity	Splint of PIP in extension for 6 weeks
IV	Proximal phalanx	May be closed primarily Tendon adhesion to periosteum is a common complication	PIP splinted in extension for 6 weeks
V	Metacarpophalangeal joint	Commonly secondary to human "fight bites" Practitioner should have a high index of suspicion as patient may deny event	Hand surgery consultation Burkhalter splint with wrist in 45° extension and MCP, PIP, and DIP in extension Consider early referral for dynamic splinting
VI	Metacarpals	Very superficial May be repaired in emergency department	Splint wrist in 30° to 45° of extension, MCP, PIP, and DIP in extension Consider early referral for dynamic splinting
VI	Carpals	Often have associated extensor retinaculum lacerations	Hand surgery referral
	Proximal wrist and distal forearm		If hand surgeon chooses delayed repair, close skin and splint in 35° wrist extension and MCP, PIP, and DIP in extension Early referral for dynamic splinting

emergency practitioner, but should be done so only in communication with a hand surgeon who is willing to provide follow-up. There are eight anatomic zones into which the hand, wrist, and forearm are divided. Table 19-2 shows considerations and treatment recommendations for injuries in each of the specific zones.[6]

TENDON AVULSION INJURIES

Exposure to extreme torque leads the distal phalanx to be prone to tendon avulsion injuries. Mallet finger is classically described as a sports injury but is also reported as a result of household activities. It consists of an avulsion of the extensor tendon that may be associated with break of a bone fragment off the dorsal distal phalanx. The patient presents with edema and is unable to extend the DIP joint (Figure 19-5).[9] Mallet finger is treated with pain control, splinting the DIP joint in full extension for 6 weeks, and follow-up by a hand surgeon. Those with large bone fragments may need operative repair.

Jersey finger is the other type of common avulsion injury and is the most common closed flexor tendon injury. This occurs when the flexed finger is forcibly extended leading to rupture of the FDP and

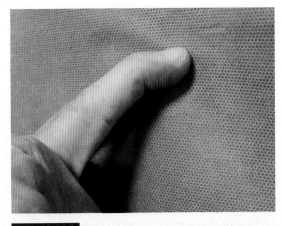

FIGURE 19-5
Mallet finger.

inability to actively flex the DIP joint. This occurs commonly to football players classically when a player grabs another's jersey during a tackle[9] and is most often seen in the ring finger. Jersey finger is defined as a blunt force avulsion of the FDP from its insertion.[5] Patients present complaining of pain and swelling with the inability to flex the DIP joint. As in mallet finger, treatment in the ED consists of pain control, splinting, and early follow-up with a hand surgeon as these injuries need operative repair. The splinting should be done with the wrist in 45° of flexion, MCP joint in 70° degrees of flexion, and the PIP and DIP joints in extension.

SUBUNGUAL HEMATOMAS AND NAIL BED INJURIES

A subungual hematoma is a painful condition caused by bleeding under the nail and presents most often after a crush injury with painful fingertip and discoloration under the nail (Figure 19-6, upper). In the evaluation of a subungual hematoma, x-rays should be obtained to rule out distal tuft fractures.[10] If a fracture is found on radiography it should be considered an open fracture and treated with antibiotics and referred to a hand specialist for follow-up.[11] These are usually comminuted and do not generally need reduction.[9] The treatment of subungual hematoma includes drainage of the hematoma via electrocautery or a heated paper clip (Figure 19-6, lower). If the hematoma involves greater than 50% of the nail bed, consider removing the nail plate to evaluate and repair the nail bed if necessary.[9] Resulting complications of these injuries include nail loss, paronychia, and osteomyelitis.[10]

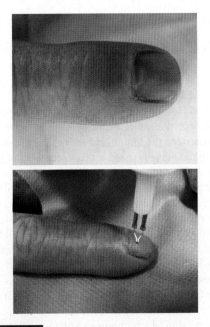

FIGURE 19-6
Subungual hematoma (upper). Nail trephination using hand held electrocautery device (lower).

Large subungual hematomas are often associated with a nail bed laceration. Patients with nail bed lacerations also require x-rays to rule out tuft fractures. Nail bed lacerations require removal of the nail to suture the laceration. This is accomplished by blunt dissection of the nail plate from the nail bed. The nail plate can then be grasped with a hemostat and removed with firm traction. An absorbable small suture (6-0 or 7-0) should be used. Often the removed nail is then cleaned and sutured back into position to act as a splint to maintain space for the new nail growth. The old nail should remain in place for 2 to 3 weeks.[9,12]

NERVE INJURIES

Emergency practitioners should consider the possibility of nerve injury with all hand wounds as optimal outcomes result from early diagnosis and treatment.[13] The sensory examination can be unreliable in the acute setting as can the patient's reporting of numbness or subjective testing for numbness. The report of significant or pulsatile bleeding with a volar laceration implies digital artery laceration. Because the nerve is dorsal to the artery, it has probably been lacerated as well. Two-point discrimination (2PD) is an objective way to test sensation in the digit with normal 2PD being between 3 mm and 5 mm. A 2PD greater than 8 mm in someone with otherwise normal sensation should raise concern for a digital nerve laceration. Loss of sweating distal to the site of the injury or failure of the skin to wrinkle after soaking the digit of concern in warm water can also signal a digital nerve injury.[1] Sensory assessment of the median nerve can be checked on the volar aspect of the thumb, index, long, and radial aspect of the ring fingers. Sensation is verified for the radial nerve by examining the web space between the thumb and index finger. Sensation of the ulnar nerve is tested at the volar aspect of the tip of the small and ulnar aspect of the ring finger.[13]

Motor function may be tested in the following ways. For ulnar function, palpation of contraction of the first dorsal interosseus, abduction and adduction of the digits, and flexion of the FDP of the small finger shows that the ulnar nerve is intact. The Froment's test, which consists of maintaining a sheet of paper between thumb and index finger also tests for ulnar nerve function (Figure 19-7). If the thumb IP joint flexes to maintain the paper, it is considered a positive Froment's sign which signifies adductor pollicis weakness secondary to ulnar nerve damage.[1]

Median nerve function is tested by assessment of abduction of the thumb and flexion of the thumb, index, and long finger flexor tendons and FDS tendons of the fingers. Clean-cut lacerated nerves should be repaired acutely (i.e., within 2 weeks and preferably within 48 hours). Open nerve avulsion injuries are repaired between 3 weeks and 3 months depending on the nature of the injury as they will usually require nerve grafting. Closed nerve injuries or gunshot wounds with nerve injuries are followed clinically for spontaneous recovery. If no recovery occurs within 3 months the nerve is explored and grafted if needed. Immediate consultation with a hand surgeon is recommended with any nerve injury. Complications of neural repair include chronic paresthesias, neuromas, and sympathetic dystrophy as well as loss of sensory and motor function.[13,14]

AMPUTATIONS

In the pre-hospital setting, every attempt should be made to preserve the amputated digit. Amputated parts can be wrapped in saline-soaked gauze, and placed in a plastic bag in an ice slurry. Ice should not directly come into contact with the amputated part. Cooling to 4 °C is beneficial as it doubles the potential ischemic time. The initial ED care, of course, should be aimed at stabilizing the patient as blood loss may be substantial. General guidelines for replantation include single-digit amputation between the PIP and DIP, amputated thumbs, multiple digits, any amputation in children, and higher level amputations.[1] Even if the patient does not fit one of these categories, care should still be taken to preserve the amputated part as the final decision should be made by the surgeon and the part may also be a source of tissue for the surgeon. Amputations tend to be tetanus-prone wounds and, thus, tetanus toxoid should be administered.[15] Prophylactic antibiotics should be given in the ED. They should include coverage for staph but also consideration must be given to methicillin-resistant *Staphylococus aureus* (MRSA) coverage as several studies show the recent rise of MRSA particularly in certain geographic areas.[16]

For patients who require transfer to a referral center for potential replant, the referral center should be called immediately as the referral center will help to direct care of the amputated part during transit. Large dressings should be avoided as the transport team might not be able to appreciate the volume of blood being actively lost.[15]

Fingertip Amputations

Fingertip amputations are classified by the place at which they are lacerated, identified as zones I to III from distal to proximal (Figure 19-8). Zone I is distal to the phalanx, zone II is distal to the lunula of the nail bed, and zone III involves the nail matrix.[13] Zone I fingertip amputations can be treated by the emergency practitioner and entail débridement, wound care, and antibiotic ointment. Zones II and III, however, will require repair by a hand surgeon. Important principles in their repair include the preservation of length especially in the thumb and index finger to preserve function.[9] A practical way to look at fingertip amputations is by the angulation of the injury (volar, dorsal, and

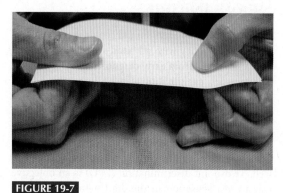

FIGURE 19-7
Froment's test.

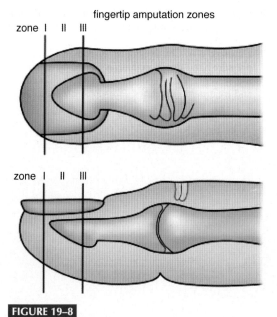

fingertip amputation zones

zone I II III

zone I II III

FIGURE 19–8
Zones of fingertip avulsion.

transverse) and loss of tissue (skin, subcutaneous, bone). A wound that involves less than 1 cm² of skin loss with minimal subcutaneous tissue loss can usually be treated with simple dressing changes and allowed to heal by secondary intention.

HIGH-PRESSURE INJECTION INJURIES

High-pressure injection injuries of the hand are uncommon with an estimated incidence of 600 per year presenting to EDs.[18] A pressure of only 100 psi is required to cause damage to skin. High-pressure injection injuries are generally work-related and result from inexperience with the equipment. The majority of these injuries (57%) are caused by grease guns; however, spray guns and diesel injectors are also frequent causes. The damage caused depends not only on the material injected but also on the velocity of the material and the location on the affected hand.[3] Once recognized, the emergency practitioner must act quickly as these injuries are associated with a high rate of amputation.[19] The initial injury can be deceiving in that it may appear to be only a small puncture wound if the patient presents early, but it will quickly progress.

In the past, the phases after injury have been described as acute, intermediate, and late stages. The acute phase is characterized by swelling, pain, and vascular insufficiency. If not properly treated, this can progress to necrosis within a short period of time. The intermediate stage is characterized by the formation of granulomas secondary to foreign-body reaction. The danger of their presence is that they are associated with functional loss. During the late stage there is breakdown of skin leading to ulcers and draining sinus in the areas of the oleomas. Successful management hinges on early recognition of the potentially severe injury. Pain control, radiographic evaluation, and consultation with a hand specialist for emergent surgical drainage and débridement are key. Prophylactic broad-spectrum antibiotics should be given and tetanus prophylaxis has been recommended by some.[20]

REFERENCES

1. Harrison B, Holland P. Diagnosis and management of hand injuries in the ED. *Emerg Med Pract.* 2005; 7(2):1–28.
2. Lehfeldt M, Ray E, Sherman R. MOC-PS(SM) CME article: treatment of flexor tendon laceration. *Plast Reconstr Surg.* 2008;121(4 suppl):1–12.
3. Steele MT, Tran LV, Watson WA, Muelleman RL. Retained glass foreign bodies in wounds: predictive value of wound characteristics, patient perception, and wound exploration. *Am J Emerg Med.* 1998; 16(7):627–630.
4. Hart RG, Uehara DT, Kutz JE. Extensor tendon injuries of the hand. *Emerg Med Clin North Am.* 1993; 11(3):637–649.
5. Hart RG, Uehara DT, Wagner MJ. *Emergency and Primary Care of the Hand.* Dallas, TX: American College of Emergency Physicians; 2001.
6. Hart RG, Kutz JE. Flexor tendon injuries of the hand. *Emerg Med Clin North Am.* 1993;11(3): 621–636.
7. Rohrbough JT, Mudge MK, Schilling RC. Overuse injuries in the elite rock climber. *Med Sci Sports Exerc.* 2000;32(8):1369–1372.
8. Verdan CE. Primary repair of flexor tendons. J Bone Joint Surg Am. Jun 1960; 42-A:647–57.
9. Wang QC, Johnson BA. Fingertip injuries. *Am Fam Physician.* 2001;63(10):1961–1966.
10. Hart RG, Kleinert HE. Fingertip and nail bed injuries. *Emerg Med Clin North Am.* 1993;11(3):755–765.
11. Coyle MP Jr, Leddy JP. Injuries of the distal finger. *Prim Care.* 1980;7(2):245–258.
12. Strauss EJ, Weil WM, Jordan C, Paksima N. A prospective, randomized, controlled trial of 2-octyl-cyanoacrylate versus suture repair for nail bed injuries. *J Hand Surg Am.* 2008;33(2):250–253.
13. Sloan EP. Nerve injuries in the hand. *Emerg Med Clin North Am.* 1993;11(3):651–670.
14. Dagum AB. Peripheral nerve regeneration, repair, and grafting. *J Hand Ther.* 1998;11(2):111–117.
15. Schlenker JD, Koulis CP. Amputations and replantations. *Emerg Med Clin North Am.* 1993;11(3):739–753.
16. Moran GJ, Krishnadasan A, Gorwitz RJ, et al. Methicillin-resistant S. aureus infections among

patients in the emergency department. *N Engl J Med.* 2006;355(7):666–674.

17. Jackson EA. The V-Y plasty in the treatment of fingertip amputations. *Am Fam Physician.* 2001;64(3): 455–458.

18. Dailiana H, Kotsaki D, Varitimidis S, et al. Injection injuries: seemingly minor injuries with major consequences. *Hippokratia.* 2008;12(1):33–36.

19. Schoo MJ, Scott FA, Boswick JA Jr. High-pressure injection injuries of the hand. *J Trauma.* 1980;20(3): 229–238.

20. Gutowski KA, Chu J, Choi M, Friedman DW. High-pressure hand injection injuries caused by dry cleaning solvents: case reports, review of the literature, and treatment guidelines. *Plast Reconstr Surg.* 2003; 111(1):174–177.

CHAPTER 20

Soft Tissue Infections of the Hand

Breena R. Taira, MD, MPH, Guy Cassara, RPAC, and Mark Gelfand, MD

Hand wounds and infections are very common,[1] and the compartmentalized anatomy of the hand predisposes to development of infection.[2] Certain risk factors increase the propensity to develop hand infections including diabetes mellitus,[3] immunocompromised states, intravenous drug use, exposure to an aquarium, and sexually transmitted diseases. Immunocompromised states include both patients on immunosuppressive therapy and those with disease processes leading to immunosuppression such as HIV and AIDS[4].

Despite the frequency with which patients present with infections of the hand, most of the standard practices are based on tradition, expert opinion, and case reports. Few prospective trials have been performed to evaluate the current treatment of hand infections.

As in other infections of the skin, hand infections are often caused by *Staphylococus* and *Streptococcus* species. However, of note is the recent concern with methicillin-resistant *Staphylococcus aureus* (MRSA) that has been found to be a causative agent in hand infections as well. A review of 761 patients with hand infections over 3 years confirmed the rising incidence of MRSA hand infections.[5] A 2009 study in an urban center reported the prevalence of community-acquired MRSA in their hand infection patients to be 55%.[6] Some now routinely culture all hand abscesses during drainage and choose antibiotic coverage with

adequate coverage of MRSA empirically.[5] Specific risk factors include history of intravenous drug injection,[7] living in close quarters, and recent antibiotic usage.[9] History of previous temporally unrelated hand infection and felon type infection have also been cited as risk factors.[7] MRSA is a growing problem in patients from the community without any obvious risk factors and, thus, coverage of MRSA should be considered whenever antibiotics are prescribed for hand infections.[9] A recent review by Imahara and Friedrich revealed a steady increase of community-acquired MRSA hand infections as well to the extent that in 2007 more than 50% of patients treated for hand infections in their study had community-acquired MRSA.[7] Although many resources still list antistaphylococcal penicillins as first-line therapy, many hand surgeons now use vancomycin empirically for hand infections because of the rise of MRSA.

In children, Harness and Blazar reported that because of the high number of mixed aerobic and anaerobic infections without risk factors, pediatric hand infections should be treated with broad-spectrum antibiotic coverage.[10] Other populations to be aware of include those with exposure to fish tanks, salt water, or fresh water, in whom *Mycobacterium marinum* of the hand has been reported.[11] Other less common organisms responsible for hand infections that have been reported in the literature include *Streptococcus milleri*,[12] *Mycobacterium* species,[13,14] and *Vibrio* species.[15]

General principles of hand infection treatment include thorough and rapid drainage, débridement, irrigation, antibiotics, hand elevation, immobilization in "intrinsic plus" position, and, once inflammation has decreased, rapid mobilization to preserve function. The intrinsic plus position of the hand is also known as the safe position. In the intrinsic plus position, the metacarpophalangeal (MP) joints are flexed at 60-70°, the interphalangeal (IP) joints are fully extended, and the thumb is in the fist projection. The wrist is held in extension at 10° less than maximal. The remainder of this chapter will focus on the identification and treatment of specific types of common soft tissue infections of the hand.

PARONYCHIA

Paronychia is defined as an infection of the epidermis adjacent to the nail[2] and can be either acute or chronic. Causes of paronychia are usually trauma to the nail or nail fold[16] including manicure, artificial nail application, ingrown nail, nail biting, or thumb sucking.[2,16] Paronychia appears as erythema and swelling next to the nail bed (Figure 20-1). The two most common bacteria that cause paronychia are *S aureus* and *Streptococcus pyogenes*.[1] Antibiotics should be given to cover these organisms such as first-generation cephalosporins or antistaphylococcal penicillins. In the very early stages the infection may respond to oral

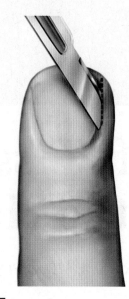

FIGURE 20-2

Drainage of a paronychia: An incision is made below the perionychial fold with the blade directed away from the nail bed and matrix.

antibiotics, soaks, and rest. Once an abscess forms, drainage is mandatory. The procedure can be performed under digital block with care to keep the scalpel directed away from the nail bed to prevent its injury. Drainage is accomplished by using a No. 11 blade scalpel (Figure 20-2). If infection extends under the nail plate then nail removal becomes necessary.[17] When paronychia is a chronic problem the most likely cause is *Candida* and treatment with a topical antifungal is appropriate.

FELON

When an abscess forms within the pulp of the distal finger or phalanx pad it is referred to as a felon (Figure 20-3). Because the pulp of the finger is divided by multiple septae an abscess collection can result in significant discomfort and eventual tissue necrosis. A felon does not extend proximal to the distal interphalangeal (DIP) joint. If infection appears to continue proximal to the DIP joint, deeper space infections must be considered. Predisposing factors include penetrating trauma to the fingertip including fingersticks for blood glucose, pieces of glass, and splinters. The most common causative organisms are the same as those for paronychia and, thus, antibiotic choices also include first-generation cephalosporins and antistaphylococcal penicillins. Final antibiotic selection should be dictated by cultures. If MRSA infection is

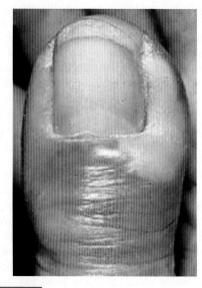

FIGURE 20-1

Paronychia.

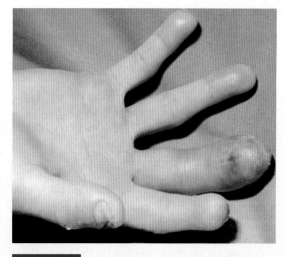

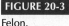
FIGURE 20-3
Felon.

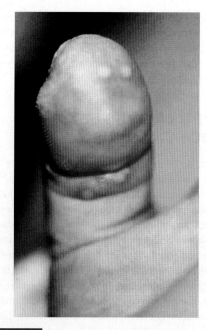

FIGURE 20-5
Whitlow.

suspected treatment with intravenous (IV) van-comycin is appropriate and should be continued until cultures are available.

Although felon in the early stages might also be amenable to antibiotic treatment and warm soaks, they usually require incision and drainage. Two tech-niques for drainage include a single midvolar incision or a unilateral longitudinal incision (Figure 20-4).[18,19] The incisions are carried to 5 mm distal to the DIP crease. Care should be taken to ensure that any locula-tions are broken up with a small hemostat. The wound is then irrigated and packed with sterile gauze. The hand should be elevated and the gauze should be removed in 48 hours.[18] Afterward the hand should be elevated and splinted in "intrinsic plus" position. The wound should be re-examined on the following day and twice-daily soaks or whirlpool therapy can be ini-tiated. Untreated felon can lead to such complications as osteomyelitis, secondary suppurative tenosynovitis, and flexor tendon rupture.[20]

WHITLOW

Herpetic whitlow is one of the rare viral infections of the hand and is caused by herpes simplex virus. Those whose work exposes them to oral secretions are at increased risk such as dental hygienists, dentists, other health care workers, and wrestlers. Herpetic whitlow must be distinguished from felon because the treat-ment differs. Drainage is not indicated for whitlow and the treatment is antiviral medications. Whitlow is usu-ally abrupt in onset and consists of edema, erythema, and severe localized tenderness of the infected finger. Clear vesicles may be seen and whitlow is sometimes associated with fever and lymphadenopathy (Figure 20-5). The vesicles appear between 2 and 14 days after exposure and coalesce as the infection progresses.

FIGURE 20-4
Drainage of a felon: The pus may be drained via an incision through the volar (left), or lateral aspect (middle) of the distal finger pulp. A curved hemostat is then inserted through the incision to break down all involved septal compartments (right).

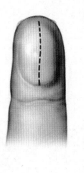
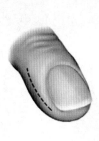
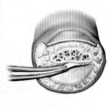

The diagnosis is often made clinically but can be confirmed with Tzanck prep or viral culture. Antivirals such as acyclovir and valacyclovir can be used to shorten the duration of symptoms.[21] Lesions remain contagious until they are re-epithelialized.

SUPPURATIVE FLEXOR TENOSYNOVITIS

Suppurative flexor tenosynovitis occurs when the flexor tendon sheath of the fingers becomes infected.[18] The flexor tendon sheath extends from the DIP joint to the distal metacarpal. There is synovial fluid between the two layers of the sheath that provides a medium in which it is easy to propagate infection. In addition, the radial and ulnar bursas are contiguous with the forearm, which allows the spread of infection quickly from the fingers to the forearm. In most cases the patient will recall some trauma to the hand; however, hematogenous spread to the flexor tendon sheath is possible.

The classic 1939 work of Kanavel on flexor tenosynovitis describes four signs including symmetric digital swelling, digits held in partial flexion at rest, excess tenderness along the entire tendon sheath, and pain along the tendon sheath with passive digit extension (Figure 20-6).[22] If infection is not treated it may spread to the deep hand spaces, joint spaces, or bone. Very rarely, if the patient presents in the early stage of infection, it is possible to treat such early infection with IV antibiotics, elevation, splinting, and close inpatient follow-up; however, most will require immediate surgical intervention consisting of drainage and irrigation in the operating room. Early consultation with a hand surgeon is mandatory for all patients.

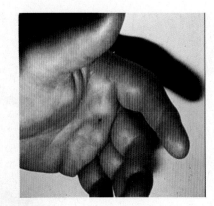

FIGURE 20-6

Flexor tenosynovitis.

Cultures should be obtained at the time of surgery. Until results are obtained the patient can be placed on IV cefazolin to cover *S aureus* and *Streptococcus*.[23] The threshold for empiric coverage of MRSA should be very low. If a bite is the initial causative trauma, however, the coverage must be broadened to include anaerobes. In addition, immunocompromised patients may be susceptible to disseminated gonococcal infections[24] and *Candida*[25] as causes of flexor tenosynovitis. Acute gonococcal tenosynovitis has been shown to be present in more than two thirds of patients with disseminated gonococcal infections.[26] In general, hospital admission with intravenous antibiotic therapy is needed, and most will require surgical intervention.

DEEP SPACE INFECTIONS

The hand contains several potential subfascial spaces also referred to as "deep" spaces (Figure 20-7). Usually

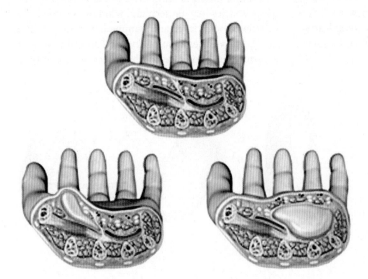

FIGURE 20-7

Deep spaces of the hand.

an infection of the deep space is secondary to a penetrating wound. Although its appearance can be similar to a cellulitis of the dorsum of the hand, it can be distinguished by the presence of extreme tenderness on extension of the digits. When deep space infection is suspected, immediate consultation with a hand surgeon is required as treatment requires an incision and drainage through the dorsal surface of the hand. These infections can be severe and require hospitalization and IV antibiotics postdrainage. The initial antibiotic choice should be broad-spectrum, and again the possibility of MRSA infection should be kept in mind. After drainage the incisions are typically left open to heal by secondary intention.

SEPTIC ARTHRITIS

Septic arthritis commonly results from a penetrating wound that enters the joint space inoculating it with an infectious agent. Hematogenous spread can also bring infectious agents into the joint. When these agents

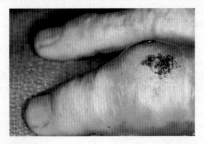

FIGURE 20-8
Septic arthritis.

begin to affect the articular cartilage, which can occur as soon as 24 hours after the injury, the result is septic arthritis.[18] The immune reaction to the infectious agent leads to an increase in white blood cells within the joint fluid and subsequent increase in pressure within the joint. This is common among patients with other medical comorbidities including diabetes or cancer, renal patients, and those who abuse alcohol. Clenched fist injuries or "fight bite" injuries may also increase susceptibility to septic arthritis. (Bites are covered extensively in Chapter 15.)

The initial appearance of septic arthritis is erythema, edema, and marked tenderness of a joint that is usually held in a position that maximizes the volume of the joint space so as to reduce the pressure within the joint (Figure 20-8).[1] Diagnosis is made by aspiration of the joint fluid. Fluid should be sent for gram stain, cell count, and culture. Characteristic results of infected fluid include a turbid appearance, high white blood cell count, and low glucose. Gram stain can be very helpful in guiding choice of antibiotic coverage if positive, but if negative the patient must still be covered with antibiotics. Antibiotics should be initiated immediately after the sample of fluid is obtained. Coverage traditionally includes antistaphylococcal penicillin; however, as in other infections, the rising rate of MRSA should be considered. In addition, those whose initial insult was a human bite must be covered for *Staphylococcus, Streptococcus,* and *Eikenella corrodens*, which can be accomplished via a beta-lactamase–inhibitor combination or penicillin G with a first-generation cephalosporin.[2]

Below is a summary of common soft tissue infections of the hand, the likely causative organisms, predisposing factors and treatment. (Table 20-1).

TABLE 20–1	Summary of Hand Infections		
Infection	**Likely Organisms**	**Predisposing Factors**	**Treatment**
Paronychia	*Staphyloccus aureus,* MRSA, anaerobes	Thumb sucking, professional dishwasher	Antistaphylococcal penicillin or first-generation cephalosporin,* incision and drainage
Felon	*Staphylococcus aureus, Streptococcus,* MRSA	Glucose monitoring via finger sticks, splinters, embedded glass	Antistaphylococcal penicillin or first-generation cephalosporin,* incision and drainage
Whitlow	Herpes simplex virus	Exposure to oral secretions	Acyclovir, valacyclovir
Flexor tenosynovitis	*Staphylococus, Streptococcus,* MRSA	Diabetes, disseminated gonococcal infection	Surgical drainage, IV cefazolin*

(Continued)

TABLE 20–1	Summary of Hand Infections (Continued)		
Infection	**Likely Organisms**	**Predisposing Factors**	**Treatment**
Deep space infections	Staphylococcus, Strepto-coccus, MRSA, gram-negative bacilli, anaerobes	Penetrating hand wounds	IV beta-lactamase inhibitor together with a penicillin or first-generation cephalo-sporin with penicillin,* surgical drainage
Septic Aarthritis	Staphylococcus, Streptococ-cus, MRSA, Eikenella if secondary to human bite	Penetrating hand wounds, medical comorbidities	Incision and drainage, IV antistaphylococcal penicillin*

Note. MRSA = methacillin-resistant Staphylococcus aureus.

*Strongly consider antibiotic coverage for MRSA based on location and risk factors.

REFERENCES

1. Moran GJ Talan DA. Hand infections. Emerg Med Clin North Am. 1993;11(3):601–619.
2. Clark DC. Common acute hand infections. Am Fam Physician. 2003;68(11):2167–2176.
3. Sidibe AT, Dembele M, Cisse IA, et al. The diabetic hand [in French].Mali Med. 2006;21(3):1–4.
4. Ching V, Ritz M, Song C, De Aguir G, Mohanlal P. Human immunodeficiency virus infection in an emergency hand service. J Hand Surg Am. 1996; 21(4):696–699.
5. LeBlanc DM, Reece EM, Horton JB, Janis JE. Increasing incidence of methicillin-resistant Staphylococcus aureus in hand infections: a 3-year county hospital experience. Plast Reconstr Surg. 2007;119(3): 935–940.
6. O'Malley M, Fowler J, Ilyas AM. Community-acquired methicillin-resistant Staphylococcus aureus infections of the hand: prevalence and timeliness of treatment. J Hand Surg Am. 2009;34(3):504–508.
7. Imahara SD, Friedrich JB. Community-acquired methicillin-resistant Staphylococcus aureus in surgically treated hand infections. J Hand Surg Am. 35(1):97–103.
8. Skiest DJ, Brown K, Cooper TW, Hoffman-Roberts H, Mussa HR, Elliott AC. Prospective comparison of methicillin-susceptible and methicillin-resistant community-associated Staphylococcus aureus infections in hospitalized patients. J Infect. 2007;54(5): 427–434.
9. Moran GJ, Krishnadasan A, Gorwitz RJ, et al. Methicillin-resistant S. aureus infections among patients in the emergency department. N Engl J Med. 2006;355(7):666–674.
10. Harness N, Blazar PE. Causative microorganisms in surgically treated pediatric hand infections. J Hand Surg Am. 2005;30(6):1294–1297.
11. De Smet L. Mycobacterium marinum infections of the hand: a report of three cases. Acta Chir Belg. 2008;108(6):779–782.
12. Lunn JV, Rahman KJ, Macey AC. Streptococcus milleri infection.J Hand Surg Br. 2001;26(1):56–57.
13. Vigler M, Mulett H, Hausman MR. Chronic Mycobacterium infection of first dorsal web space after accidental Bacilli Calmette-Guérin injection in a health worker: case report. J Hand Surg Am. 2008; 33(9):1621–1624.
14. Hellinger WC, Smilack JD, Greider JL Jr, et al. Localized soft-tissue infections with Mycobacterium avium/Mycobacterium intracellulare complex in immunocompetent patients: granulomatous ten-osynovitis of the hand or wrist. Clin Infect Dis. 1995; 21(1):65–69.
15. Huang KC, Hsieh PH, Huang KC, Tsai YH. Vibrio necrotizing soft-tissue infection of the upper extremity: factors predictive of amputation and death. J Infect. 2008;57(4):290–297.
16. Rigopoulos D, Larios G, Gregoriou S, Alevizos A. Acute and chronic paronychia. Am Fam Physician. 2008;77(3):339–346.
17. Green D, Hotchkiss RN, Pederson WC, Wolfe SW. Green's Operative Hand Surgery. 5th ed. Churchill Livingstone; 2005:59.
18. Hart RG, Uehara DT, Wagner MJ. Emergency and Primary Care of the Hand. Dallas, TX: American College of Emergency Physicians; 2001.
19. Jebson PJ. Infections of the fingertip. Paronychias and felons. Hand Clin. 1998;14(4):547–555, viii.
20. Watson PA, Jebson PJ. The natural history of the neglected felon. Iowa Orthop J. 1996;16:164–166.
21. Schwandt NW, Mjos DP, Lubow RM. Acyclovir and the treatment of herpetic whitlow. Oral Surg Oral Med Oral Pathol. 1987;64(2):255–258.
22. Kanavel A. Infections of the Hand. A Guide to the Surgical Treatment of Acute and Chronic Suppurative Processes in the Fingers, Hand and Forearm. 7th ed. Philadelphia, PA: Lea & Febiger; 1939.
23. Hausman MR, Lisser SP. Hand infections. Orthop Clin North Am. 1992;23(1):171–185.
24. Krieger LE, Schnall SB, Holtom PD, Costigan W. Acute gonococcal flexor tenosynovitis. Orthopedics. 1997;20(7):649–650.
25. Townsend DJ, Singer DI, Doyle JR. Candida tenosynovitis in an AIDS patient: a case report. J Hand Surg Am. 1994;19(2):293–294.
26. Schaefer RA, Enzenauer RJ, Pruitt A, Corpe RS. Acute gonococcal flexor tenosynovitis in an adolescent male with pharyngitis. A case report and literature review. Clin Orthop Relat Res. 1992;(281):212–215.

CHAPTER 21

Burns

Harry S. Soroff, MD, and Steven Sandoval, MD

Each year between 1 and 2 million burns are sustained in the United States alone.[1] Fortunately, most are small and the care of victims focuses on local wound care.[2] Initial care of the burn victim should address life-threatening injuries that compromise vital functions including the airway, breathing, and circulation. For optimal follow-up, one should refer all but the most minor burns to a burn center if one is available. The response to burns is determined by the total area of the body surface burned and the depth of the burns. Accurate assessments of burn extent and depth are required to determine the appropriate therapy for the burn injury. Avoiding infection and further damage to the injured tissues will help optimize healing and result in the most aesthetically pleasing and functional scar.

GENERAL PRINCIPLES OF CARE

Immediate Evaluation

Before caring for a burn injury, it is important to identify and treat any associated injuries; some burn victims may have other life- or limb-threatening injuries. The immediate evaluation of a patient who has sustained a burn injury includes the following: (See later in the chapter for full explanation of some terms.)

1. Was the patient burned in an open space or in an enclosed space such as a house? If burns are sustained in a closed space, determine the carboxy-hemoglobin level.
2. Is there evidence of smoke inhalation and is the airway clear?
3. What was the causative agent of the burn (for example, water, oil, kerosene, gasoline, or an explosive gas such as propane) and is there any evidence of an electrical or chemical injury?
4. What is the extent of the burn, expressed as percentage of the body surface area (BSA)?
5. How much of the body surface has sustained a partial-thickness injury, either superficial or deep, and how much has sustained a full-thickness injury?

Precautionary Measures

Precautionary ancillary measures in the care of moderate and major burns (all second-degree burns over 15% **BSA** in adults and over 10% BSA in children) include:

- A nasogastric tube to prevent gastric ileus and to decompress the stomach from swallowed air.
- Intravenous analgesics, such as morphine sulfate, as needed for pain.
- Tetanus prophylaxis (tetanus toxoid 0.5 mL) if full-thickness burns cover more than 10% BSA. If the immunization history is not known or more than 10 years have elapsed since the most recent booster, tetanus immunoglobulin (250 units) is also given.

The Effects of Patient Age on Burn Morbidity and Mortality

As with other forms of injury, the very young and the elderly experience a higher morbidity and mortality rate from burns. When burns occur in children who are less than 24 months of age, the possibility of either neglect or abuse should always be considered. Burns in which there is a sharp line of demarcation between the burned and the unburned area suggest immersion, which is suspicious for neglect or abuse.

Patients aged older than 60 years are at high risk, even with a moderate burn, and should be admitted to the hospital. This is especially true for patients with preexisting diseases such as diabetes mellitus, strokes, or cardiac or respiratory insufficiency. The burn wound itself presents special problems, because the thickness of the skin decreases with age. This makes the diagnosis of the depth of the burn more difficult. In elderly patients, one should assume that the burn is deep.

Transfer to a Burn Center?

Criteria for transfer to a burn center are:

- Third-degree burns over 5% BSA
- Second-degree and/or third-degree burns over 15% BSA (10% in children aged younger than 10 years)
- Electrical burns
- Inhalation injury
- Patient is elderly (>60 years) or has severe comorbidity
- Burns involve the face, hands, feet, joints, or genitalia

PHYSIOLOGIC ALTERATIONS FOLLOWING BURNS

Early Changes

Burns are caused by the conduction of thermal energy to the skin from a hot substance such as water, oil, or burning clothing. The effect on the skin will depend on both the temperature to which the skin is heated and the time period during which the hot substance is in contact with the skin. Moritz and Henriquez[3] studied these effects in pigs. The early changes, at temperatures between 40°C and 44°C, are denaturation of protein and interference with the function of cellular enzyme systems. The sodium pump is one of the most important functions of the cellular membrane that is adversely affected, allowing a high intracellular sodium concentration to develop, which leads to intracellular

swelling. Oxygen free radicals and proinflammatory mediators are also produced and further aggravate the abnormalities of cell membrane function.[4] As the injury progresses, the cellular proteins become severely altered and eventually progress to cell death or necrosis.

The burn injury is not limited to the surface of the skin; penetration of the heat produces a three-dimensional injury.[4] At the skin surface, there is cell destruction and necrosis. This area is called the zone of coagulation. Clinically, this is manifested by the eschar of the full-thickness injury. Beneath the zone of coagulation is a zone of stasis. Here the cells are initially viable. As the circulation to the area becomes progressively diminished, however, the early ischemia within the zone of stasis may progress to necrosis and the death of cells that were previously viable. With optimal therapy, the circulation improves in the entire zone of stasis, and recovery can occur in 7 to 14 days. During this recovery period, the tissues are very susceptible to injury and infection, however, and must be protected. There is a third, outer zone of hyperemia surrounding the ischemic zone of stasis. In this outer zone there is minimal cell destruction and the tissues receive an increase in blood flow, secondary to regional vasodilatation.

Formation of Edema

Injury to the capillaries in the burned area impairs their integrity, thus permitting proteins to escape from the serum into the wound.[5] The increased permeability is aggravated by the release of a large number of inflammatory mediators. Even though the edema is most marked in the area of contact with heat, it extends far into the surrounding tissues and interferes with the delivery of oxygen and other nutrients to the injured area, thus aggravating the effect of the ischemia. However, the capillaries retain a selective permeability that keeps large molecules such as fibrinogen and globulin within the vessel while allowing smaller molecules such as albumin to escape into the edema fluid.

The formation of edema begins rapidly, within the first 2 to 3 hours after injury. It then increases, reaches its maximum at about 12 to 24 hours, and persists until 48 to 72 hours. Thereafter, recovery begins with a slow reabsorption that usually takes as long as 7 to 10 days to be completed. The amount of the edema and its duration depend upon the severity of the injury. In an extensive or deep burn, the edema becomes massive and continues for a longer period. Fluid therapy (discussed later) is required to prevent the resulting decrease in vascular and intracellular volume from impairing organ function. The suggested formulas for replacing the intravascular and extracellular volume lost into the burn edema are largely based upon the weight of the patient and the extent of the burn, which is measured as the percentage of BSA involved.

DETERMINATION OF THE EXTENT OF THE BURN

The extent and the depth of the burn set the stage for the physiologic, metabolic, and anatomic changes that ensue, and are the major determinants of the chances for the patient's survival. The percentage of BSA that is burned can be roughly estimated in an adult by the "rule of nines,"[6] in which the head and each upper extremity each comprise 9% of the body surface, each lower extremity and the anterior and posterior trunk each comprise 18%, and the genitalia are 1% (Figure 21-1). A good estimate can be made by using the chart developed by Lund and Browder,[7] which takes into account the differences in relative surface areas of the body that exist in infants and how they change with growth (Figure 21-2). In the adult, the area of the palm

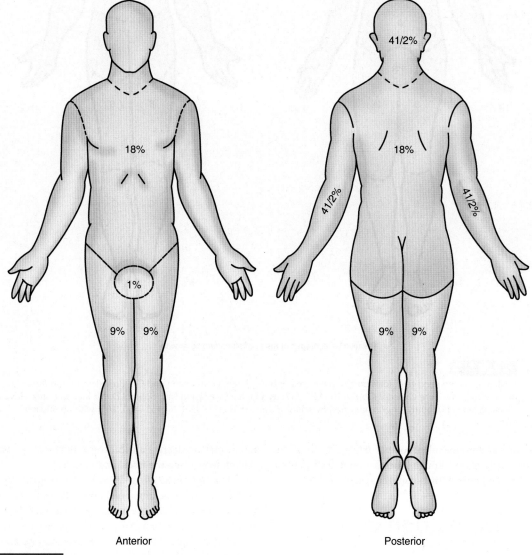

Anterior   Posterior

FIGURE 21-1

Estimating the percentage of total body surface area of burns in adults. From Lund CC, Browder NE. The estimation of areas of burns. *Surg Gynecol Obstet,* 1944;79:357; as adapted by Clayton MC, Solem LD. No ice, no butter. Advice on management of burns for primary care physicians. *Postgrad Med.* 1995;97(5):151–160, 165, with permission.

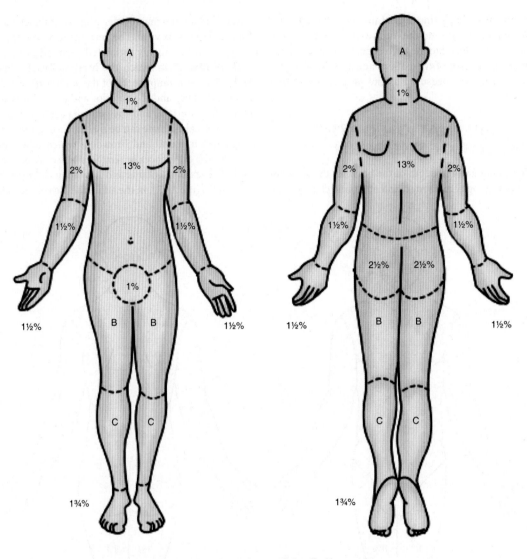

Relative percentages of areas affairs affted by growth

FIGURE 21-2

Estimating the percentage of total body surface area of burns in children. From Lund CC, Browder NE. The estimation of areas of burns. *Surg Gynecol Obstet.* 1944;79:357; as adapted by Clayton MC, Solem LD. No ice, no butter. Advice on management of burns for primary care physicians. *Postgrad Med.* 1995;97(5):151–160, 165, with permission.

of the hand is equivalent to approximately 1% of the body surface area. Rough "guesses" often lead to both under- and overestimation of the size of the burn.

DETERMINATION OF BURN DEPTH

Burns are usually classified either as partial- or full-thickness burns based on the degree of damage to the dermis. Partial-thickness burns may be either

superficial or deep. Full-thickness burns may also extend deeper into the fascia and muscle.

The *superficial (first-degree) burn* is most commonly caused by the ultraviolet rays of the sun. It may also be caused by a brief exposure to heat, such as the heat that occurs in an explosion of propane gas. Even though first-degree burns are painful and may be associated with minimal edema, they almost always heal in 3 to 5 days.

The *superficial partial-thickness (second-degree) burn* is characterized by the presence of blisters and a

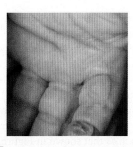

FIGURE 21-3

Photograph of superficial partial thickness burn: Presence of blisters on hand and fingers indicate its superficial nature.

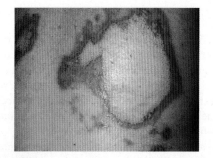

FIGURE 21-4

Photograph of deep partial-thickness burn: The white tissue represents denatured collagen.

weeping, erythematous skin surface (Figure 21-3). Because the nerve endings are intact, this type of burn is associated with a great deal of pain. Burns of this depth, which usually result from exposure to hot water or steam, are very common. Patients with superficial second-degree burns should be followed carefully. The burned area should be checked frequently to determine whether the depth of the injury is progressing. The injured surface contains many viable exposed nerve endings, so that dressing changes are extremely painful despite the use of analgesics.

Probably the most difficult burn to diagnose is the *deep partial-thickness* (second degree) or *deep dermal burn*. The wound should be observed and dressed daily to determine whether the depth becomes more severe with the passage of time. Laser Doppler flow measurements have been shown to be useful in predicting whether the deep dermal burn will heal or will progress to a full-thickness injury.[8] Deep dermal burns that do not heal in 21 days should definitely be excised and grafted, because when healing does occur at a later time, scarring is common. This is especially true in children. The surface of the deep dermal burn is comprised of denatured collagen, which is light tan or white in color and adheres to the deeper tissues (Figure 21-4). Over a period of days, as the dead collagen of the injured dermis is gradually débrided, it exposes a normal hyperemic layer of dermis, which contains numerous epithelial papillae or islands from which new epithelium grows to resurface and heal the burned area. This new epithelium should be protected by dressings because it is friable and liable to injury for some time.

The diagnosis of *full-thickness* or *third-degree burns* is usually obvious on presentation. The burned surface is dry and leathery in texture and is insensate. There are no viable hairs in the injured area. If the destruction is severe, the area may actually be charred, with thrombosed vessels that are visible within the

eschar (Figure 21-5). It is more difficult, however, to diagnose a full-thickness injury that evolves over time from a deep dermal injury. This diagnosis may be complicated if the amount of heat applied to different portions of the body is not uniform; in such a situation an area of deep dermal injury that will heal may be side-by-side with an area of full-thickness burn that requires excision and grafting.

Deeper burns can involve muscle, fascia, nerves, and even bone. The most common cause of such a devastating injury is the passage of high-voltage electricity through the body, or the prolonged exposure of portions of the body to heat of a high intensity, which can occur when gasoline ignites clothing or the person is trapped in a closed space.

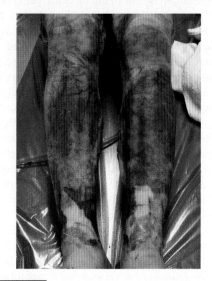

FIGURE 21-5

Photograph of full-thickness burn: The presence of vessel thrombosis beneath the burn eschar is pathognomonic of full-thickness burns.

FLUID THERAPY

The rationale for providing fluid therapy is to replace the intravascular, extracellular, and intracellular fluid that has translocated into the burn wound in the form of edema. If this fluid is not replaced, then the resulting decrease in vascular, extracellular, and intracellular volume following a large burn will result in impaired organ function and, ultimately, death.

Lactated Ringer's solution is the most commonly used form of fluid replacement. It has a sodium content of 130 mEq/L and its composition approximates that of the extracellular fluid that has translocated into the edema. The most popular formula for fluid administration is the Parkland formula—4 mL × body weight in kilograms × percentage of BSA burned. Because the burn wound edema forms most rapidly in the first 8 hours after injury, it has been recommended that half of the first day's fluid budget be administered during this period, and the third and fourth quarters should be given during each of the ensuing 8-hour periods. This formula also included a fourth 8-hour period during which plasma or albumin should be given at a rate of 0.3 to 0.5 mL/kg percentage of total BSA burned. During the remainder of the second 24-hour period, dextrose and water should be given.[9]

The adequacy of the fluid replacement can be gauged from the volume of urine output. In an adult, if the hourly urine output is 30 mL to 50 mL per hour (or about 0.5 mL/kg body weight in children), it reflects an adequacy in the fluid volume replacement. However, if the urine output falls to 10 mL to 15 mL per hour, the rate of fluid administration should be accelerated. A urine output that exceeds 60 mL per hour indicates that the rate of fluid administration should be adjusted downward to prevent the accumulation of an excessive amount of burn wound edema. Excessive fluid resuscitation also carries with it the danger of overloading the heart as the fluid is resorbed in the ensuing postburn course. The administration of colloid during the second 24-hour period, and the judicious administration of crystalloid solution in the initial resuscitation period, appear to decrease the likelihood of the occurrence of "fluid creep" or gradual accumulation of excessive tissue edema, which may result in acute abdominal compartment syndrome.[10]

Alvarado et al at the Army Institute for Surgical Research have recommended the use of a simplified resuscitation formula named "The Rule of Ten" in which the estimated burn size in percentage total BSA is multiplied by 10 to derive the initial fluid rate in mL/hr. An additional 100 mL is added to this rate for every 10 kg in weight above 80 kg.[11]

In children, the surface areas of the various parts of the body are different from those of adults. For example, a child's head represents a larger percentage of the surface area than the child's limbs. The relationship between surface area and weight in adults does not pertain to growing children. The fluid requirements for resuscitation of children should be based upon surface area, which can be determined from a nomogram such as that shown in Figure 21-6. During the first 24 hours, the volume of lactated Ringer's solution should be 5000 mL per square meter of body surface burn. Children should also be given 2000 mL of 5% glucose in water per square meter of body surface to make up for insensible losses.

A patient who has suffered a crush or electrical injury may produce dark red urine owing to myoglobin or hemoglobin. Sodium bicarbonate should be added to the intravenous fluids to alkalinize the urine.

INHALATION INJURY

It has been estimated that about 20% to 30% of patients exposed to fires experience an element of smoke inhalation injury and carbon monoxide intoxication. The possibility of such an inhalation injury must be evaluated in every burn patient, because it is one of the major determinants of morbidity and mortality. Fire and the combustion products of a wide variety of materials create heated gases containing particulate matter as smoke. The history of where the fire occurred is important because the smoke and heated gases are the most concentrated when they are in a closed space. Direct heat is injurious to the upper airway; it initiates the formation of edema, which obstructs the free movement of air. For this reason it is recommended that all burn victims should receive humidified oxygen at a concentration of 100% at the scene of a fire.[12]

The symptoms that should alert the clinician to inhalation injury are hoarseness, stridor, a severe barking cough, and wheezing. The presence of carbonaceous material in and around the mouth and singed nasal hairs is clear evidence that smoke inhalation has occurred. In addition to the examination of the status of the airway, the expansion of the patient's chest should also be observed. Radiographic changes typical of inhalation injury are often delayed (Figure 21-7). If there are full-thickness circumferential burns of the chest, which compromise respiratory excursions, emergent escharotomies should be planned. In the presence of a face or neck burn and evidence of smoke inhalation, endotracheal intubation should be

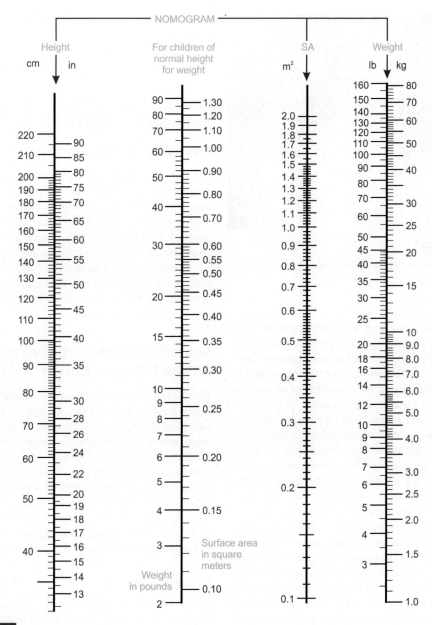

NOMOGRAM

Height	For children of normal height for weight	SA	Weight
cm in		m²	lb kg

FIGURE 21-6

Nomogram for determining surface area based on height and weight in children. From: Herndon DN, Rutan RL, Alison WE Jr, Cox CS Jr. Management of burn injuries. In: Eichelberger MR, ed. *Pediatric Trauma: Prevention, Acute Care, Rehabilitation*. St Louis, MO: Mosby Year Book; 1993:572, with permission.

considered. This should be carried out in the emergency department before the development of edema begins to obstruct the airway, creating difficulties for intubation. It is preferable to insert an endotracheal tube of an adequate caliber that will enable frequent lavage, suctioning, and bronchoscopy. Once the patient has been stabilized, fiberoptic bronchoscopy should be performed, and should be repeated until the inhaled particles of soot are removed. When in doubt, fiberoptic laryngoscopy (when available) may be helpful in determining the need for endotracheal intubation.

In young children, the small caliber of the airway makes them especially vulnerable to any narrowing

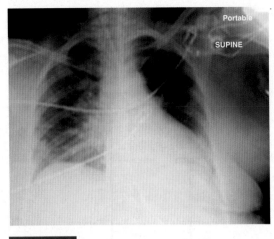

FIGURE 21-7

Radiograph of the chest demonstrating early changes of inhalation injury.

that would be caused by edema; even a small decrease in the cross-sectional area of the airway can result in a significant increase in airway resistance. Direct laryngoscopy and bronchoscopy allow the clinician to determine whether soot is present in the trachea and permits lavage and the concurrent placement of an endotracheal tube. If these measures cannot be performed because of severe edema, then an emergent cricothyroidotomy or tracheostomy should be carried out.

Carbon monoxide is produced from the partial oxidation of carbon-containing compounds; it forms when there is not enough oxygen to produce carbon dioxide. When patients are burned in a closed space, the air may become deficient in oxygen and contain a high level of carbon monoxide. Carbon monoxide in the blood shifts the oxygen dissociation curve to the left, which inhibits the release of oxygen to the tissues, so that the patient develops neurologic or cardiac abnormalities. A carboxyhemoglobin concentration greater than 15% is toxic and a concentration greater than 50% can be lethal. The patient may exhibit symptoms of headache, irritability, visual disturbances, and impaired judgment.[12,13] The treatment for carbon monoxide toxicity is delivery of a high concentration of oxygen. Patients with severe exposures are administered 100% oxygen in a hyperbaric chamber at 2.5 atmospheres for 30 minutes. More than one session may be required.

When polymers containing nitrogen are burned, they may produce hydrogen cyanide. The presence of hydrogen cyanide should be suspected in patients in whom an odor of bitter almonds is detected. The symptoms include lethargy, nausea, and headache, and may progress to coma. The treatment includes intra-venous sodium thiosulfate 125 mg/kg to 250 mg/kg and hydroxycobalamin 4 g, as well as 100% oxygen. Cyanide poisoning should always be considered in burn victims with severe metabolic acidosis.

LOCAL CARE OF THE BURN WOUND

First-Degree Burns

The patient with a first-degree burn requires only symptomatic care. Patients are more comfortable if the burn is covered with an ointment such as petrolatum or aloe vera, or an ointment containing an analgesic (such as diclofenac acid) to relieve the local pain caused by the movement of air over the wound. There is no need for topical antibiotics. Bed rest and analgesics are recommended for 24 to 48 hours, depending upon the extent of the burn. This type of injury resolves itself in that period.

Superficial Partial-Thickness Burns (Second-Degree Burns)

The most striking manifestation of a superficial second-degree burn is the formation of blisters. The blister is formed by the leakage of serum into the stratum spinosum layer of the epidermis. Plasma proteins and other products of the injured skin are contained within the blister fluid and these draw more serum into the blister, so that it increases in size over the first 24 hours and sometimes breaks. The presence of blisters usually indicates that the burn is fairly superficial and that it will heal spontaneously by reepithelialization within 10 days to 2 weeks, providing that no infection occurs.

Management

Studies in human volunteers and animals suggest that leaving the burn blisters intact results in more rapid reepithelialization than when the blisters are débrided.[14,15] Most blisters should be left intact to allow the outer layer of the blister to function as a biologic dressing.[16] However, large or tense blisters may be aspirated using sterile technique to facilitate their care. After the blisters break, the desquamated skin dries and can be cut away, uncovering the new epithelium that has grown over the surface of the burned area.

The burned surface can be managed in one of several ways. The burn is gently washed with soap and water, and then a topical antimicrobial agent is applied to the surface. The most commonly used topical treatment is 1% silver sulfadiazine (SSD), which is washed off and replaced twice daily. However, recent data suggest that the use of SSD delays reepithelialization.[16] Bacitracin or triple antibiotic ointment may be used instead, especially in superficial burns, and on the face. The ear lobes and the nose are especially vulnerable to infection because the skin overlying the poorly vascularized cartilage of these structures is thin. Mafenide acetate (Sulfamylon) should be applied topically, twice daily, to the ear lobes and the tip of the nose. Use of this agent should be limited to small areas, however, because patients often complain of local pain. This agent is also a carbonic anhydrase inhibitor, so if it is used on large burns for long periods, hyperchloremic metabolic acidosis can occur. Its spectrum of activity is against most gram-negative pathogens and most gram-positive bacteria. Sulfamylon also has an excellent capacity for penetrating the eschar of a full-thickness burn.

The use of SSD as a 1% cream is painless and it has in vitro activity against a wide range of organisms, including *Staphylococcus aureus, Escherichia coli, Klebsiella, Pseudomonas aeruginosa, Enterobacter*, and *Proteus* species. The most common toxic side effect of this agent is a transient leukopenia, which can manifest after several days of therapy as a marked decrease in the neutrophils. The leukopenia tends to correct itself after the use of the cream is stopped. A small number of patients experience a maculopapular rash, which also disappears after the SSD is stopped. As noted, the use of SSD has been falling out of favor because of evidence that suggests that SSD may delay reepithelialization.

Alternative burn dressings for superficial partial-thickness burns

In the past several decades, a number of synthetic wound coverings have become available. The theory behind the use of such materials is that they do not have to be changed several times daily, they protect the wound, and they decrease the local pain it causes. Epithelialization can then proceed under the moist environment of the synthetic dressing and heal the partial-thickness wound. Indeed, a moist environment has been shown to enhance reepithelialization.[17] Biobrane (Bertek Pharmaceuticals, Morgantown, WV) was one of the earliest of these dressings. It is a fabric made up of an inner layer of knitted nylon fibers coated with collagen, and an outer layer of silicone. Opsite (Smith & Nephew, Hull, UK) and Tegaderm (3M, St Paul, MN) are transparent films of polyurethane that have an adhesive coating. Once the wound is cleaned, these synthetic dressings are applied and

fitted snuggly to the surface of the wound. If necessary, they can be held in place with an outer layer such as Flexinet (Derma Sciences Inc, Princeton, NJ). The wound is then inspected daily, and if fluid collects it can be aspirated with a needle. The synthetic material is left in place until reepithelialization occurs; then it is gently removed, exposing the healed surface.

In the past several years, Acticoat (Acticoat, Smith & Nephew), a silver-impregnated absorbent dressing, has been found to be useful in the treatment of partial-thickness burns. Its advantage is that the silver that is released provides antimicrobial activity against both gram-negative and gram-positive organisms.[18] It does not have to be changed more frequently than every 3 days. The Acticoat dressing is placed on the wound and is kept moist with application of sterile water, which activates the release into the wound of the silver ions in nanocrystalline form. An outer layer of gauze bandage such as Kerlix (Curad [Beiersdorf USA], Wilton, CT) or Kling (Johnson & Johnson Medical, Arlington, TX) is used to protect the wound and keep the Acticoat in place. A large number of silver-based advanced dressings are now available on the market with comparable results.[19]

Use of dressings

Burn wound dressings should be applied snugly to the injured area and should extend above and below the burn. They should be occlusive and have sufficient thickness or layers of gauze so that all the secretions are absorbed into the dressings. The purpose of the dressing is to protect the wound from bacterial contamination from the outside, and to prevent the wound from rubbing against clothing or other objects. The frequency of dressing changes varies, depending on the amount of secretions. When antimicrobial creams are used, which require washing and reapplication, the dressings are changed once or twice daily. In the case of the synthetic dressings such as Acticoat or Biobrane, however, dressing changes are required only once every several days as needed. The advantage to the patient of this type of dressing is the decrease in the frequency of dressing changes to once every 3 days or longer.

Deep Partial-Thickness (Dermal) Burns

Deep partial-thickness burns result from exposure to agents such as very hot water or hot oil. Upon presentation, the wound surface is less moist than in a superficial second-degree burn, and is usually covered with an orange or light tan crust composed of dead collagen, which is very adherent to the underlying wound (Figure 21-4). The dead collagen must be completely débrided before healing can take place. Depending upon their depth, these burns may require from 14 to 35 days to heal. Sometimes infection of the wound may destroy the remaining viable epithelium and cause conversion of the partial-thickness burn to a full-thickness injury. Deep partial-thickness burns should be cared for by a burn specialist, because enzymatic[20] or surgical débridement followed by grafting is often required.[1]

Full-Thickness (Third-Degree) Burns

The dead skin covering the full-thickness burn is called an *eschar*. After several days, the eschar of the full-thickness injury becomes permeable and loses the ability to control the rate of evaporation of water from the body.[21] An even more serious consequence of a full-thickness injury is that the skin ceases to function as a barrier against infection, and bacterial growth inevitably occurs in the deeper layers of the eschar. Depending upon the extent of the full-thickness injury, as the bacterial growth proceeds it may become invasive and life-threatening septicemia may ensue.

Patients who sustain circumferential full-thickness burns of an extremity should be carefully observed. As edema forms in the subcutaneous tissues, a great deal of pressure is exerted against the eschar, which is stiff and unyielding. This may result in partial or even total occlusion of the blood flow to the extremity. The vessels to the distal extremities such as the hands and feet are especially vulnerable. The adequacy of the pulses to the extremities should be frequently monitored by a Doppler flowmeter.

If there is any question concerning the quality and adequacy of the pulses in a patient with a circumferential extremity burn, escharotomy should be performed. Escharotomies can be performed at the patient's bedside with intravenous sedation. An electrocautery device is used to reduce the amount of bleeding (Figure 21-8). The incisions are made over the lateral and medial aspects of the extremities and of the digits to release the pressure exerted upon the vessels by the edematous subcutaneous tissues (Figure 21-9). When the chest is involved by a circumferential full-thickness injury, escharotomies should be performed to improve the ease and completeness of ventilation. These incisions are carried out in both anterior axillary lines. The incision of eschar should be carried out through the depth of the eschar into the subcutaneous tissues. When the compression is

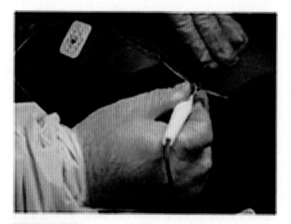

FIGURE 21-8

Performance of escharotomy by using cautery.

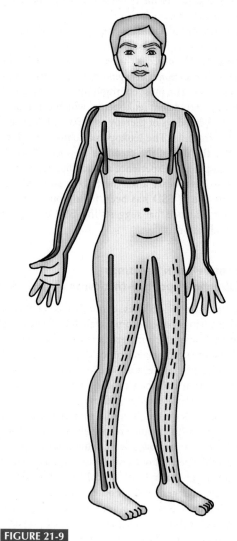

FIGURE 21-9

Locations for incisions when performing escharotomies.

relieved, the subcutaneous tissue will pout out from the wound, and the arterial pulses will return to their normal levels. If they do not, and the burn is deep, or if there is a concomitant crush injury, a compartment syndrome is possible. In that case, the tissue pressures in the deeper compartment of the limbs should be measured directly. If the tissue pressures are elevated, they can be relieved in the operating room by releasing the fascia from its osseous attachments. All patients with full-thickness burns should be managed by a burn specialist, because the necrotic tissue will need to be surgically excised and grafted. The proper timing of excision of the eschar is largely dependent on the overall condition of the patient.

ELECTRICAL BURNS

Electrical injury is caused by the passage of the current through the body. As the electric current encounters the resistance of the tissues of the body, it is converted to heat. The amount of heat produced is a function of both the amperage of the current and the resistance that that portion of the body offers to its passage. Thus, the smaller the size of the part of the body affected, and the more bone there is in relation to the soft tissue, the more intense the heat becomes and the more damage occurs.[22] Thus, fingers, feet, lower legs, and forearms suffer more extensive and devastating injury. Usually the points of entrance and exit may be identified as necrotic areas, often several millimeters in diameter, which will heal by themselves. If they involve an area around the mouth or the fingers, however, an excision and extensive grafting may be required, or an amputation. Delayed sloughing of the eschar at the corner of the mouth may result in significant bleeding from the labial artery in children who have bitten an electrical cord. A typical electrical burn is demonstrated in Figure 21-10.

The systemic effects caused by an electrical current depend on its voltage. A low-voltage current is defined as one that is less than 1000 volts. Patients sustaining a low-voltage injury are in danger of developing an arrhythmia such as ventricular fibrillation. Following such an injury, there may be nonspecific ST-T wave abnormalities of the electrocardiogram, and arrhythmias also may develop.

High-voltage injuries cause the most destructive tissue injuries. The muscles, fascia, and even bone are severely injured in the current's path. Such injuries are often life-threatening and usually require amputations and very extensive operative excision of the injured tissues.

CHEMICAL BURNS

Chemical burns destroy the skin in such a manner that the depth of injury is difficult to assess. It is important to identify the causative agent, because the destruction of the tissue can continue until the chemical is inactivated. Acid burns tend to be more limited in their depth than burns caused by alkali, which reacts with the fats in the skin to cause progressive injury. A typical chemical burn is demonstrated in Figure 21-11.

Treatment of chemical burns begins with removing the causative agent as soon as possible. The chemical should be brushed off and washed by copious lavage with water for up to 1 hour or until the pain subsides. Chemical burns should be observed carefully for 4 to 7 days because, even though the injury initially may appear to be superficial, it may become deeper after a few days.

Burns caused by hydrofluoric acid are commonly encountered in industrial areas where it is used in the etching process because of its ability to dissolve glass and metals. The danger associated with its use is its ability to penetrate tissue such as skin. Because hydrofluoric acid interferes with nerve function, the burns may not be painful initially.[23] If a substantial amount of hydrofluoric acid is absorbed into the body, it can cause arrhythmias as a result of the binding of the fluoride ion to calcium. The treatment is to inject

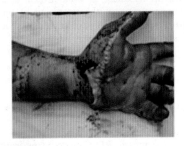

FIGURE 21-10
Photograph of an electrical burn.

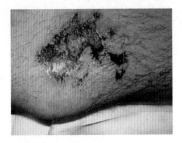

FIGURE 21-11
Typical appearance of chemical burn.

calcium ions intraarterially into the artery that perfuses the area that is affected. If this is not possible, then the injured tissue should be injected directly with calcium gluconate. For superficial injuries, calcium gluconate can be applied topically as a 2.5% calcium gluconate gel.

Wet cement is capable of causing a deep chemical burn.[24] Inexperienced workers sometimes kneel in wet cement for long periods without protecting their knees, or the cement may enter their clothing and not be noticed for several hours. The wet cement converts to calcium hydroxide, and it is the alkaline hydroxyl ion that produces the injury. The resultant burn is treated in the standard manner.

Exposure to hot tar and asphalt causes severe burns. If the patient is exposed to hot tar directly from the container in which the tar is heated, it will cause a full-thickness injury. However, if an accident occurs from exposure to heated tar that has already been spread, the adherent tar must first be removed. It can be dissolved by applying a petrolatum-based ointment such as De-Solv-it. Débridement of the wound is accomplished by changing the dressings every several hours until the tar is dissolved and the wound becomes clean. The depth of the wound can then be properly assessed and treated following the treatment regimens used in other burns.

REFERENCES

1. Brigham PA, McLoughlin E. Burn incidence and medical care use in the United States: estimate, trends, and data sources. *J Burn Care Rehabil.* 1996; 17(2):95–107.
2. Saffle JR, Davis B, Williams P. Recent outcomes in the treatment of burn injury in the United States: a report from the American Burn Association Patient Registry. *J Burn Care Rehabil.* 1995;16(3 pt 1): 219–232.
3. Moritz AR, Henriques FC. Studies of thermal injury: II. The relative importance of time and surface temperature in the causation of cutaneous burns. *Am J Pathol.* 1947;23(5):693–720.
4. Kramer GC, Lund T, Beckum OK. Pathophysiology of the burn wound. In: Herndon DN, ed. *Total Burn Care.* 3rd ed. Philadelphia, PA: WB Saunders; 2007:93–107.
5. Arturson G. Microvascular permeability to macromolecules in thermal injury. *Acta Physiol Scand Suppl.* 1979;463:111–122.
6. Evans EI, Purnell OJ, Robinett PW, Batchelor A, Martin M. Fluid and electrolyte requirements in severe burns. *Ann Surg.* 1952;135(6):804–817.
7. Lund CC, Browder NC. The estimate of area of burns. *Surg Gynecol Obstet.* 1944;79:352–358.
8. Jaskille AD, Ramella-Roman JC, Shupp JW, Jordan MH, Jeng JC. Critical review of burn depth assessment techniques: part II. Review of laser doppler technology. *J Burn Care Res.* 2010;31(1):151–157.
9. Baxter C. Fluid resuscitation, burn percentage and physiologic age. *J Trauma.* 1979;19(suppl 11): 864–865.
10. Saffle JI. The phenomenon of "fluid creep" in acute burn resuscitation. *J Burn Care Res.* 2007;28(3): 382–395.
11. Alvarado R, Chung KK, Cancio LC, Wolf SE. Burn resuscitation. *Burns.* 2009;35(1):4–14.
12. Traber DL, Herndon DN, Enkhbaatar B, Maybauer MO, Maybauer DM. Physiology of inhalation injury. In: Herndon DN. *Total Burn Care.* 3rd ed. Philadelphia, PA: WB Saunders; 2007:248–261.
13. Nugent N, Herndon DN. Diagnosis and treatment of inhalation injury. In: Herndon DN, ed. *Total Burn Care.* 3rd ed. Philadelphia, PA: WB Saunders; 2007:262–273.
14. Gimbel NS, Kapetansky DI, Weissman F, Pinkus HK. A study of epithelialization in blistered burns. *AMA Arch Surg.* 1957;74(5):800–803.
15. Wheeler ES, Miller TA. The blister and the second degree burn in guinea pigs: the effect of exposure. *Plast Reconstr Surg.* 1976;57(1):74–83.
16. Burd A, Kwok CH, Hung SC, et al. A comparative study of the cytotoxicity of silver-based dressings in monolayer cell, tissue explant, and animal models. *Wound Repair Regen.* 2007;15(1):94–104.
17. Hinman CD, Maibach H. Effect of air exposure and occlusion on experimental human skin wounds. *Nature.* 1963;200:377–378.
18. Wright JB, Hansen DL, Burell RE. The comparative efficacy of two antimicrobial barrier dressings: in-vitro examination of two controlled release of silver dressings. *Wounds.* 1998;10:179–188.
19. Gravante G, Caruso R, Sorge R, Nicoli F, Gentile P, Cervelli V. Nanocrystalline silver: a systematic review of randomized trials conducted on burned patients and an evidence-based assessment of potential advantages over older silver formulations. *Ann Plast Surg.* 2009;63(2):201–205.
20. Soroff HS, Sasvary DH. Collagenase ointment and polymyxin B sulfate/bacitracin spray versus silver sulfadiazine cream in partial-thickness burns: a pilot study. *J Burn Care Rehab.* 1994;15:253–260.
21. DeLuca M, Albanese E, Bondanza S, et al. Multicenter experience in the treatment of burns with autologous and allogeneic cultured epithelium, fresh or preserved in a frozen state. *Burns.* 1989;15: 303–309.
22. Sances A Jr, Myklebust JB, Larson SJ, et al. Experimental electrical injury studies. *J Trauma.* 1981; 21(8):589–597.
23. Anderson WJ, Anderson JR. Hydrofluoric acid burns of the hand: mechanisms of injury and treatment. *J Hand Surg Am.* 1988;13(1):52–57.
24. Early SH, Simpson RL. Caustic burns from contact with wet cement. *JAMA.* 1985;254(4):528–529.

CHAPTER 22

Evaluating and Treating Skin Ulcers

Charlene M. Morris, MPAS, PA-C, and Adam J. Singer, MD

Chronic ulcers such as diabetic foot ulcers, pressure ulcers, and venous leg ulcers are a worldwide problem. Venous stasis ulcers account for more than half of all leg ulcers affecting somewhere between 1% and 2% of the world's population.[1] They are more common in women than in men and increase in incidence with age. It has been estimated that approximately 15% of all diabetic patients will develop lower-extremity ulcers and, of those, nearly one in four will ultimately require limb amputation during their leftime.[2,3] Pressure ulcers are especially prevalent in elderly and debilitated patients and are estimated to affect 1 to 3 million people in the United States.[4]

In most patients, an accurate diagnosis of the ulcer can be made on the basis of a medical history and physical examination. Often knowledge of the underlying diseases and the location and appearance of the ulcer will suffice to make a diagnosis and treatment plan (Table 22-1). In some patients, ulcers may be of mixed etiology. Because the treatment of venous ulcers and arterial ulcers differs, it important to exclude underlying arterial disease in all patients with venous stasis ulcers.

A thorough history should be obtained in all patients regarding the onset, duration, location, and prior management of ulcers. Intermittent claudication suggests an arterial origin. The presence of underlying diseases such as diabetes, peripheral arterial disease, deep venous thrombosis (DVT),

hypertension, coronary artery disease, cerebrovascular disease, and hyperlipidemia should be also noted. Local infection is suggested by the presence of increased swelling, redness, and drainage and systemic infection is suggested in patients with fever and chills.

On physical examination the patient's vital signs and presence of peripheral arterial pulses are noted. The location, size, depth, and margins of the ulcer are noted. The presence of malodorous exudate and surrounding warmth, redness, and swelling suggests infection. The ankle–brachial index (ABI) is measured by dividing the arterial pressure in the arm by that in the ankle. An index less than 0.9 suggests arterial insufficiency. Duplex ultrasound should be considered to assess the underlying venous and arterial structures and to rule out a DVT. Plain radiography or magnetic resonance imaging (MRI) should be considered when osteomyelitis is suspected. Osteomyelitis is also suggested when probing of the ulcer bed with a sterile probe comes into contact with bone.

The general principles of wound care are similar for all ulcers. All devitalized or necrotic tissue should be removed and any infection or bacterial bioburden should be controlled with topical or systemic or topical antibiotics, respectively. Wound dressings should maintain a moist healing environment optimal to wound healing while avoiding maceration. In addition, control of underlying

TABLE 22–1	Comparison of Ulcer Types			
	Venous	**Arterial**	**Neuropathic**	**Pressure**
Underlying conditions	Venous insufficiency and hypertension Deep venous thrombosis Women more than men	Tissue ischemia, peripheral vascular disease, hypertension, diabetes, coronary or cerebrovascular disease, hyperlipidemia, smoking	Diabetes	Debilitated, bed-ridden, paralyzed, malnourished
History	Rapid onset, edema, trauma, pain worse with dependency	Intermittent claudication, pain worse on elevation	Insensate foot, paresthesias	Prolonged immobilization
Location	Ankle, medial malleolus, lower calf, stocking distribution	Toes, heel, bony prominences, lateral malleolus, anterior shin	Pressure points, plantar foot, metatarsal heads	Bony prominences, sacrum, ischium, hips
Ulcer characteristics	Irregular border, shallow, granulation tissue at base, weeping	Deep, well demarcated, punched-out appearance Pale or white base	Thin, unclear margins Black, yellow, or gray base	Depends on staging (Table 22–3)
Associated findings	Edema, varicosities, hyperpigmentation, hyperkeratosis, stasis dermatitis, inverted bottle appearance Normal ABI (≥0.9)	Pale, cyanotic, pulseless foot, dependent rubor Shiny, hairless toe skin Low ABI (<0.9), delayed capillary refill, pallor with elevation and rubor with dependency, prolonged venous filling	Calluses, pallor, hammertoes, Charcot's deformity Pulses usually present With diabetic ulcers, mixed neuropathic and vascular findings	Malnutrition, limited mobility, excessive moisture, incontinence
Treatment	Compression, débridement, occlusive dressings, infection control Consider venous repair, growth factors, pentoxifylline, skin replacements	Smoking cessation and control of underlying conditions, occlusive dressings, infection control Consider revascularization or amputation, antiplatelet agents, rheologic agents	Control diabetes, débridement, occlusive dressings, infection control May require amputation	Pressure relief, débridement, occlusive dressings, infection control, nutrition Consider excision of bone and flap coverage

ABI = ankle–brachial index.

conditions should be achieved whenever possible. With venous ulcers, compression forms the mainstay of therapy whereas revascularization may be required with arterial ulcers. Tight glycemic control and relief of pressure are necessary in diabetic and pressure ulcers, respectively. Healing is defined as 100% reepithelialization and no exudates nor need for dressings. After skin ulcers have occurred, speedy identification, classification, recognition of comorbidities and their ramifications, and subsequent team effort, family or caretaker education, and involvement with directed therapies and surveillance can improve mortality and morbidity.

VENOUS STASIS ULCERS

Etiology and Pathogenesis

The fundamental underlying cause of venous stasis ulcers is chronic venous insufficiency as a result of damage to the valves in the veins of the legs.[5] The venous insufficiency leads to an increase in the hydrostatic pressure in the peripheral circulation in the lower extremities. Venous hypertension then leads to vessel damage and leakage of fibrinogen into the extravascular tissues forming fibrin cuffs that limit the diffusion of oxygen and nutrients to the surrounding tissue. Chronic venous insufficiency may also result in chronic inflammation, repeated cycles of ischemia-reperfusion, and oxidative stress contributing to ulceration and impaired healing. Increased local expression of proteolytic enzymes further contributes to poor healing and chronic ulceration. Because treatment may differ significantly in the presence of associated peripheral arterial disease, ABI should be measured to exclude arterial disease. The presence of sickle cell disease should also be excluded.

Diagnosis

The diagnosis of venous stasis ulcers is suggested by the clinical history and physical examination.

Patients with venous ulcers commonly complain of swelling and aching of the legs, often worse at the end of the day, which may be exacerbated by dependency and improved by leg elevation. A history of ulcer recurrence, especially at the same location, is characteristic. Despite prior beliefs that venous ulcers were painless, most venous ulcers are painful and can adversely affect the patient's quality of life.

Signs of venous insufficiency include telangiectasia, varicose veins, and edema of the lower extremity. Reddish-brown discoloration of the leg is the result of

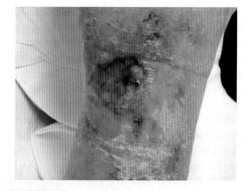

FIGURE 22-1

Venous stasis ulcer on the lower leg.

extravasation of blood with subsequent breakdown to hemosiderin. Eczematous changes include redness, scaling, and itching. Venous ulcers are typically located over the medial malleolus of the ankle. They may also be seen on other areas of the ankle and the lower calf, often in a stocking distribution. The ulcers may be single or multiple, sometimes involving the entire leg circumference. Venous ulcers usually have irregular, flat, or only slightly steep borders (Figure 22-1). The ulcer bed is usually shallow with granulation tissue, as well as some fibrinous material. In long-standing venous disease, the skin develops an induration and fibrosis of the dermis and subcutaneous tissue that results in an inverted bottle appearance termed lipodermatosclerosis.

Although the history and physical examination can identify most cases of venous ulcers, color duplex ultrasonography is the gold standard in evaluating venous disease. Duplex ultrasonography is a noninvasive yet accurate study that helps provide important information regarding the anatomy and function of both the arterial and venous systems.

In patients with a venous ulcer that fails to heal for more than 3 months or that does not respond to treatment within 4 to 6 weeks, a tissue biopsy should be obtained to exclude underlying conditions such as malignancy, vasculitis, and collagen vascular disease. If osteomyelitis is suspected, plain radiography, bone scanning, MRI, or a bone biopsy may be required.

Treatment

The cornerstone of therapy for ulcers caused by venous stasis is compression. A recent systematic review conducted by the Cochrane Collaboration reviewed 39 randomized controlled trials evaluating compression for venous ulcers.[6] Compression therapy increased ulcer healing rates compared with no compression. In addition, multicomponent compression systems containing an elastic bandage and absorbent layers were more effective than single-component compression. The most supportive systems are high-compression systems containing three or four layers such as the paste containing bandages (e.g., Unna's boot, Duke boot).[7] Although the optimal pressure necessary to overcome venous hypertension is not well defined, an external pressure of 35 mm Hg to 40 mm Hg at the ankle is probably necessary to prevent capillary exudation in the legs.[8]

Care should be taken to avoid excessive pressures that may further impair dermal perfusion leading to pressure ulcers. Because even moderate pressures may be harmful in patients with underlying arterial insufficiency, all patients with venous ulcers should be screened for arterial disease with Doppler measurement of the ABI. Intermittent pneumatic pressure may be considered in patients who do not tolerate compression dressings. Compression therapy with dressings and elastic bandages should continue until the ulcers are healed. After healing, patients should wear compression stockings to prevent ulcer recurrence.

Infection of venous ulcers is common and contributes significantly to impaired and delayed healing. Because the presence of necrotic tissue and exudate promotes infection, all necrotic or devitalized tissue should be removed with sharp, enzymatic, mechanical, biological, or autolytic débridement. Sharp débridement is usually achieved with a scalpel, forceps, scissors, or curette. With sharp débridement the devitalized tissue is removed until normal tissue is apparent by brisk bleeding. Proteolytic enzymes, such as collagenase may also be used for slow débridement. With autolytic débridement the necrotic tissue is allowed to slough off slowly in a moist environment. A deep-tissue biopsy should be performed to determine the type and level of infection in patients who fail to show signs of healing within 2 weeks of débridement. Topical antimicrobial agents should be used in patients with beta hemolytic streptococci or high burdens of bacteria ($>1 \times 10^6$ CFU/g of tissue). Patients with surrounding cellulitis (most commonly caused by streptococci or staphylococci) should be treated with systemic bactericidal antibiotics aimed at gram-positive organisms. Proper nutrition is also necessary to improve wound healing.

Dressings are often applied underneath the compression dressings to control exudate and aid healing. A systematic review of dressings for healing of venous ulcers including 42 randomized trials concluded that ulcer healing was not affected by the type of dressing.[9] In addition, healing was similar with hydrocolloid dressings and low-adherent dressing. Any dressing that maintains a moist wound healing environment while avoiding maceration can be used under the compression dressing. Wound location, patient activity, and the quality of the skin surrounding the ulcer should all be taken into consideration when one is choosing a dressing. In the absence of evidence for healing benefit with any specific dressing, cost should be a factor in the choice of dressings.[10] Wet-to-dry dressings do not maintain continuous moisture and should not be used. At each dressing change the ulcer should be cleansed with a nonirritating substance such as saline or sterile water. Tap water from a reliable source may also be used to irrigate the wound.

Large or persistent ulcers may require a skin graft and should be evaluated by a plastic surgeon. However, because this does not address the underlying etiology, they are likely to recur. Recalcitrant ulcers may sometimes require treatment with a free skin flap. There is currently insufficient evidence to support the use of local growth factors and oxygen free radical scavengers. Systemic pentoxifylline in conjunction with compression has been shown to improve healing.[11] Patients with healed or surgically treated venous ulcers should wear compression stockings indefinitely. All patients with venous ulcers should see a surgical specialist to evaluate the need for surgery.

Prevention

As with most conditions, efforts to prevent the development of venous ulcers should always be made in those with risk of venous stasis ulcers including patients with a history of DVT, incompetence of the direct calf and ankle perforating veins, venous hypertension, calf pump dysfunction, edema, cellulitis, and lipodermatosclerosis. Patients with signs of venous hypertension and/or the postphlebitis syndrome (after DVT) should be treated indefinitely with compression stockings.[12] Exercises to increase calf muscle pump function may also be helpful in preventing ulcers. A patient with a DVT should be treated with venous thromboembolism prophylaxis to reduce the risk of recurrent DVT, the postphlebitis syndrome, and venous ulceration. Subfascial endoscopic perforator surgery should be considered to prevent backflow of blood from the deep to superficial venous system in patients with severe venous hypertension. Less extensive surgery (superficial venous ablation, endovenous laser ablation) can also help reduce venous hypertension when used in combination with compression. Finally, cellulitis of the lower extremity should be treated with appropriate systemic antibiotics, especially in patients with underlying edema.

DIABETIC ULCERS

Etiology and Pathogenesis

Diabetic ulcers are usually multifactorial in origin. They are the result of various combinations of small and large vessel diseases (atherosclerosis), poor glycemic control, neuropathy, and minor trauma. By definition, any ulcer in a diabetic patient is considered a diabetic ulcer. Sensory neuropathy leads to loss of the protective sensations to pain, temperature, and pressure. Charcot's neuropathy leads to wasting of the intrinsic muscles of the foot and a resulting deformity with prominence of the metatarsal heads that are subject to pressure from improper gait or poorly fitting footwear. Autonomic neuropathy can cause vasodilatation and decreased sweating of the skin with loss of the skin's integrity and the risk of bacterial infection. Peripheral arterial disease leading to stenosis of large vessels and reduced perfusion is common in those with diabetes. Early revascularization may help prevent subsequent limb amputation. Even in the absence of large vessel disease, small vessel disease and impaired angiogenesis may result in local ischemia.

Diagnosis

Diabetic ulcers are diagnosed when a nonhealing wound or ulcer develops in a patient with diabetes. Many of these patients have sensory neuropathy leading to an insensate foot and paresthesia that is best confirmed using the Semmes–Weinstein filament test.[13] If light touch from the microfilament is not perceived, then check for sharp, cold, and warm perception, as well as the patient's perception of toe position.

A history of intermittent claudication suggests the presence of peripheral arterial disease. Motor neuropathy may result in typical foot deformities including hammertoes (flexion of the toes) and Charcot's deformity (flattening of the medial longitudinal arches of the foot). With autonomic neuropathy the skin may appear dry and shiny often with fissuring. Typically, diabetic ulcers occur on the plantar surface of the foot or over pressure sites such as the heels and bony prominences (Figure 22-2). The base of the ulcer appears black, gray, or yellow and its margins are thin and ill defined. Diminished or absent pulses may be noted in patients with concomitant peripheral vascular disease. All patients with a diabetic ulcer should have a formal determination of their ABI with Doppler.

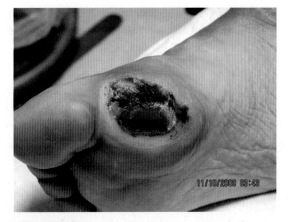

FIGURE 22-2

Diabetic foot ulcer.

Diabetic ulcers are commonly classified on the basis of the extent of the lesions according to a system proposed by Wagner (Table 22-2).[14]

Treatment

Whenever possible tight glycemic control, with hemoglobin A1C level below 6.2, or an average daily glucose level of less than 125 should be achieved and patients should stop smoking. All patients should be examined for callus formation that may be a sign of impending ulceration. Removal of calluses may reduce local pressure and prevent ulcers. Fungal infections are common in diabetic patients and may lead to skin breakdown and bacterial infections. Oral or topical therapies should be administered in diabetic patients with fungal infections of the foot. Patients with an ABI less than 0.9 or a transcutaneous oxygen pressure of less than 40 mm Hg should be referred to a vascular surgeon for possible revascularization. Patients must be educated about the importance of good foot care and frequent examination of their foot, especially in the presence of sensory deficits. Patients should also be encouraged to stop smoking.

Débridement of necrotic or devitalized tissue and any calluses should be performed, usually with a scalpel or scissors.[15] The tissue should be débrided until the margins of the ulcer appear healthy as suggested by the presence of bleeding and soft skin. After débridement, the ulcer should be covered with a cost-effective dressing that provides a moist wound healing environment. A recent systematic review of various dressings for diabetic ulcers concluded that hydrogels increase the healing rates of diabetic foot ulcers compared with gauze dressings or standard care.[16] The

TABLE 22–2	Classification and Treatment of Diabetic Foot Ulcers	
Grade	**Appearance**	**Treatment**
Grade 1	No ulcer, high-risk foot	Preventive foot care
Grade 2	Superficial ulcer involving the full thickness of the skin but not involving the underlying tissues	Extensive débridement, local wound care, infection control, pressure relief
Grade 3	Deep ulcer penetrating down to the ligaments and muscle, but with no bone involvement	Evaluate for bony involvement and arterial insufficiency Débridement, infection control, pressure relief, revascularization when appropriate Generally requires hospital admission
Grade 4	Localized gangrene	Urgent hospital admission Surgical consultation Amputation may be required
Grade 5	Extensive gangrene involving the whole foot	Urgent hospital admission Surgical consultation Amputation may be required

same study did not find evidence to support surgical débridement over standard treatment. Despite the widespread use of dressings and topical agents that contain silver for diabetic foot ulcers, there is little high-quality evidence to support their use.[17]

The Wound Healing Society has recently published guidelines for the treatment of diabetic ulcers.[18] If infection is suspected or if healing of the ulcer fails to progress within 2 weeks of treatment a tissue biopsy should be performed to determine bacterial type and load. If beta hemolytic streptococci or a bacterial burden of greater than 10^6 CFU/g are present, topical antibiotics should be prescribed. To prevent bacterial resistance or toxicity, topical antibiotics should be stopped once the bacterial load is lowered. Systemic antibiotics should be given to patients with surrounding infection or systemic toxicity. Infection is often polymicrobial and should be aggressively treated with broad-spectrum antibiotics and adjusted based on bacterial antibiotic susceptibility testing.

Probing of the wound with a sterile cotton-tipped applicator and specialized imaging (plain radiography, MRI, computed tomography (CT), bone scans) should be conducted when osteomyelitis is suspected. If osteomyelitis is present, the infected bone should be removed by a surgeon followed by 2 to 4 weeks of antibiotics. Platelet-derived growth factor (PDGF) has been shown to be effective in treating diabetic neuropathic ulcers.[19] The use of other topical growth factors for diabetic ulcers is not yet supported by the evidence.[18] Negative pressure wound therapy with a vacuum-assisted closure device may be of benefit for nonhealing diabetic ulcers.[20] The role of living skin equivalents, electrical stimulation, and hyperbaric oxygen is unclear but these may be of benefit for recalcitrant ulcers.[15,21]

Prevention

The recurrence rates of diabetic foot ulcers range from 8% to 59%. As a result, protective footwear should be used after the ulcer heals to prevent recurrence.[22] Good foot care and daily inspection of the feet should be encouraged in all patients with diabetic foot ulcers. Offloading of any pressure to the foot should be achieved with casting or orthotics.[23] Other acceptable methods of offloading include crutches, walkers, and wheelchairs. Patient self-monitoring, when possible, is also effective in prevention or early detection and intervention of skin lesions. This can be accomplished with mirrors either on the floor or those made with handles for this purpose, newer infrared temperature monitoring, and episodic clinical exams.[24-26]

ARTERIAL ULCERS

Etiology

Arterial leg ulcers are the result of insufficient blood supply to the skin, generally secondary to atherosclerosis. Impaired perfusion results in susceptibility to minor trauma and impairs wound healing. Peripheral arterial disease resulting in foot ulcers may be seen in diabetic patients as well as in patients with venous insufficiency. A history of coronary artery disease, cerebrovascular disease, hypertension, diabetes, and hyperlipidemia should raise the suspicion for arterial disease. A family history of arterial disease and smoking also increases the risk of peripheral arterial disease. Additional disorders that may cause arterial disease include Raynaud's disease, Buerger's disease, arteriosclerosis obliterans, arterial emboli or thrombi, and cutaneous vasculopathies.

Diagnosis

Intermittent claudication, or pain with exertion that is relieved with rest, is commonly reported. Pain at rest suggests more severe vascular occlusion. The ulcer is often painful and the pain is exacerbated with elevation of the extremity. Physical examination may reveal a cool lower extremity with diminished or absent distal pulses and delayed capillary refill. Arterial ulcers are typically round with sharply demarcated borders. These ulcers often occur over bony prominences. The surrounding skin may be hairless, shiny, and atrophic.

As noted previously, all patients with suspected arterial ulcers should have a formal Doppler ultrasound to evaluate the status of the peripheral venous and arterial systems in both lower extremities. Arterial disease is diagnosed in the presence of an ABI less than 0.9 and/or a transcutaneous oxygen tension of less than 40 mm Hg. Formal arteriography may also be indicated. Other diagnostic modalities include magnetic resonance arteriography and CT angiography.

Treatment

Lifestyle modification including control of hypertension, diabetes, and hyperlipidemia are required and patients should be strongly encouraged to stop smoking. Multiple methods and strategies for tobacco cessation exist and should be mentioned and encouraged at every patient encounter.[27] Graded exercise (such as walking until pain appears) may help slow the progression of arterial disease. Patients with arterial ulcers should be urgently evaluated by a vascular surgeon for surgical or endovascular revascularization. Compressive therapy should not be used in patients with arterial disease. As with other ulcers, local wound care that promotes a moist healing environment and controls local infection is indicated. Amputation may be the final option to prevent intractable ulceration or infection.[28]

PRESSURE ULCERS

Etiology and Pathogenesis

Most skin ulcers are preventable if not modifiable with respect to contributing to the development of pressure and stasis ulcers. Pressure ulcers are caused by impaired perfusion and tissue malnutrition of the skin resulting from prolonged pressure on the skin. In general, local ischemia and skin necrosis occur when the tissue pressure exceeds the capillary pressure (approximately 30 mm Hg) for at least 2 hours. Areas of the skin that are over bony prominences (e.g., sacrum, hips, or malleoli) are typically involved (Figure 22-3).[29] Pressure skin ulcers, as alluded to previously, are largely seen in the immobile, higher risk groups. In as little as 1 week, early lesions may be identified in a bed-bound patient. If in a hospital or long-term facility, there is further incentive to prevent these from occurring, by insurance disallowing reimbursement for incidental care of newly developed skin ulcers. Patients who have developed contractures may benefit from range-of-motion exercises performed continuously as well as the aforementioned surveillance and therapies.

Diagnosis

Pressure ulcers are classified on the basis of a system proposed by the National Pressure Ulcer Advisory Panel for Pressure Ulcers (Table 22-3).[30]

Treatment

Treatments for pressure ulcers are many and need not be complex to be effective. First and foremost, the wound must be cleaned. Normal saline is effective and inexpensive, and if no specific cleansers are available or necessary, this will suffice. Other options include Technicare (when no infection exists), CC-500, SAF-Clens or MicroKlenz directly to the area may

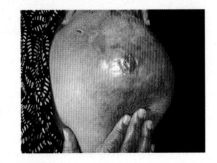

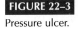
Pressure ulcer.

Progression of decubitis ulcer

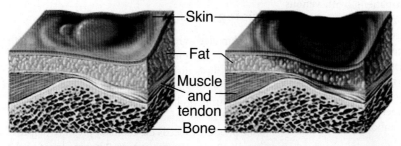

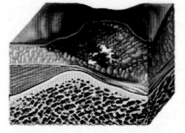

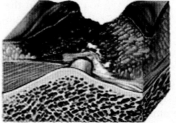

FIGURE 22-4

Classification of pressure ulcers.

TABLE 22–3	Classification and Treatment of Pressure Ulcers	
Stage	**Manifestations**	**Treatment**
Stage I	Nonblanchable erythema with intact skin may indicate the start of skin ulceration With darker pigmented tissue, a discoloration, warmth, edema, induration, or localized firm skin are the important indicators.	Transparent dressings and increased vigilance to progression and escalating prevention
Stage II	Partial thickness skin loss involves the epidermis, dermis, or both The ulcer is superficial and presents clinically as an abrasion, blister, or shallow erosion at the center	Occlusive semipermeable dressings that provide a moist wound situation
Stage III	Full-thickness skin loss involves damage or necrosis of subcutaneous tissue that can extend down to, but not through, underlying fascia Clinically, this may appear as a crater with or without undermining or damage of adjacent tissue.	Often require infection treatment Débridement must be considered if necrosis is present at the periphery, based on ulcer characteristics Dressings are chosen appropriate to wound type Surgical management may be necessary in some full-thickness skin ulcers
Stage IV	Full-thickness skin loss with extensive destruction, tissue necrosis, or damage and exposure of muscle, bone, or supporting structures (e.g., tendon, joint capsule) Undermining and sinus tracts also may be associated with these pressure ulcers May manifest or progress to osteomyelitis	As for stage III above

be used. The specific wound care based on staging of the pressure ulcer is noted in Table 22-3. All necrotic or devitalized tissue should be débrided. Infected wounds need to be cultured and treated appropriately. Skin wounds may grow several organisms, making treatment decisions more difficult. A broad-spectrum antibiotic such as amoxicillin-clavulanate (Augmentin) or clindamycin may be effective. Still, with the emergence of methicillin-resistant *Staphylococcus aureus* (MRSA), reverting to older, but effective trimethoprim– sulfamethoxazole or doxycycline is effective and low cost. For more serious infections and for hospitalized patients with skin ulcers, vancomycin or some of the newer antimicrobials—piperacillin–tazobactam or dubromycin—may be considered.[31]

Wet-to-dry dressings are no longer considered effective treatments of skin ulcers. Polyurethane films (e.g., Tegaderm) or similar occlusive dressings allow a protective barrier and self-monitoring and are easily changed and effective for mild wounds. Ulcers with extensive exudates require absorptive barriers. These include calcium alginates, foams, and hydrofibers. For ulcers that do not exhibit moisture or fluids, wet dressings are indicated to promote healing. Saline dressings are effective and inexpensive, yet require intensified nursing care and must be kept moist to prevent further wound desiccation. Film dressings can be used as adjuncts with another choice for stage III and IV ulcers or as primary coverage of stage II on to progression to healing. Skin that is adjacent to the pressure ulcer should be treated with hydrating lotions such as Lac-Hydrin, which not only provides occlusion, allowing second-intention healing, but also provides lubrication for xerotic tissue.

A recent systematic review of more than 100 randomized clinical trials concluded that there was little evidence to support the use of specific support surfaces or dressings over other alternatives. In addition, there is little evidence to support the routine use of nutritional supplements or adjuvant therapies in patients without malnutrition.[32] According to the guidelines issued by the Wound Healing Society all patients with pressure ulcers should be screened for nutritional deficiencies and treated accordingly and adequate dietary intake should be maintained to prevent malnutrition.[33] Distant infection should be treated with appropriate antibiotics in all patients at risk of pressure ulcers. Cost-effective dressings that control exudate while maintaining moisture balance and minimizing damage to surrounding tissues are recommended. Irregular wound extensions forming sinuses or cavities should be explored and unroofed. Underlying bony prominences may need to be re-moved and nonhealing ulcers often will require surgical procedures such as local flaps. Use of local growth factors (PDGF) and negative-pressure wound therapy should also be considered in nonhealing wounds, especially when surgery is contraindicated.[33]

Pain levels in the skin ulcer patient must be addressed and appropriate medication administered, as skin ulcers can be painful. Oral analgesia may be adequate in some patients, with respect to renal function and gastrointestinal bleed and polypharmacy consideration. Opioids with antiemetics when appropriate may be necessary to achieve relief. Patches and other delivery systems such as intramuscular and intravenous may be considered when other systems are ineffective.

Nutrition has often been disregarded as a factor in wound healing, yet addressing nourishment as curative adjunct will result in robust improvement of skin rejuvenation. Assessed are not only caloric intake, but protein amounts as well as fluid and electrolyte status. When oral intake is not possible, enteral (nasogastric tube) or parenteral (total parenteral nutrition—or TPN) may become necessary to correct the catabolism state. Other nutritional supplementations include multi- and solitary vitamins, and zinc may be helpful.

Depression is treatable in the outpatient setting and may serve as a worthy adjunct for a chronically ill patient's treatment. When patients participate in their care, illnesses and wounds are more effectively treated. Music has been studied and found useful in decreasing depression as well as enhancing patient quality of life and self- empowerment. Music chosen by the patient may aid his or her healing process, regardless of living arrangement or treatment center.[34,35]

Prevention

Prevention tools aid the clinician in preventing hospitalization and should be utilized at every opportunity.[36] Patient positioning and methods to reduce pressure-related tissue damage are essential to help prevent recurrence of pressure ulcers. A recent systematic review of support surfaces for pressure ulcer prevention concluded that higher specification foam mattresses should be used in patients at high risk for pressure ulcers whereas the relative merits of constant low or alternating pressure mattresses remain unclear.[36] Medical grade sheepskins can be used to reduce the development of pressure ulcers in those at risk. Patients at risk of ischial pressure ulcers should avoid prolonged sitting and should use pressure-relieving seat cushions.

COMPLEMENTARY AND ALTERNATIVE MEDICINE

Patients or their families may be interested in or utilizing therapies unfamiliar to allopathic clinicians. Open communication allows those in clinical practice to identify those treatments that may be harmful or not helpful while monitoring progress or deterioration of wound management. The onus of identifying complementary and alternative medicine and beliefs of the patients and their families must also be taken into consideration for these patients.

Unripe papaya is used as skin ulcer therapy, and has been reported to enhance desloughing, granulation, and healing, and to diminish odor.[37] Additionally, it is available and cost-effective and regarded to be as effective as other therapies in skin ulcer treatment. A more recent study utilizing honey on burns and leg ulcers revealed enhanced healing of thermal injuries, yet no appreciable difference for chronic leg ulcers.[38] Of interest, patients with diabetes were not mentioned in this study. Draconian and originating from ancient medical interventions, maggot therapy on leg ulcers was found to be both effective in débridement and to promote healing. The actual time to heal after larval therapy was not improved compared with hydrogel dressings and patients treated with maggots experienced more associated pain.[39]

PATIENT DISPOSITION

Hospitalization may be required for those severely ill patients with skin ulcers. These include septic or febrile, infected, and severely debilitated cases that cannot be managed on an outpatient basis, or have not progressed despite intensive nonhospital-directed therapies. Associated primary diagnoses of sepsis, urinary tract infections, and pneumonia will also more likely require discharge to a skilled nursing facility or other long-term domiciliary care.

Hospitalizations for skin ulcers have increased 80% in the past decade, resulting in increased levels of patient care, worsening disease, and death. More than half of patients admitted to hospitals for a primary ulcer in 2006 were aged older than 65 years. Three out of four hospitalizations reported in 2006 for secondary pressure ulcers in 2006 were, similarly, in patients aged older than 65 years. Those same hospitalizations of patients diagnosed with pressure ulcers required payments of $11 billion in the same time period. In younger patients, the primary diagnosis shifts to paralysis and spinal cord injury as the primary justification. Fluid and electrolyte imbalance in both groups is more likely associated with inadequate nutrition with two primary variables: patients' inability to feed themselves and caretaker abilities or resources.

REFERENCES

1. Trent JT, Falabella A, Eaglstein WH, Kirsner RS. Venous ulcers: pathophysiology and treatment options. *Ostomy Wound Manage.* 2005;51(5):38–54.
2. Reiber GE. The epidemiology of diabetic foot problems. *Diabet Med.* 1996;13(suppl 1):S6–S11.
3. Consensus Development Conference on Diabetic Foot Wound Care:7-8 April 1999, Boston, Massachusetts. American Diabetes Association. *Diabetes Care.* 1999;22(8):1354–1360.
4. Hirshberg J, Coleman J, Marchant B, Rees RS. TGF-beta3 in the treatment of pressure ulcers: a preliminary report. *Adv Skin Wound Care.* 2001;14(2):91–95.
5. Chen WY, Rogers AA. Recent insights into the causes of chronic leg ulceration in venous diseases and implications on other types of chronic wounds. *Wound Repair Regen.* 2007;15(4):434–449.
6. O'Meara S, Cullum NA, Nelson EA. Compression for venous leg ulcers. *Cochrane Database Syst Rev.* 2009;(1):CD000265.
7. Robson MC, Cooper DM, Aslam R, et al. Guidelines for the treatment of venous ulcers. *Wound Repair Regen.* 2006;14(6):649–662.
8. Fletcher A, Cullum N, Sheldon TA. A systematic review of compression treatment for venous leg ulcers. *BMJ.* 1997;315(7108):576–580.
9. Palfreyman SJ, Nelson EA, Lochiel R, Michaels JA. Dressings for healing venous leg ulcers. *Cochrane Database Syst Rev.* 2006;(3):CD001103.
10. Palfreyman S, Nelson EA, Michaels JA. Dressings for venous leg ulcers: systematic review and meta-analysis. *BMJ.* 2007;335(7613):244.
11. Jull A, Waters J, Arroll B. Pentoxifylline for treating venous leg ulcers. *Cochrane Database Syst Rev.* 2002;(1):CD001733.
12. Robson MC, Cooper DM, Aslam R, et al. Guidelines for the prevention of venous ulcers. *Wound Repair Regen.* 2008;16(2):147–150.
13. Mayfield JA, Sugarman JR. The use of the Semmes-Weinstein monofilament and other threshold test for preventing foot ulceration and amputation in persons with diabetes. *J Fam Pract.* 2000;49(11 suppl):S17–S29.
14. O'Neal LW, Wagner FW. *The Diabetic Foot.* St Louis, MO: Mosby; 1983:274.
15. Brem H, Sheehan P, Rosenberg HJ, Schneider JS, Boulton AJ. Evidence-based protocol for diabetic foot ulcers. *Plast Reconstr Surg.* 2006;117(7 suppl):193S–209S.
16. Edwards J. Debridement of diabetic foot ulcers. *Cochrane Database Syst Rev.* 2002(4): CD003556.
17. Steed DL, Attinger C, Colaizzi T, et al. Guidelines for the treatment of diabetic ulcers. *Wound Repair Regen.* 2006;14(6):680–692.

18. Bergin SM, Wraight P. Silver based wound dressings and topical agents for treating diabetic foot ulcers. *Cochrane Database Syst Rev.* 2006;(1):CD005082.

19. Robson MC, Payne WG, Garner WL, et al. Integrating the results of Phase IV (postmarketing) clinical trial with four previous trials reinforces the position that Regranex (becaplemin) gel 0.01% is an effective adjunct to the treatment of diabetic ulcers. *J Appl Res.* 2005;5:35–45.

20. Eginton MT, Brown KR, Seabrook GR, Towne JB, Cambria RA. A prospective randomized evaluation of negative-pressure wound dressings for diabetic foot wounds. *Ann Vasc Surg.* 2003;17(6):645–649.

21. Hinchliffe RJ, Valk GD, Apelqvist J, et al. A systematic review of the effectiveness of interventions to enhance the healing of chronic ulcers of the foot in diabetes. *Diabetes Metab Res Rev.* 2008;24(suppl 1):S119–S144.

22. Steed DL, Attinger C, Brem H, et al. Guidelines for the prevention of diabetic ulcers. *Wound Repair Regen.* 2008;16(2);169–174.

23. Spencer S. Pressure relieving interventions for preventing and treating diabetic foot ulcers. *Cochrane Database Syst Rev.* 2000;(3):CD002302.

24. Self-management to prevent ulcers in veterans with SCI (spinal cord injury) [clinical trial]. Available at: http://clinicaltrials.gov/ct2/show/results/NCT00763282.

25. Stasis dermatitis information for adults [Skinsite Web page]. Available at: http://www.visualdxhealth.com/adult/stasisDermatitis-selfCare.htm.

26. Armstrong DG, Holtz-Neiderer K, Wendel C, Mohler MJ, Kimbriel HR, Lavery LA. Skin temperature monitoring reduces the risk for diabetic foot ulceration in high-risk patients. *Am J Med.* 2007;120(12):1042–1046.

27. Anczak JD, Nogler RA II. Tobacco cessation in primary care: maximizing intervention strategies. *Clin Med Res.* 2003;1(3):201–206.

28. Surgical treatment options [Cleveland Clinic Web page]. Available at: http://my.clevelandclinic.org/disorders/atherosclerosis/vs_surgical_treatment_options.aspx.

29. Bansal C, Scott R, Stewart D, Cockerell CJ. Decubitus ulcers: a review of the literature. *Int J Dermatol.* 2005;44(10):805–810.

30. National Pressure Ulcer Advisory Panel for Pressure Ulcers. Ulcer classification [Web page]. Available at: http://www.woundcare.org/newsvol2n1/ulcer1.htm.

31. Community-associated methicillin resistant *Staphylococcus aureus* (CA-MRSA) [Centers for Disease Control and Prevention Web page]. Available at: http://www.cdc.gov/ncidod/dhqp/ar_mrsa_ca.html.

32. Reddy M, Gill SS, Kalkar SR, Wu W, Anderson PJ, Rochon PA. Treatment of pressure ulcers: a systematic review. *JAMA.* 2008;300(22):2647–2662.

33. Whitney J, Phillips L, Aslam R, et al. Guidelines for the treatment of pressure ulcers. *Wound Repair Regen.* 2006;14(6):663–679.

34. Siedliecki SL, Good M. Effect of music on power, pain, depression and disability. *J Adv Nurs.* 2006; 54(5)553–562.

35. Maratos AS, Gold C, Wang X, Crawford MJ. Music therapy for depression. *Cochrane Database Syst Rev.* 2008;23(1):CD004517.

36. McInnes E, Bell-Syer SEM, Dumville JC, Legood R, Cullum NA. Support surfaces for pressure ulcer prevention. *Cochrane Database Syst Rev.* 2008;(4):CD001735.

37. Hewitt H, Whittle S, Lopez S, Bailey E, Weaver S. Topical use of papaya in chronic skin ulcer therapy in Jamaica. *West Indian Med J.* 2000;49(1):32–33.

38. Jull AB, Rodgers A, Walker N. Honey as a topical treatment for wounds. *Cochrane Database Syst Rev.* 2008;(4):CD005083.

39. Dumville JC, Worthy G, Bland JM, et al. Larval therapy for leg ulcers (VenUS II): randomized controlled trial. *BMJ.* 2009;338:b773.

CHAPTER 23

Postoperative Care of Wounds

Judd E. Hollander, MD

Postoperative wound care should optimize healing. It must be tailored to both the type of wound and method of wound closure. Sutured or stapled lacerations should be covered with a protective, nonadherent dressing for 24 to 48 hours. Maintaining a warm, moist environment increases the rate of reepithelialization. Hinman and Maibach[1] studied experimental split thickness wounds in human volunteers who served as their own controls. They found that occluded wounds healed faster than those exposed to air, although after 1 week both groups were similar. On the other hand, leaving lacerations exposed to air does not affect the infection rate. Howells and Young[2] showed that lack of postoperative dressings in 105 patients did not result in an increased infection rate. Therefore, maintenance of a moist wound environment with a dressing may improve healing but it does not decrease the infection rate. Details of the various dressing options are addressed in Chapter 8, Wound Dressings.

Topical antibiotics can be used to maintain a moist environment in sutured or stapled lacerations but not in lacerations repaired with tissue adhesive. Topical antibiotic ointments may help reduce infection rates and prevent scab formation. Dire and coworkers[3] compared topical antibiotics to petrolatum gel in 465 patients. They found that the infection rates with postoperative topical triple antibiotic or bacitracin were one third the infection rate of patients treated with petrolatum alone.

Therefore, maintenance of a moist environment in sutured or stapled lacerations might be best accomplished by using topical antibiotics. However, patients whose lacerations are closed with tissue adhesives should not use topical ointments because they will loosen the adhesive and may result in dehiscence. Additionally, tissue adhesives serve as their own antimicrobial barrier.

Semipermeable films are manufactured from transparent polyurethane or similar synthetic films, coated on one surface with a water-resistant hypoallergenic adhesive. They are highly elastic, conform easily to body parts, and are generally resistant to shear and tear. They are permeable to moisture vapor and oxygen but impermeable to water and bacteria. These films are sometimes used to cover sutured or stapled wounds without any topical antibiotics. The disadvantages of many of these materials are that they cannot absorb large amounts of fluid and exudate and they do not adhere well in very moist states. They are generally more appropriate for covering elective surgical incisions and not traumatic lacerations.

When possible, the site of injury should be elevated above the patient's heart to limit the accumulation of fluid in the wound interstitial spaces. Wounds with little edema heal more rapidly than those with marked edema. Pressure dressings can be used to minimize the accumulation of intercellular fluid in the dead space.

ANTIBIOTICS

Prophylactic oral antibiotics should not be used except for specific indications. Several studies and a meta-analysis have all found no benefit to prophylactic antibiotics for routine laceration repair.[4] Use of antibiotics should be individualized based upon the degree of bacterial contamination, the presence of infection-potentiating factors (e.g., soil), the mechanism of injury, and the presence or absence of host predisposition to infection.[5] In general, decontamination is far more important than antibiotics. Antibiotics should be used for most bites by humans, dogs, or cats; intraoral lacerations; open fractures; and exposed joints or tendons.[5] Additionally, patients with dirty soft-tissue lacerations who are prone to the development of infective endocarditis, patients with prosthetic joints and other permanent "hardware," and patients with lymphedema should receive antimicrobial therapy. Patients at high risk for systemic complications such as endocarditis can be given intravenous antibiotics before wound care.

PREVENTION OF TETANUS

Tetanus status should be assessed prior to discharge. Two thirds of the recent tetanus cases in the United States have followed lacerations, puncture wounds, and crush injuries. For every wounded patient, information about the mechanism of injury, the characteristics of the wound and its age, previous active immunization status, history of a neurologic or severe hypersensitivity reaction after a previous immunization treatment, and plans for follow-up should be recorded in a permanent medical record.

Proper immunization plays the most important role in tetanus prophylaxis. Recommendations on tetanus prophylaxis are based on the condition of the wound and the patient's immunization history.[6] A summary guide to tetanus prophylaxis of the wounded patient is outlined in Table 23-1. Passive immunization with tetanus immune globulin (TIG) must be considered for each patient.

Contraindications to tetanus and diphtheria toxoid (Td) and the reduced diphtheria toxoid and acellular pertussis (Tdap) is a history of neurologic or severe hypersensitivity reaction after a previous dose. Local side effects do not preclude repeated use. Local reactions, generally erythema and induration with or without tenderness, are common after the administration of vaccines containing diphtheria, tetanus, and pertussis antigens. These reactions are usually self-limited and require no therapy. If a systemic reaction is suspected to represent allergic hypersensitivity, immunization should be postponed until appropriate skin testing is undertaken. If the use of a tetanus toxoid is contraindicated, passive immunization against tetanus should be considered in a tetanus-prone wound.

POSTOPERATIVE WOUND CLEANING

Sutured or stapled wounds can be gently cleansed within 12 hours. Goldberg and colleagues[7] demon-

TABLE 23–1	Recommendations for Tetanus Prophylaxis			
History of Tetanus Immunization	**Clean Minor Wounds**		**All Other Wounds**[a]	
	Administer Td or Tdap[b]	**Administer TIG**	**Administer Td or Tdap**[b]	**Administer TIG**
< 3 or uncertain doses	Yes	No	Yes	Yes
≥ 3 doses				
Most recent dose within 5 yrs	No	No	No	No
Most recent dose within 5 to 10 yrs	No	No	Yes	No
Most recent dose > 10 yrs ago	Yes	No	Yes	No

Notes. Td = tetanus–diphtheria toxoid; Tdap = reduced diphtheria toxoid and acellular pertussis; TIG = tetanus immune globulin.

[a]For example, contaminated wounds, puncture wounds, avulsions, burns, crush injuries.

[b]Adolescents and adults who require a tetanus toxoid–containing vaccine as part of wound management should receive Tdap instead of Td if they have not previously received Tdap. If Tdap is not available or was administered previously, Td should be administered. Tdap is not licensed for use among adults aged 65 years and older, as it has not been studied in this population.[6]

strated that the use of soap and water to cleanse lacerations was not associated with an increased infection rate. Heal et al. randomized 857 patients to keeping the wound dry for 48 hours compared with wetting the wound within 12 hours and found no difference in infection rate.[8] When the wound is wet, gentle blotting should be used to dry the area. Wiping could result in dehiscence. Daily cleansing ensures that the patient examines the laceration for early signs of infection. Patients should be instructed to observe the wound for redness, warmth, swelling and drainage, as these findings may indicate infection. Use of standardized wound care instructions improves patient compliance and understanding.[9]

Reapplication of topical antibiotics will continue to decrease scab formation, improving the likelihood of continued wound-edge apposition. Patients with tissue adhesives may shower but they should avoid bathing and swimming because prolonged moisture will loosen the adhesive bond.

FOLLOW-UP

Patients should be told when and with whom to follow-up for suture removal or wound examinations. Sutures or staples in most locations should be removed after approximately 7 days (Table 23-2). Facial sutures should be removed within 3 to 5 days to avoid formation of unsightly sinus tracts and hatch marks.[10] Sutures subject to high tensions (on the joints or hands, for instance) should be left in place for 10 to 14 days. When one is removing sutures, care should be

TABLE 23–2	Time From Wound Closure Until Removal of Sutures or Staples
Location	**Number of Days**
Face	3–5 days
Scalp	7 days
Chest	8–10 days
Back	10–14 days
Forearm	10–14 days
Fingers	8–10 days
Hand	8–10 days
Lower extremity	8–12 days
Foot	10–12 days

taken to avoid applying tension in a direction that would tend to cause dehiscence. The suture should be cut on one side of the knot and then pulled out through the skin in the same direction. (Figure 23-1). One should not attempt to remove the suture by passing the knot through the wound, as this may result in wound dehiscence. Use of a specialized curved stitch cutter and fine forceps helps ease removal of fine sutures. Any scab or crusting over the sutures may be débrided prior to suture removal by gently applying hydrogen peroxide with gauze.

To remove staples, the double-sided jaw of the staple remover is inserted beneath the exposed

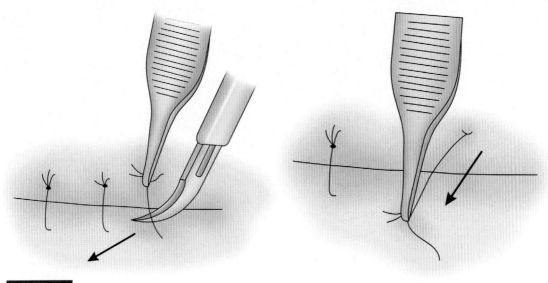

FIGURE 23-1
Method of removing sutures.

cross-limb of the staple, and the upper jaw is closed over the staple, elevating the ends of the staple and removing the staple from the skin (see Figure 11-3).

Tissue adhesives will slough off on their own within 5 to 10 days of application. They do not require removal by a health care practitioner. When a topical skin adhesive is used, the patient should be careful to avoid picking at it or scrubbing the area or exposing it to water for more than brief periods until healing has occurred. When tissue adhesives remain on the skin for prolonged periods, antibiotic ointment, petrolatum or bathing can accelerate removal, although delayed sloughing is not necessarily a disadvantage. Acetone can be used when more rapid removal is required.

Healing lacerations and abrasions should not be exposed to the sun; exposure can result in permanent hyperpigmentation.[11] Abraded skin should be protected with a sun-blocking agent for at least 6 to 12 months after injury.

REFERENCES

1. Hinman CD, Maibach H. Effect of air exposure and occlusion on experimental human skin wounds. *Nature.* 1963;200:377–378.
2. Howells CH, Young HB. A study of completely undressed surgical wounds. *Br J Surg.* 1966;53(5): 436–439.
3. Dire DJ, Coppola M, Dwyer DA, Lorette JJ, Karr JL. Prospective evaluation of topical antibiotics for preventing infections in uncomplicated soft-tissue wounds repaired in the ED. *Acad Emerg Med.* 1995; 2(1):4–10.
4. Cummings P, Del Beccaro MA. Antibiotics to prevent infection of simple wounds: a meta-analysis of randomized studies. *Am J Emerg Med.* 1995;13(4): 396–400.
5. Singer AJ, Hollander JE, Quinn JV. Evaluation and management of traumatic lacerations. *New Engl J Med.* 1997;337(16):1142–1148.
6. Kretsinger K, Broder KR, Cortese MM, et al. Preventing tetanus, diphtheria, and pertussis among adults: use of tetanus toxoid, reduced diphtheria toxoid and acellular pertussis vaccine recommendations of the Advisory Committee on Immunization Practices (ACIP) and recommendation of ACIP, supported by the Healthcare Infection Control Practices Advisory Committee (HICPAC), for use of Tdap among health-care personnel. *MMWR Recomm Rep.* 2006;55(RR-17):1–37.
7. Goldberg HM, Rosenthal SA, Nemetz JC. Effect of washing closed head and neck wounds on wound healing and infection. *Am J Surg.* 1981;141(3):358–359.
8. Heal C, Buettner R, Raasch B, et al. Can sutures get wet? Prospective randomized controlled trial of wound management in general practice. *BMJ.* 2006;332(7549):1053–1056.
9. Austin PE, Matlack R II, Dunn KA, Kesler C, Brown CK. Discharge instructions: do illustrations help our patients understand them? *Ann Emerg Med.* 1995; 25(3):317–320.
10. Crikelair GF. Skin suture marks. *Am J Surg.* 1958; 96(5):631–639.
11. Ship AG, Weiss PR. Pigmentation after dermabrasion: an avoidable complication. *Plast Reconstr Surg.* 1985;75(4):528–532.

Index

Information in figures and tables is indicated by *f* and *t*.